TRUE LOVE

Integral Lifework Theory & Practice

T.Collins Logan

First Edition, May 2009
ISBN 978-0-9770336-3-8

Published by the Integral Lifework Center
PO Box 221082
San Diego, CA 92192
www.integrallifework.com

For seekers who become answers

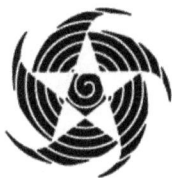

SPECIAL THANKS

A heart-felt *thank you* goes out to the many folks who helped in some way with this book. First and foremost to those intrepid souls who slogged through early drafts and provided valuable feedback; these include Andrew H., Bill E., Bill J., Ken C., Mollie K., Pauline H. and Robin H. Thanks also to Bill J., Ken C. and Rhonda L. for always being willing to share the wellness perspectives, approaches and philosophies they explore in their own work. To Elizabeth M. and Terry L. for encouragement and opportunities in other areas of my journey that have allowed me the time and resources to pursue my writing. To Mollie K., as always, for holding me accountable to my own ideals. To Scott G.-S. for providing excellent resources on corporate America. To Tracy C. for tales of Odin. And of course I am eternally grateful to my students and *Integral Lifework* clients of past, present and future whose curiosity, courage and personal victories make this effort worthwhile.

TABLE OF CONTENTS

INTRODUCTION

This book is about the power of relationship. The relationship we have with ourselves and the relationships we have with others, with society at large, the natural systems of the Earth, and ultimately with the Universe itself. The exchanges that take place at all of these levels are what nourish us and everything around us. And at the center of all relationships, shaping and facilitating each exchange, is love. Love is the unitive force behind every concept and practice illuminated here, and the perfection of love as it indwells each of us, as it is expressed through every one of us in the world, is both the guiding context and the intended outcome of each chapter. What we love and how we love defines who we are. So loving kindness, compassion, charity, devotion, affection and the many other faces of love are both a conscious discipline we invoke from a place of wholeness and effective self-nourishment, and a governing influence constantly at work in our lives, even when we are least aware of it.

There are four basic steps in the cultivation of authentic love, and each one has many facets and variations to consider:

1) Discovering and experiencing authentic love.

2) Cultivating and dwelling in love-consciousness.

3) Being skillful, courageous and discerning in how love is expressed and received.

4) Regularly appreciating and renewing love as nourishment in all its forms.

These steps are possible when willingness, insight and follow-through combine with know-how. So this book is not just about intellectual knowledge, but about the ways in which we can enlarge our insight and understanding on every level – emotional, physical, social, spiritual and so on. That is in fact a theme you will see repeated many different ways as you explore these pages; a holism that incorporates love is a holism that infuses every corner of our being – no matter how obscure or elusive – with warming light. To love fully and skillfully is to nurture every level of existence throughout widening circles of influence, beginning with interior dimensions of self and radiating out to the farthest reaches of our imagination. Love is the foundation of healing, growth and transformation, and so love's conscious cultivation naturally becomes essential to any systemized approach to well-being.

How can we best love ourselves, each other and the world around us? This has been a recurring question in my own journey and is centerpiece of my daily practice. It is how *Integral Lifework* came into being as a holistic self-care modality. In the following pages I will draw upon both theory and many real world examples to illustrate a truly transformative type of love. We will explore how to nurture every aspect of self, and the qualities of relationship necessary for compassionate affection to flourish within and without. Which thoughts, feelings and actions most skillfully support love that is true? Which modes of consciousness or being energize love and inspire individual and even cultural evolution? *Integral Lifework* attempts to answer all of these questions.

That said, those with a deep understanding of the essence of love know that words alone cannot convey that essence. As a writer and teacher, there is always a challenge in this regard. Likewise, reductionism, historicism, cultural egocentrism, intellectualism, exclusivity or inflexible idealism often intrude on many of the most seminal and well-meaning contributions to our culture's dialogues about love. So I will try to avoid these pitfalls even as I shape a huge, ineffable topic with carefully chosen words. To be realistic, the power of true love is experiential in nature, and all that can be accomplished in the following pages is a gentle nudge toward personal encounters with love that edify more effectively than any book ever could.

True love demands courage. Returning to our natural proclivities and unlearning much of our cultural programming is an important part of discovering authentic love. As we progress through a process of replacing unhelpful patterns with helpful ones, we will inevitably encounter resistance from a society and relationships that still value those old patterns. We will also encounter ambivalence within ourselves, a result of those same cultural and interpersonal habits that have taken root in our psyche. But if we never encountered such challenges or resistance, we would never grow. A little personal and social discomfort – a little realignment of our priorities and the dynamics of our relationships – is a reliable indicator of healthy growth. The consequence of that growth is harmony and joy within ourselves and in every arena we lavish with genuine affection. Beyond that, when harmony and joy flourish in our lives, lies the realm of substantive transformation.

Brokenness

Only through brokenness
    can I feel the whole truth
Opening myself to life
    real substance fills the voids
    where ego once fed
I am bereft
    from forgetting
      who I am
    looking outward
      instead of inward
Now
    I see a path clearly
    and joy lights the way
      through all of my illusions

Integral Practice, Integral Lifework

You will come across the term *integral practice* frequently here. There are many ways to define this term, but in this book it will mean the holistic disciplines we consciously employ to nurture ourselves and others, and most specifically those practices that both inspire and sustain growth in many dimensions at once. For instance, what might nourish spirit, mind and body at the same time? Or what could satisfy my heart while reinforcing my sense of purpose? Is there a way I can nurture compassion within myself while offering healing and encouragement to others around me? Although the specific emphasis of personal practice is often different for each person, the solutions presented here can be used by anyone to create an integrative, interdependent and multidimensional approach to wholeness and effective living. And this essential nourishment is what the integral practice among these pages encourages you to synthesize.

Integral Lifework includes integral practice, but it also encompasses a broader methodology. I came up with the term to describe a therapeutic model that took a decade to develop. It involves careful evaluation of self-nourishment and barriers to self-nourishment, which then informs a *Lifework Plan* that aims to heal, grow and ultimately transform us through personalized integral practice. The goal of *Integral Lifework* is to provide insight and empowerment so that anyone can nourish themselves in twelve essential dimensions. A lot has gone into this model, and we will cover most of the major components, but this book is really about the core principles of integral practice as implemented under a *Lifework* umbrella.

As an *Integral Lifework Practitioner* (ILP), my role over the past five years has been to facilitate an initial nourishment and barrier self-assessment for my clients, and then provide them with tools and resources to nourish themselves in multidimensional ways. You could think of an ILP as a primary care provider for the entire being. But the most critical role of an ILP is to help someone liberate themselves from dependence on anyone else for their own wellness. Chief among those tools is learning how to love self, others and the surrounding environment in far-reaching and transformational ways.

For context, it may be helpful to briefly summarize how all of this came into being, especially since my own journey passed through many different places and phases to arrive at an integral approach. At times I have acted as a patient advocate in the traditional medical establishment, which has shown me both the value and incompleteness of conventional medicine.   When training in various alternative healing arts, my eyes were opened to a more integrative model of healing and wholeness, as well as the decisive roles that somatic awareness and intuition play in the healing process.   In positions as a personnel manager and then spiritual counselor, I gained appreciation for what motivates and energizes people, as well as the criticality of compassionate relationships in sustaining well-being on any level.   When I worked through my own physical and emotional crises over time, it not only became clear how a unique combination of tools worked well for me, but also how empathic care and therapy should be modeled, as I had some excellent teachers throughout my healing process.   And while studying martial arts, I quickly discovered the essential interdependence of mind, body and spirit.   I have immersed myself in spiritual traditions in most of my life, ultimately settling back where I most naturally began – as a devoted mystic, which means that I seek to integrate a spiritual dimension into my life and thereby encourage the ongoing evolution of my spiritual being.   This has played a major role in the inclusion of spiritual energy exchanges in any integral approach.   Also, in teaching classes on mysticism, it became obvious that a system of holistic self-care was required to support and sustain balanced spiritual exploration.

Throughout this journey, I was also introduced to helpful literature that hinted at the interrelationship between all the disciplines I was exploring. Books like *Chop Wood, Carry Water*; *Conscious Loving*; *Anatomy of the Spirit*; *7 Habits of Highly Effective People*; *The Mind of Light*; *Full Catastrophe Living*; *The Life We Are Given*; *One Taste* and so on.   These works seemed to be saying "Yes! Keep going down this road, you're definitely onto something...."   This sentiment was reinforced by the music I listened to, the movies I watched, the friends I made, the mystical insights of my spiritual practice, new research I stumbled upon in everything from neurophysiology to macrobiology to quantum physics, and so on. So in many ways I feel I did not discover anything new, but observed what was already there, arranging it in a way that made sense to me.   And without really trying to, all those disparate elements abruptly coalesced into a delightful *aha*:   the essential nourishment model.   And that is how *Integral Lifework* was born.

How does true love fit into this model?   Love is nourishment, and nourishment is love.   As we delve into nourishment theory and its supportive processes, you will see that love is an inextricable part of that matrix – something that exists without our being aware of it, as well as something we want to consciously cultivate. It is the cofactor for all essential nourishment. I frequently emphasize the importance of a governing intentionality for integral practice. True love is that governing intentionality, while at the same time it is a product of integral effort. It is not possible to separate the qualities of empathy, kindness, compassion, affection or generosity from the fabric of *Integral Lifework*. They intersect persistently throughout all of its methods and intended outcomes.

A Suggested Approach to This Book

Life is by nature a constant reinvention. But writing something down imbues ideas with permanence and solidity, giving us an opportunity to appreciate the newly sculpted object from multiple vantage points. "Oh look, here's an unfinished bit of clay waiting to be formed. And over here the surface seems very smooth and finished. See how the sculpture wobbles when we push it from this angle? Well, at least this part over here looks fairly solid...." And so a dialogue begins, and from that dialogue we gain ever greater appreciation of the power of our mind over what matters. So I would encourage you to maintain a healthy skepticism as you read this book, one that brings you right up to the brink of disbelief while still leaving a little ledge of hope to perch upon. For in that tiny space where you entertain improbable possibilities, I will offer what I think is true, nourishing and empowering. And then, if and when you decide to step off that ledge to test your wings, you'll find out for yourself whether these concepts really fly.

As a quick overview, *True Love* is organized into six parts:

Part I, Theoretical Foundations, discusses the conceptual underpinnings of *Integral Lifework,* and why love is such a critical factor in the quality of our existence.

Part II, Essential Nourishment, explores the twelve dimensions of energy exchange in the *Integral Lifework* model, along with the most important characteristics of these nourishment centers.

Part III, All About Love, differentiates love that is authentic and effective from other patterns of affection and action, capturing what true love looks like from as many angles as possible.

Part IV, Understanding and Managing Barriers to Wholeness, uncovers the nature of personal barriers and provides ways to transform those barriers into holistic nourishment.

Part V, Love's Expansion, explores how true love expands to fill ever larger arenas of affection, suggests actions that express love effectively in each of those arenas, and examines what happens when love fails.

Part VI, An Integral Life, enumerates the benefits of a lifetime of integral practice and the step-by-step process of creating an *Integral Lifework Plan.*

Since I have already alluded to some of the writings that influenced me, I should clarify that this book has very few quotes, references or citations. This was a deliberate decision on my part. When I make certain claims, such as that a practice might lower blood pressure or produce lasting feelings of contentment and happiness, most of the time I will be speaking from direct experience or observation of my own clients rather than relying on other sources. I provide a number of real world, first-hand observations, though often names have been changed for privacy. In many cases, when I do offer external data to support my assertions, a careful web search with reputable sources will verify its current accuracy. Sometimes, on particularly controversial topics, I might also include a reference or two. As resources for wider study, I do offer a few choice books, allude to some research I am familiar with, and encourage additional investigation using suggested terms and topics. The reality is that much of the encouraging evidence for various practices in *Integral Lifework* is either readily available with a little careful digging, or is easily experienced first-hand by those willing to commit to integral practice. Realistically, my goal here cannot be to argue my own authority or rely on the authority of others to validate my assertions; I would rather encourage you to test whatever I claim with your own integral explorations.

Before diving into the following pages, I recommend first posing this question to yourself: why are you reading this book? Spend a moment reflecting and introspecting on this question, because what you discover with such inward searching will likely determine how this book will most benefit you. Are you curious about true love? Then among these pages you will find powerful ways of experiencing and expressing love in your life. Have you suffered pain and loss to a degree that compels you to seek out healing? Then you will find tools here to help you care for yourself along that path. Do you wish to help others heal? You will find tools here to help you do so. Do you long for wholeness? Then you will encounter many doors that open onto that inward horizon. So this book is for the curious, the hurting, the healing, the helpful and anyone yearning to be whole. But it has also been written for those who feel a distinctive call emanating from their innermost being, a call to harmony and unity; a call to radical transformation and the promise of spiritual evolution. I believe this call is universal, but it is sometimes difficult to hear. When we have opened ourselves to it, its voice sweeps all other concerns aside and grounds us in a greater purpose. If this description seems alien to you, you may find that by reading this book and practicing the techniques suggested here, this transformative imperative will unveil itself to you. But regardless of your experiences and orientation, by immersing yourself in these pages I suspect you will shift your consciousness in a direction it already longs to go.

Concept, Then Practice

When exploring love, I frequently touch upon the idea that critically important concepts are transmitted or absorbed experientially, and you will notice a pattern throughout the book that reflects this. After discussing a topic, there will often be an exercise relating to that topic. Concept is just a preamble for practice, because to fully grasp the breadth of any idea, we must integrate that idea through action. Although we may comprehend something intellectually, we cannot truly know something in a complete, holistic way without investing in it experientially. A conceptual framework must be paired with experiential validation. You could call this integral education, where our whole being is allowed to weigh the importance of any new information before we accept it or incorporate it into our lives. I have relied on this teaching method in all of my classes and with each of my clients, and it has always proven more powerful and penetrating than intellectual discourse alone. I hope you will take advantage of this approach as you absorb each chapter. I also suggest that you obtain a journal with lots of blank pages to track your progress.

Our first example of concept, then practice involves the diagram below, which explores parts of the theoretical foundation of *Integral Lifework*. These are some core concepts that relate specifically to motivation, the main topic of Part I. By the end of the book, you should have a thorough understanding of the diagram and all of its components. Immediately following this diagram is an exercise.

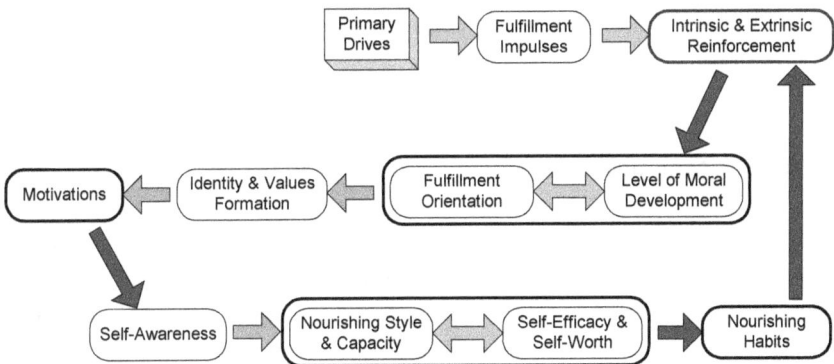

Exercise: What Motivates You? Take a moment to look over the diagram, beginning with the Primary Drives box and following the arrows from one box to the next. Just get a general feel for it, knowing that a more complete explanation will be provided later on. Now experiment with the following introspection. Find a quiet place to sit with your hands resting quietly in your lap. Close your eyes and breathe slowly through your nose, deep down into your belly. With your mental attention focused inward around the air filling and emptying your lungs, silently ask yourself the following questions, one at a time:

- "What drives me?"

- "What motivates me?"

- "What fulfills me?"

Without forcing anything particular to happen, just rest quietly in that inward focus and see what arises as you ask these questions of yourself. If nothing seems to be happening, ask the questions again, this time paying closer attention to the sensations in your body and any emotions that surface in response to each phrase. Every half minute or so, ask one of the questions again and try to maintain that inward focus, letting whatever bubbles up within you expand through your awareness, then dissipate as you ask the next question. Relax into that rhythm for about ten minutes. When you are finished, capture the results in your journal and reflect on what you observed.

Reading Techniques

There are many methods to absorb the information presented here, linear chapter-by-chapter reading being just one of them. Here are some less conventional recommendations for you to consider:

- Look through the table of contents, and then let the words draw you where your heart wants to go. If you see a chapter heading that intrigues you right away, go there first, then expand out into other sections.

- If you hit any speed-bumps, such as a description or idea that doesn't make sense to you, just skip over it. Move on to another section and come back later.

- Read small amounts, and – especially if you encounter ideas that are completely new – mull over what you've read for a day or more before trying to push further. There is a lot that interrelates to everything else, so it likely won't be beneficial to rush or force your way through this book.

- Try being random: just open up and read a paragraph or two, then close the book, think about what you've read, and repeat the exercise.

- Find a friend – or start a group – with whom you can discuss each topic or chapter over a period of time.

- Read actively – mark up the pages, underline phrases, write notes in the margins, etc. Make reading more of a dialogue than a one-way communication.

I myself enjoy skimming through books to get a feel for what they have to share before I delve in. You can get a lot out of skimming, but it usually only gathers a little heavy cream, a little tasty fat to titillate the senses; it does not provide a rich, multidimensional meal. For that we need to shift from one mode of being into other modes of being, to forms that require different amounts of time and space, and call upon different styles of perception and interior processing. Words have entirely different weight and meaning depending on their context, and unless we allow our personal context to shift from what is familiar and comfortable to what is inherently new and different, we will undoubtedly miss important revelations. For instance, remaining in a fast-paced, intellectual mode of information gathering will keep us on the surface; it will prevent us from experiencing the emotional, spiritual and somatic depths of transformative information. Which is likely why so many wisdom traditions teach with proverbs, poetry, koans, parables – or without using words at all. So, in addition to the exercises, along the way you will find encouragement to shift out of a traditionally Western, Cartesian, analytical mode of information processing to something new. Here a poem, there a story and so on...each is an opportunity to shift gears. Spend some time with these and see what they offer you. Unless you pause to stretch your wings and trust the rising currents just beyond the reach of thought, flying may prove an impossible challenge.

Lastly, I would encourage you to explore the different impact this material will have when it is re-read after a few months of integral practice. Through personal experience you will inevitably gain insights that transcend the written word, and through which complex or abstract ideas become concrete, integrated knowledge. Once concept leads to practice, practice leads to wisdom. Then an entirely new level of understanding becomes available.

Intended Audience

This book is really for anyone who wishes to cultivate a greater connection with themselves, others and the good of All, and who desires to develop ever more skillful and effective means of exercising loving kindness. However, as you read through each chapter you will notice that some of the material is technical or abstract, and some is more concrete and easier to process. The first section, Theoretical Foundations, covers what is likely familiar ground for those immersed in healing modalities, but may be somewhat overwhelming to general readers. Other sections, such as Love's Expansion, offer ways to apply Lifework principles that may add little value for readers who are already experts in those areas, while still providing inspiration for non-experts. There is, I hope, something for everyone here, so feel free to seek it out rather than relying on sequential reading. On the one hand, anyone already on a path of self-discovery and growth will be able to incorporate many of the concepts and practices into their own journey. On the other, I am also hopeful that health practitioners – from traditional medicine to psychotherapy to alternative healing modalities – will find applications in their own practice. One healthcare professional suggested *True Love* be used as a reference for residential treatment programs. I myself plan to use it as a teaching reference for classes and seminars.

The theory and techniques are also intended to be of interest to those involved in health advocacy and health care policy development. As is already widely recognized, healthcare in the U.S. is a sophisticated landscape of highly specialized disciplines, which are often professionally isolated and sometimes working at odds or in competition with each other. Primary care physicians can find themselves struggling to coordinate a chaos of options for an ever-increasing number of patients, and weigh an extremely complex matrix of factors within very brief patient visits. This landscape is mainly the result of tectonic pressures from continually escalating health care costs, and is a contributing factor to some of the worst health outcomes of any developed country.   The alternative model proposed in this book encourages a vision of what primary care could become if physicians were empowered to provide truly comprehensive, holistic services.   In other words, to provide multidimensional triage of the whole person – not only throughout the healing process, but also into higher stages of health, growth and personal and societal transformation.

PART I

THEORETICAL FOUNDATIONS

WHAT IS LOVE?

Love sustains life. On an emotional level, it is the felt experience of affection for someone or something in the present moment. This is not a feeling that exists because we felt it once in the past, or because we anticipate or depend upon it in the future, it is what indwells us and inspires us right here, right now. This felt experience is naturally and immediately accompanied by three reactions: the desire to communicate the felt experience with the object of affection; the desire for the well-being of the object of affection; and a desire to personally contribute in some way to the well-being of the object of affection. In other words, a desire to nourish in love even as we are nourished by love. So by its nature love involves the impulse to communicate and act in accordance with effective nourishment. These feelings and reactions might remain recognized or unrecognized, shared or unshared, reciprocated or rebuffed, but many different nourishment processes are activated and supported the instant love takes root. In this way, love sustains and amplifies itself; it could be described as a self-sustaining energy.

In a spiritual sense, we can also be so infused with love that it controls our every thought and deed – a sort of spiritual possession and reformation of identity. I call this love-consciousness. And of course love has a broad spectrum of intensity and modes of expression. There is friendship love, romantic love, puppy love, material love, sibling love, unconditional love, parental love, divine love...and a hundred other nuances of affection. So love can encompass every aspect of our being, every type of relationship, every impulse of our will and every possible mode of action that contribute to nourishing outcomes. In and of itself, then, love facilitates and permeates the well-being, growth and evolution of our species.

And love is even more, because it also evolves and changes shape. In relationship, when the mutuality of loving feelings, reactions and intentions is discovered, a cycle of affection and reinforcing actions is initiated that becomes larger than the sum of its parts. Once again how that love is contextualized or expressed depends on the nature of the relationship – it might be platonic, or romantic, or devotional, etc. – but when first kindled, the felt affection in the present moment expands beyond the boundaries of that relationship. A door to broader perception is opened, and we allow ourselves to fall in love with everything and everyone; we fall in love with life itself, so that we are full of hope and certainty that all is well in the world.

Over time, the felt experience of affection inevitably transforms into different emotional forms and new kinds of action, but if love is present, high quality energy exchange and self-perpetuation will continue in some fashion. As just one example, consider how initial excitement and connection can eventually become loyalty, commitment or self-sacrifice in a loving relationship. The high-soaring sentiment of "I would do anything for this love" translates into unpredictable situational challenges, difficult decisions, and constant but incremental effort. And love can really encompass every emotion, from warmth and elation to somber duty to insistent confrontation, with all sorts of gradations along the way. What I want to emphasize here is that love is first and foremost a felt experience in the present, which is quickly followed by reinforcing communication and action, even though the characteristics of each of these changes over time.

What is true love, then? In the following chapters, true love will be a way of describing intentions, communications and actions that effectively and skillfully convey the felt experience of love, are nourishing across multiple dimensions, and ultimately create physically healthy, emotionally supportive and spiritually constructive relationships. True love is an answer to the question: "Okay, I feel a profound affection in the present moment...now how can I translate that into meaningful action?" I am confident that we all have a great capacity for love, perhaps more than we have yet experienced or imagined, and we certainly all have the ability to love truly. Over the course of my life and work I have heard expressions like "I never knew this kind of love was possible," or "this love has changed me forever" from countless individuals. Someone describing how they feel about their first child. Someone discovering their first healthy and supportive romantic relationship. Someone entering a new phase of healing and wholeness or who has fallen deeply in love with life. Someone who has experienced a life-changing spiritual connection for the first time. The list is endless. And so the love itself is always within us, just waiting for such moments to spring forth – it just needs us to have the courage to create helpful opportunities. And creating or inviting those opportunities is something we will discuss in a bit. But once that love is set free, what do we do with it? How do we release it into our lives and the lives of others? True love is devoted to the most effective answers to these questions.

Looking in the opposite direction, it is easy to observe that a miscommunication of love through unskillful words and actions has led to much suffering. Even when our intentions are sincere and our aim is to enhance the well-being of those we care about, ineffective love can cause more harm than good. That is, instead of supporting and strengthening our connections, we inadvertently undermine and disrupt them. A lover who becomes overly demanding or controlling. A parent who is unconsciously crushing their child's spirit. A sibling who is compulsively competitive. A friend who sabotages our joy without realizing it. A child who misbehaves to get attention. A relative who angrily lashes out to protect their family from imaginary wrongs. Someone whose religious fervency alienates those they are trying to help. These situations do not necessarily reflect a lack of love. The felt experience of love may be present, but it is being expressed and acted upon in ineffective or inappropriate ways. Unskillful love happens all the time. I would even generalize that the vast majority of my *Integral Lifework* clients seek me out when they have arrived at a painful, grief-filled situation in which natural reactions of love have become distorted, misdirected or depleted through unskillful action. This manifests as everything from chronic illness to breakdowns in close relationships to anxiety or depression over successive failures. Yet people know, instinctively, that there is a better way. A way to feel more freely, to share more freely, to thrive more freely, to transform pain and suffering into joy and laughter. And of course all of this is possible…through love that is true.

A central tenet in *Integral Lifework* is the necessity of liberating all that powerful, nourishing and transformative love within us. We cannot, in fact, love anyone else in a nourishing or even satisfying way until we have learned to fully love ourselves. Earlier in my own life, confusion about the nature of love and how to express it appropriately led me down some dark, despairing roads. So I have plenty of first-hand experience with unskillful loving, and plentiful observations and realizations to share from counseling others. It seems that the barriers to loving effectively are as common as the desire to love itself, perhaps because, as conscious and inquisitive beings, we are easily distracted from what we know to be fulfilling, and can be inadvertently but deeply wounded by those distractions. We can feel trapped in ignorance, in a lack of loving examples or caring relationships, and in a perceived inability to love ourselves. And yet we need nourishment, so we find it any way we can. But what drives these patterns of nourishment and the frustration of nourishment within us? Why do we struggle to comprehend the nature of love even as we long for it? The answer, I believe, lies in our fundamental drives and fulfillment impulses – that is, in the underlying currents that form our motivations and our efforts to self-nourish. Examining those currents will, I think, help clarify how love operates, how it can sometimes appear to be thwarted, and how we can ignite a beacon of light within to guide our way.

Before we explore that motivational framework, I want to briefly cover some of the fertile ground in which love takes root. That is, the operational parameters within which true love can flourish once the spark of affection is ignited. This covers much of the conceptual groundwork and vocabulary that will be used in subsequent chapters.

A Proposed Maturity Model

To understand the nature of love and how to love effectively, we must explore what it means to mature. Why? Because our level of overall maturity determines our capacity to love and the compassionate skillfulness we bring to our efforts. Reflecting for a moment on the different kinds of love can help clarify this principle. The kind of intense affection and compulsive attachment that a young child has for their favorite toy or pet could be categorized as love, but it is inspired primarily by the pleasurable rewards of interaction, a limited understanding of reciprocation and interdependence, and unmitigated impulses and assessments rooted in emotional reasoning. When an adolescent becomes infatuated with a peer, role model or cultural idol, they likewise scarcely involve rationality in their assessments and have little management over impulses; the process of devotion, obsession or being "in love" often overwhelms healthy boundaries and undermines the best interests of all parties. That is not to say that children and adolescents don't experience intense love, or that the outcome of their loving interactions isn't positive or healthy in some ways. But, from a developmental standpoint, the very young simply have not fully learned or integrated the complex concepts of mutual commitment, constructive self-sacrifice, healthy emotional boundaries, appropriate progressions of intimacy, disciplined self-management, the interdependent nature of relationships, or compassion without attachment. They are still exploring and experimenting. And these are just some of the measures of maturing love; as we examine these and many other metrics for assessing our own levels of maturity, it will become clear that love's perfection is a continual, organic cycle of growth and interior revolution.

What, then, are the measures of maturity or of maturing love? Allow me to propose a few areas for initial self-examination. Many of these will relate back to the foundations of self-nourishment so pivotal to *Integral Lifework*. Others may at first seem unrelated to either nourishment or love, but in fact reflect the fruits of interior growth that are necessary for skillful loving. And although some maturity factors may – as we attempt to address them – tug at our attention and resources in superficially competing ways, they are ultimately complimentary and interdependent, building on each other into an amalgam much greater than the sum of its parts. In order for our expression of love to be authentic, skillful and nourishing, that amalgam must exist within a special environment, an environment created by a narrow band – a finely balanced range – of mature function within each area. To begin, let's explore how each part in that amalgam is defined, and what its optimal band of function looks like.

The Fulcrum's Plane

The idea that there is a range of operation within which something is most efficient or effective is not new. Hesiod encouraged moderation in all things. The Buddha advocated a middle way of thought and action between extremes. Goldilocks preferred her porridge not too hot and not too cold, her bed not too hard and not too soft...everything had to be "just right." When we test our cholesterol levels, measure our heart rate or check our weight, again there is an optimal range – relating to our age, gender, height and so forth – which correlates with overall health. The maximum horsepower in an engine occurs within a specific bracket of rpm – not too fast, and not too slow. When exploring the conditions that led to life on Earth – and the conditions that continue to support life – it quickly becomes clear that a narrow band of variables is necessary; without a consistent temperature range, just the right amount of water, a balanced composition of atmospheric gases, the precarious interrelationship between evolving species and so on...life could not exist. Applying this principle to both energy exchanges and personal maturity, *Integral Lifework* asserts that there is a narrow band of optimal function within each dimension of nourishment that facilitates health, healing, growth and transformation. What is "optimal" is defined both quantitatively and qualitatively. Outside of that band, each process can be impeded and even retrograded. Within that band, love flourishes.

The following chart begins to define the optimal range of operation for several *maturity factors*. The list captures only a portion of these, dividing them into a few digestible categories, but those listed here have a direct bearing on our capacity and skillfulness in loving ourselves and others. Why is this the case? Because they shape our ability to nourish and be nourished, and in *Integral Lifework*, nourishment is the language of love. This initial fly-by is a lot to assimilate in one reading – and I will elaborate on many of these factors in later chapters – so for now I encourage you to just look it over and familiarize yourself with the general ideas and categories, getting a feel for the variety of behaviors, reactions and patterns represented here. Also note that the optimal range is just that – a continuum of function rather than a confining specificity; the fulcrum of this balancing act has a very broad plane.

	Foundational Factors for Effective Loving		
MATURITY FACTOR	**DEPLETION ←**	**OPTIMAL RANGE**	**→ EXCESS**
Values Alignment	Inauthentic – either unaware of an apparent disconnect between one's values and beliefs and one's thoughts and actions, or a lack of commitment to aligning them (laziness)	Authentic – tolerance of paradox and ambiguity with relaxed acceptance, while committed to aligning thoughts and actions with values and beliefs as closely as possible	Exaggerated – excessive effort to rationalize thoughts and actions that contradict values and beliefs (i.e. cognitive dissonance)
Integrity	Inability to harmonize intentions, thoughts, words and deeds and/or high tolerance of failure, with little interest in or commitment to self-betterment	Thoughtful harmonization of intentions, thoughts, words and deeds with low tolerance of failure and realistic commitment to self-betterment (example: what I intend I think about, talk about and do).	Obsessive effort to harmonize intentions, thoughts, words and deeds at any cost, with extreme intolerance for failure and unrealistic ideal of integrity
Morality	Amoral – rejecting moral framework for intentions and actions and/or a disregard for the same	Moral – conscious effort to evolve moral standards of intention and action within a framework constantly reassessed according to its effectiveness (i.e outcomes reflecting values)	Legalistic – rigid adherence to moral code without evaluating outcomes and efficacy of our approach
Fulfillment Orientation	Protective – unable or unwilling to engage in nourishing exchanges with others in one or more areas, forcefully rejecting any perceived dependence	Self-reliant – fully individuated from family of origin, peers, tribe and society and able to support and maintain own well-being through comfortably interdependent, mutual exchanges	Dependent– a strong identification with and reliance on environment, parents, peers tribe or society for all nourishment and sense of well-being (i.e. lack of individuation)

	DEPLETION ←	OPTIMAL RANGE	→ EXCESS
Identity	Unformed or insecure identity – unable to maintain clear and solid sense of self around other strong influences	Interdependent and inclusive - strong sense of self, expanding to include wider arenas of affection, spiritual unfolding, growth and interdependent connection	Over-identification with self-limiting descriptors – i.e. tribe, survival personas, ego, etc.
Spiritual Grounding	Disconnected from spiritual experience, with little or no access to spiritual realm and own spiritual essence (often with an overemphasis on material experience)	Open and persistent connection with the spiritual realm (ground of being, essence, Divine, etc.) with an unrestrained expression of spiritual essence and nature, balanced with material existence	So immersed in spiritual experience that effective interface with material plane is disrupted or disabled
Arenas of Affection	Affection response has not fully developed or is not active in several arenas – not even towards self	Balanced effort to expand love-consciousness into as many arenas as possible, while still sustaining affection and compassion for self	Overextension or fixation of affection in one or more arenas to the depletion of all others and especially self

Strengthening Factors for Effective Loving

MATURITY FACTOR	DEPLETION ←	OPTIMAL RANGE	→ EXCESS
Self-Concept	Low self-worth and lack of belief in own skillfulness or abilities	Healthy, balanced sense of self-efficacy and self-worth, both as a general self-concept and with respect to each dimension of nourishment	Exaggerated self-confidence and self-worth, and exaggerated belief in own skillfulness or abilities
Self-Awareness	Unskilled, unaware or in denial about one or more aspects of self, which debilitates overall effectiveness	Realistic and regular self-awareness about strengths and limitations, patterns of thought and behavior, identity, values, beliefs, etc. that facilitates increased effectiveness	Absorbed in or obsessed with self-awareness to the exclusion of all other input, resulting in decreased effectiveness
Intentionality	Reactive or unformed – absence of clear intentions or love-consciousness	Golden intention – clear and ever evolving love-consciousness directed toward the good of All, inclusive of self	Fixation on self and ego satisfaction – substitution of ego gratification for love

Mental Clarity	Suppressed – casual thoughts and creative thought process are routinely disregarded, denied or judgmentally devalued	Neutral awareness – casual thoughts and imagination process are allowed to flow freely without immediate valuation or need for action	Obsessive – thoughts or imagination process dominate all other functions, requiring immediate attention and/or action
Nourishment Discipline	Self-Depleting – inability to consistently self-nourish in one or more dimensions	Balanced – able to consistently self-nourish with a diligent but relaxed effort to progress from baseline disciplines to transformative disciplines	Overindulgent – obsessive or excessive effort to self-nourish, often resulting in addictive substitutions
Mindful Openness	Passive & closed – evaluation of meaning or importance of all information through externally defined criteria and inflexible belief system, with less willingness to suspend a sense of certainty	Active & open – evaluation of meaning or importance of new information through flexible and ongoing reevaluation of beliefs and assumptions, with a relaxed willingness to suspend a sense of certainty	Overactive & uncritical – excessive emphasis and dependence on the invented significance of all new information with an inability to critically evaluate
Discernment	Unconscious navigation of each situation based on arbitrary emphasis on either external input streams (such as advice, observed behaviors, mass media, etc.) or impulsive emotional reasoning	Consciously balanced, vigilant but relaxed assessment of input streams from all sources – internal and external, experiential and intuitive, rational and emotional, spiritual promptings and empirical observations	Fixation on one form of hyper-vigilant navigation, such as strong emotions, synchronistic events, black-and-white reasoning, or an overly stringent system of ethics

Common Barriers to Effective Loving

MATURITY FACTOR	**DEPLETION ←**	**OPTIMAL RANGE**	**→ EXCESS**
Relationship Style	Disengaged – either as indulgent pattern or neglectful/absent pattern (also can be defined as "other-depleting")	Interdependent - authoritative and egalitarian with distinct sense of "self" and "other," but with a fundamental acceptance of mutual, intrinsic sovereignty and value	Excessive engagement or enmeshment - overexertion of control, an authoritarian style, or overly attached (loss of self) resulting in "one-up" or "one-down" dynamics

Attachment Style	Destructively detached – sacrifice and denial to extreme deprivation, depletion and harm (to self and/or other) without a sense of interdependence	Compassionately detached – effortless letting go without a sense of sacrifice or denial that naturally leads to deeper connection and nourishment with a strong sense of interdependence	Compulsively attached – inability to let go to the point of dependence, over reliance and addiction, rejecting interdependence and freedom to self-nourish
Permeability (sensitivity & openness)	Impermeable, unaware, numb, unaffected by events within and without; callous and insensitive; thick-skinned to the point of either obtuseness or disinterest	Aware and able to accommodate inward and outward flows of emotional, intellectual, physical and spiritual energy without disruption or stress, as well as consciously filter or boundarize those flows when required	Excessively permeable - unable to manage adversity, stress and upheaval; less able to filter the flows of energy from any source or maintain healthy boundaries
Processing Flexibility	Inflexible and stuck – unable to move from once processing space to another	Flexible and fluid – able to move confidently and consciously between different processing spaces with ease	Sporadic – flitting from one processing space to the next without control or conscious awareness
Barrier Management, Monitoring & Resolution	Unaware – unable to recognize own barriers to well-being or repeating patterns of failure and a tendency to deny that barriers exist	Acknowledgement & compensation – able to recognize, monitor, manage and in some cases resolve own barriers to well-being without substituting for or flooding any one dimension	Overcompensation – able to recognize barriers, but a tendency to either compulsively substitute unhealthy behaviors for an impeded dimension of nourishment, or to reactively diminish the importance of that dimension
Disposition of Will	Annihilation – repression of own sovereignty and choice, expressed as a reactive, submissive or paralyzed disposition and passive inactivity	Willingness – neutrality of will preceding all thought and action while maintaining confidence in own sovereignty and freedom of choice	Willfulness – forceful imposition of will that disrupts sovereignty and choice, often manifesting as obsessive or controlling behaviors
Grief Resolution	Arrested - unaware or in denial about loss and resulting grief and pain	Acknowledgement and acceptance of loss and able to allow grieving process to take its course without suppressing or overemphasizing its importance	Fixated on loss and emotional pain to the point where these are perpetuated and amplified

To love fully and be fully loved, we must inhabit the narrow band of function in each area of maturity – or at least come close to doing so a majority of the time. How do we accomplish this? And how can we know that we have achieved balance in each area? In my experience and observation, human beings are too organic to maintain perfectly honed equilibrium across all factors all of the time. But I do believe that it is possible to dance along the top of this fence for brief periods – long enough to manifest true love in our lives. It's just that, in the normal course of living, the tensions and demands of the world around us push and pull us back out of balance again. Life is not a steady state. So we must constantly observe and adjust, celebrating those finely tuned moments in full knowledge that they are – by nature and perhaps by helpful design – fleeting ones. We will know that we are operating in the narrow band of mature function when things flow effortlessly for us in many areas at once; when we experience strong synchronicities one after another; when a sense of limitless possibility and loving empowerment coincide with profound contentment. However, the real excitement lies in how we arrive at these moments, in the skills and talents we accumulate and exercise along the way. We must first grow some wings, put some healthy feathers on them, and hop around a bit to test our budding lift.

As one brief example, consider Fernando. Fernando is a young professional who has been very successful in his career, but is feeling depressed and disconnected from his family, friends and fiancée. After discussing his situation during a brief initial visit, it rapidly becomes clear that several maturity factors are outside his optimal range. Regarding the integrity factor, Fernando struggles to be honest with himself and his loved ones about a mild substance abuse habit he has had for some time. His fulfillment orientation is also very protective – it is important for him to appear independent, masculine and strong to those he cares about, and this has prevented him from opening his heart and mind to the supportive efforts of others. Fernando appears to have found the fulcrum's plane in several other areas – notably in the well-balanced nourishment discipline he describes to me, the mental clarity he demonstrates in our interaction, as well as his realistic and humble level of self-awareness. But those first two maturity factors, where he has yet to find balance, are enough to derail his attempts to lovingly

connect with himself and others in a consistent way; his ability to love
and be loved is hampered.

After a half-hour of focused conversation, Fernando and I have only just
begun to look at his patterns of thought, emotion and interaction; we
have only touched on a few factors that influence loving exchanges.
And yet these already begin to inform an understanding of why a sense
of disconnection and depressive feelings may be occurring. And that is
really how *Integral Lifework* unfolds in both theory and practice: we
explore a few maturity factors at a time to steadily construct an overall
picture of how love functions. The order of exploration isn't all that
important, as long as we are careful to examine all factors at some point.
I am often guided by intuition in how I begin evaluating or the order in
which I touch on each area, but this could just as easily be accomplished
more methodically. As to what barriers may be present for each
maturity factor, that will be addressed in later chapters. But the key to
such exploration is empathic listening. That is, to dialogue in a language
of the heart, experiencing a person's individual reality in a felt, subjective
way. This is of course equally true when we evaluate maturity factors in
our own life.

Moving forward, the fulcrum's plane of healthy and supportive function
in each area will be discussed in more detail, and suggestions, examples
and exercises will be provided to help to define, achieve and maintain
balance. We will also touch on how these factors relate to each other –
for they are all interconnected. But before we can embrace such ideas
and practices, it is important that we ask ourselves what motivates us to
do so. The simple question of "why?" often has complex and surprising
answers, and of necessity we will root around in our interior a bit to
uncover them. Why is this important? Because if we are not clear about
our motivations and the deepest drives and desires we are serving with
our choices, we will inevitably sabotage our own efforts and fall short of
the rewards that reinforce those efforts. We should have clarity about
the reasons we or those we are trying to support seek health and well-
being, as well as clarity around what conceptions and expectations of
those ideals really look like. Once the mud settles and the water is clear,
the first steps toward healing and growth become obvious and the
energy to take those steps is readily and bountifully available.

What Drives Us?

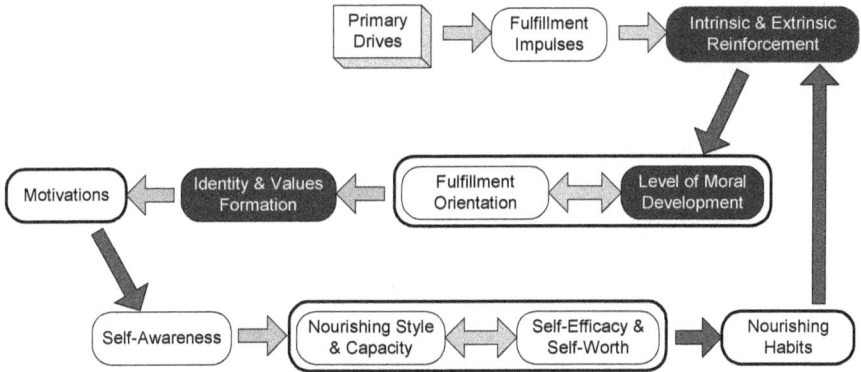

Motivation is a tricky thing, and there continues to be much speculation and debate about how motivations are formed and sustained over time. I will propose one way of looking at motivation that is useful in the context of self-nourishment and the maturation of authentic love. In *Integral Lifework*, we are mainly concerned with how the following components shape our motivation:

- Core Values & Moral Development
- Motivational Awareness & Integration Process
- Understanding Primary Drives & Fulfillment Impulses
- Motivating Change
- What "Motivational Breakdown" Represents
- The Role of Love in Motivation

Once we wrap our mind around these concepts, the path to positive transformation becomes a little clearer. As we become more conscious of our own motivational process, we can tailor that process to energize our efforts in the most positive and effective ways. We can, in fact, begin to consciously synthesize the motivation we require to reach the goals we value most.

Values & Moral Development

Our core values and the level of our moral development are inextricably linked. If I believe that the most important thing in this life is the immediate satisfaction of my own whims and impulses, this reflects a fairly early stage of moral development. If, on the other hand, I truly believe that the most important thing in this life is the welfare of the greatest number of beings possible, this indicates that some moral evolution has occurred. As our morality develops, our emphasis on which values are most important will of necessity shift, as will our ability to integrate ideal values into our actual responses and behaviors. This is an important principle, because the only reliable way to measure our level of moral development is through observing what values are consistently actualized. The proof is in the pudding, so to speak. So evaluating our core values will help us create realistic expectations around our own growth and the efficacy and sustainability of our choices. If we try to motivate ourselves with goals or intentions that don't relate to what we value most, we will almost surely fall short.

So what are core values? Core values are the idealized, hierarchical principles of importance that govern our conscious choices about how we think, feel and act. They are grounded on beliefs and assumptions about ourselves and the world around us that we hold most intimate and dear, and so they also tend to influence our unconscious reactions as well – though this is not always the case. In fact, we may highly value something, but find that our natural impulse is to tend toward its opposite. For instance, I may value cooperativeness and then frequently exhibit competitiveness instead. When this happens, it doesn't mean the sense we have of our core values is false or distorted, it just means our moral development hasn't yet caught up with the idealized principles we cherish – that and the simple fact that we are human and fallible.

This generates an interesting tension within us, too; when we observe the natural distance between what we idealize and what we have actualized, it contributes new energy and ingredients to our motivational soup. So what we value – what we believe is most important – both draws us forward towards ideal outcomes and pushes us from behind to correct our missteps.

In this way core values don't always reflect where we actually are, but rather where we want to be. This is an important distinction, and one we will return to later when we touch on cognitive dissonance. But it is important to recognize that our own learning and motivational process is dependent on the particular stage of moral development in which we reside. If I dwell in an egocentric phase that is fearful, distrusting and reactive towards anything that doesn't clearly serve my immediate wants, then a mode of being that values transpersonal love or transcendent union with the All is more likely to appear inaccessible and unattractive. If I am mainly motivated by the approval of my peers, family members or community, then complying with rules or authority because that is the "right" thing to do may likewise seem nonsensical and incompatible with my moral orientation. We need to begin wherever we are and then consciously aim a way forward. There is no shortage of examples among my own therapeutic and teaching relationships that demonstrate how someone who begins to self-nourish out of fear ends up sustaining those energy exchanges out of love. Once we experience the success of the next phase of our journey, it becomes easier to relax into that new mode of being.

What I also find interesting is that we may operate in one moral framework in one set of circumstances, and shift to another entirely in a different set of circumstances. When someone feels safe, well-loved and secure in their social status and empowerment, their choices may reflect a fairly advanced moral framework. When that same person is subjected to emotional stress, social isolation and deprivation, they may revert to a less advanced moral orientation. The gentle, generous and caring philanthropist can become a combative, callous and acquisitive criminal when all the external structures supporting their well-being are stripped away. Under stress, our core, intrinsic values may not change, but the instrumental values that serve the intrinsic ones often become more flexible. The same thing can happen when our routines are interrupted, we are subjected to unexpected challenges, or we feel threatened or vulnerable in some way. So really we do not advance from one stage to another as rungs in a ladder; instead we layer more sophisticated modes of operation over more primitive ones, but those underlying modes are still there, providing supportive functions for higher strata and waiting to reassert themselves in case we need them to survive. And, in the context of basic survival, this makes sense. Our morality has circumstantial dependencies. It is a rare and precious event when someone can sustain an advanced mode of being when all of their support systems are stripped away.

At the other extreme, overindulgence can also lead to moral regression. Instead of overtaxing stress, the eroding factor here is a lack of challenge or stimulation. To become overly secure in the infallible continuation of all of our support systems is of course a fantasy, since sweeping changes in our circumstances can occur in the blink of an eye. But that overconfidence in our position and power is just as natural a response as panic when things fall apart. It is the pendulum swinging to the opposite end of the spectrum. And so the politician whose career was spent fighting the undue influence of big corporations falls from grace in an embarrassing corporate payola scandal. Here again core values may not be entirely abandoned, but the instrumental values – the means to the end – reflect a return to more primitive moral function.

These extremes illustrate why *Integral Lifework* is focused on measuring, maintaining and adjusting a balanced, holistic form of self-care. If we can learn to dwell in the plane of the fulcrum, in the narrow band of optimal function that supports growth, we can avoid the moral pitfalls of both stress-inducing deprivation and the indolence of excess. In fact, until we experience steady and dependable nurturing that satisfies all of our nourishment centers in a balanced and holistic way, we cannot advance or sustain our values orientation. Whatever forward momentum we achieve can not be taken for granted, and requires persistent and conscious effort across inevitable plateaus and regressions. Now, you may have noticed that I haven't yet outlined a specific progression of moral development, and this is deliberate – I think it can become a distraction to dwell on that prematurely. But to clarify the general concepts, what follows is a descriptive diagram of how *moral valuation strata* are structured in *Integral Lifework*. Later on, we will discuss how these correlate with ever-expanding arenas of authentic affection, but for now they will illustrate some basic progressions in moral development.

Strata of Moral Valuation

We are born egoless, in a state of raw human need, barely aware of our own identity. Then we begin to grow, our moral compass influenced by our innate capacities, aptitudes and impulses, which are in turn shaped by the reinforcing experiences of our immediate environment. What began as insistent and fearful self-centeredness expands to include the well-being of others; what we define as beneficial, ethical and efficacious expands into larger and larger sets of interdependency. In the chart below, that process of moral expansion is broken down into recognizable strata, with each layer representing a new threshold of moral valuation. As we will later see, this evolution is tied directly to how we define our identity and how we experience and express affection. What we value most will be defined by where we are in this progression.

Take a moment to look through each definition in the following chart. Where would you place yourself in most circumstances? My observation is that different parts of us – the separate modes of operation that govern us in various kinds of relationships or levels of exchange – conform to one stratum in one situation and entirely different strata in other situations. I may operate from a place of *principled rationalism* when I enter a voting booth, in a mode of *competitive communalism* at my workplace, out of *tribal acceptance* when I join a pick-up game of basketball at the local park, from *contributive individualism* when I am beginning a romantic dating relationship, or out of *egoless raw need* when I am in profound grief over the loss of a loved one. So moral progress is not a static, step-by-step phenomenon. It is more a clustering of motivations that, if they were plotted across the entire chart, would show a denser group – a higher frequency – around one or two strata of moral valuation, while in total still being distributed across many different strata.

Applied Nonduality
Translation of mystical, nondual consciousness into unfettered being where loving kindness harmonizes with spiritual understanding; a persistent, all-inclusive love-consciousness that integrates previous value orientations and current intentions into a balanced, purposeful flow

Spiritual Universality
Through intimate connection with an absolute, universal inclusiveness of being, moral function is defined by a guiding intentionality of "the good of All" as revealed by a successive unfolding of spiritual awareness, intuition and dialectic processing

Transpersonal Holism
Appreciation and acceptance of pluralistic value system and the necessity of moral ambiguity – as guided by discernment of intentional, strategic outcomes that benefit the largest majority possible

World-Centric
Appreciation and acceptance of interdependent, globally inclusive systems and the need for individual and communal responsibility with compassionate effort in support of those systems

Principled Rationalism
Commitment to a clearly defined set of reasoned moral principles that intend to benefit all of humanity, with a corresponding individuation of identity from affinitive and beneficial communities

Cooperative Communalism
Acceptance of communal role and necessity of collaborative contribution to human welfare without a need for competition or positional authority, with facilitative conformance to a community's shared values

Competitive Communalism
Acceptance of communal role to participate in mutually beneficial community, usually in competition with others for personal positional power and influence, and without necessarily conforming to that community's shared values

Contributive Individualism
Fully individuated from tribe and committed to own well-being and wholeness, and interested in efforts that appear "good" or helpful to others as framed by (morally relativistic) individual experience and interaction

Opportunistic Individualism
In the process of individuating from tribe, morally adrift except for a sense of obligation to own well-being and wholeness, with minimal concern for the impact of that process on others

Defensive Tribalism
Championing correctness of primary social group(s) and propagating the distinct definitions of rigid rules (law & order, right & wrong, black & white) of the group(s) defines most moral function

Tribal Acceptance
Conformance with and approval or acceptance from primary social group(s) governs moral function; what is "right" or "wrong" is defined by what gains or loses social standing within the group(s)

Self-Protective Egoism
Acquisitive, consumptive, hedonistic patterns to protect and sustain ego in a self-absorbed and self-centered moral orientation with indifference to the needs of others, as moderated by fear of personal gains being lost

Self-Assertive Egoism
Aggressive promotion of own wants and whims above those of others as a moral imperative in most situations, as moderated by fear of personal pain or punishment

Egoless "Raw Need"
Naïve state: volition is centered around unrestrained basic needs fulfillment in every moment

As we mature, the more that distribution begins to center around just one stratum of moral valuation. That is, the more we pay loving attention to each and every dimension of our being, the more we evolve our whole self into the next layer of our moral development. Imagine if you will twelve spinning tops, each with a cute little propeller on its head and its own unique color. Each top represents a nourishment center in our being. When we are undernourished in any area, the corresponding top is wobbly and rotates very slowly; it is unstable and unable to stay upright. But once balanced nourishment occurs in the area the top represents, it begins to spin more quickly and evenly. And when the holistic energy exchanges provided through integral practice is achieved, all of the tops not only begin to spin smoothly and upright, but also rotate so swiftly that their propellers start generating lift. The tops then bob around, hopping here and there, up into one valuation stratum and then back down again, then higher again, and so on. Eventually, one after another, like fledgling birds leaving their nest, all the tops take flight, rising with erratic effort through successive layers of moral development. But here is the catch: they are also energetically connected to each other – none can wander too far from the others in any direction for long. The tops are loosely tethered together for their journey. Add to this that each top's rate of spin and lift capacity is affected to some degree by their immediate environment – by rain, clouds, cold, heat, dryness, light, dark and so on. That is a rough approximation of the interior processes of moral advancement, dependent as they are on nourishing every dimension of self.

Generating this hesitant, interdependent and highly changeable progress through moral valuation strata is an aim and benefit of *Integral Lifework*, and it is no simple task. Imagine trying to keep twelve tops with propellers spinning so quickly that they all remain airborne. By following the practices outlined in subsequent sections, I believe anyone will be able to accomplish this feat. I have in fact witnessed this firsthand, where it quickly becomes clear that progress depends on our passing through each successive stratum in a linear way, with each new leap dependent on our immersion in previous strata. Although we may briefly occupy a higher perspective, we can't skip any steps to dwell there consistently. But to round out the metaphor, what about the air that supports these propeller-tops as they take flight? Can you speculate what that air is made of? What facilitates lift? What makes growth and self-transformation possible?

> **Resources:**   In his book *Integral Psychology*, Ken Wilber has assembled, correlated and expounded on some of the more influential theories about moral development, including various stages and the relationship of those stages to the basic structures of his own consciousness model. For anyone who wishes to delve more deeply into the relationship between consciousness, spirituality and morality I highly recommend his work.

Motivational Awareness & Integration Process

Cognitive psychology has frequently ascribed two categories to motivation to help explain it: that which influences us to react because it is imposed on us from outside ourselves (extrinsic motivation), and that which we generate internally to compel ourselves into action (intrinsic motivation). What is really being described here is, I think, a graduated shift from motivational influences we have not yet accepted or integrated and which, consequently, we respond to in more reactive or reflexive ways, and those motivational influences we have fully accepted and integrated into our conscious way of thinking. The chart below captures the array of motivational responses that can occur when the evaluation and integration axes interact.

	Fully Accepted & Integrated ⟸	Acceptance & Integration Process	⟹ Not Integrated or Accepted
Fully Aware with Conscious Evaluation ⬆	Full awareness of motivational influence with complete acceptance & integration **(consciously intrinsic)**	Ambivalence about a motivational influence that is partially integrated, but fully aware of it & engaging in conscious processing and evaluation of that motivation	Fully aware of external motivational influence and consciously evaluating it, but tending toward rejection or non-integration of that influence **(consciously extrinsic)**
Motivational Awareness & Evaluation Process	Partial awareness of motivational influence and beginning of evaluation process with positive expectation of inclusion	Partial awareness of motivational influence with discomfort, ambivalence or avoidance regarding its acceptance & integration	Partial awareness of external motivational influence & tendency toward reflexive rejection & non-integration of that influence
Unaware, Unconscious & Reflexive ⬇	No awareness or acceptance of motivational influence, but already unconsciously integrating it **(reflexively intrinsic)**	No awareness or evaluation of motivational influence, but nonetheless unconsciously beginning to accept and integrate it	No awareness or acceptance of external motivational influence and a tendency to reflexively & unconsciously reject that influence **(reflexively extrinsic)**

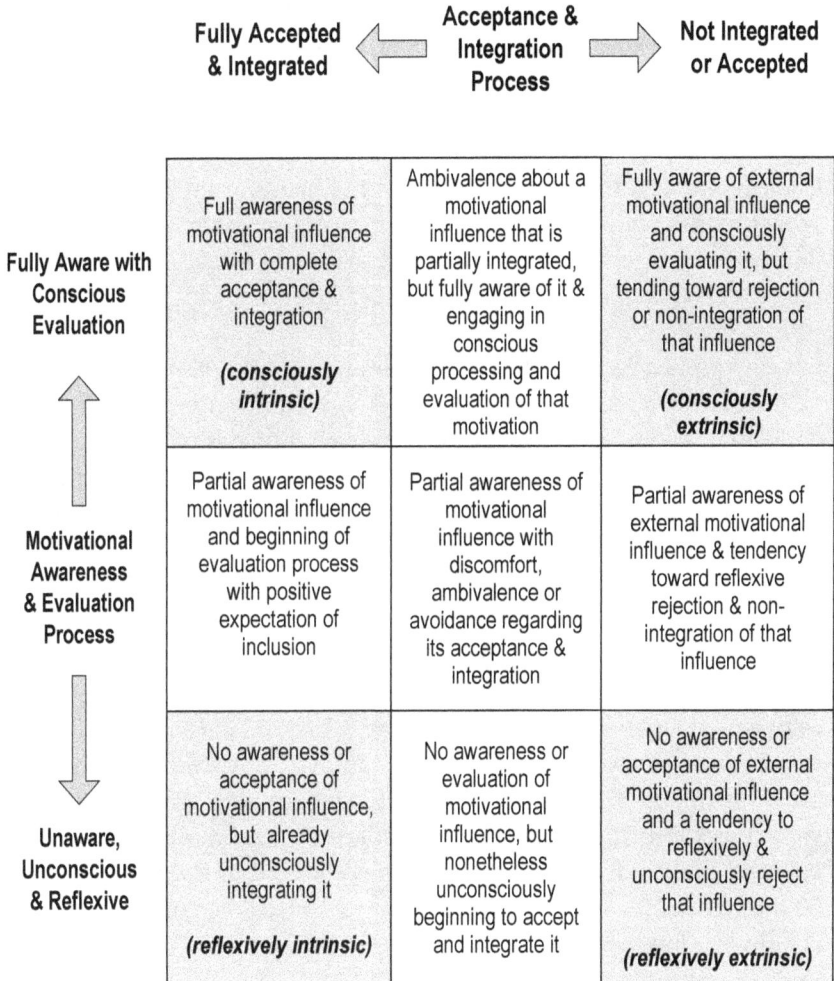

When we look at this chart, we can generate a working definition of what the extremes of the intrinsic/extrinsic spectrum really are. Either we are being driven by reflexive impulses or by conscious decisions; either our actions are governed by external influences or by internalized values. The ideal state, of course, is to be consciously aware of our motivational process, and at the same time be able to integrate what we value into our current mode of being. Am I able to find contentment and serenity within myself regardless of my circumstances from moment to moment, or am I constantly reacting to my environment in a reflexive and unconscious way? Am I able to feel compassion and affection spontaneously and without preconditions, or do I rely on others to demonstrate their feelings or fulfill certain requirements before I can express love? Have I created an interior purpose to energize me and draw me forward through my day, or do I respond to an environment's demands on me without thinking about it? Are the reasons I do things from moment to moment consciously justified and intrinsically valued, or unconsciously accepted after they have been externally imposed? I think this may be a useful model of what "extrinsic" and "intrinsic" motivations really represent.

Let me emphasize that whatever our motivational pattern is, it is not set in stone. We always have a choice to shift from reflexive and external dependencies to conscious and internal self-sufficiency. In fact, that is something we tend to do naturally over time anyway. We begin life totally dependent on the guidance of our parents and the boundaries set by our environment, but slowly we integrate that guidance and those boundaries into our self-governance. And at some point we will probably even question those integrated guidelines, synthesizing new ones from our own questioning and some new experiences. So we always have a choice. What influences us most to rely on our internal compass instead of external pressure? I think it is habit. There is tremendous comfort and security in familiar, unconscious habits, and breaking free from them can be a scary undertaking. But if we decide to consciously process how we are reacting to various situations, we can begin to challenge those habits and break free from unhealthy patterns. So the compelling question is not what motivates us, but how aware we are of what motivates us.

So the contrasts and questions persist: Are we to be governed by external pressures or internal vision? Are we paralyzed by reactive fears or liberated by our own imagination? Are we able to envision a positive, healthy and even transformative outcome, or are we trapped in a self-limiting spiral of doubts and old, self-protective patterns? Really, this line of inquiry is valid whether we are struggling to survive at the most basic level, or have bountiful resources available to us to achieve our most lofty goals. By cultivating intrinsic, self-directed motivations, we can create a different reality for ourselves and those we love. If we depend on external promptings, situational advantages or unreasoning impulse, we will inevitably become victims of that dependency. Of course, echoes of this concept are the governing principles behind decades of self-help literature in the U.S. – but perhaps this is only part of the picture of how healthy and supportive motivation is shaped and actualized.

Another aspect of reactive or habit-based motivation encompasses the external structures we create to manage our forward momentum over time. Without realizing it, we may surround ourselves with routines, commitments and familiar resources that once compelled our progress in a sensible way, but which eventually became empty habits that now interfere with the outcomes we desire. Consider the example of a romantic partnership. When two people fall in love and decide to formalize their commitment, this can result in reliance on that formalized status as sufficient proof and perpetuation of devotion. In reality, however, devotion must be renewed and reinforced daily. "I am married," is not the same qualitative statement as "today I am in love with and committed to my partner;" one relies on external structures for reinforcement, while the other is demonstrated from moment to moment and relies on internally renewed affection, openness and so on. The more we depend on the externalized status, roles or structure of a relationship to determine the quality of that relationship, the more the quality will suffer. And the same is true of all our motivations.

Without appropriate, compelling, immediate, internally generated motivation, our efforts will have oppressive and even crippling effects over time. When we push ourselves forward on autopilot, relying on decisions we made years previously or on external structures that guide our responses, our emotional life will become flat and disinterested and our efforts strained. When our responses are dependent solely on such habits or the pressures of our external environment rather than internal inspiration, we may even unconsciously create crises and conflict around us to keep ourselves reactively engaged. If we cannot frequently and actively evaluate our motivations, we will accumulate a number of negative and antagonistic results. We may sabotage our success in areas that are important to us. We may alienate loved ones. We may become depressed or physically ill. All because we resist tuning in to what we value most – what is meant to keep us focused and inspired in the current moment.

So that is our choice: to remain diligent, conscious and self-aware about our motivational landscape, or to default to unconscious impulses or automatic programming. Intrinsically generated and conscious, or extrinsically reactive and unconscious. As we differentiate between these extremes, we must ask ourselves how to best cultivate motivational awareness. How will we discern what our interior world looks like from moment to moment? How can we actively navigate it to find the motivations we require? How can we shift out of habitual reactions to more conscious modes of being? The next section begins to answer these questions. For a start, let's take a look at the first two elements of the *Integral Lifework* motivational diagram and see what we uncover.

Resources: The Internet has plentiful resources on motivational theory, including more exhaustive definitions and debates about extrinsic and intrinsic motivation. One concept that may help parse these and the other distinctions outlined in this section is *metacognition,* our ability to think about and manage our own thought processes.

Primary Drives & Fulfillment Impulses

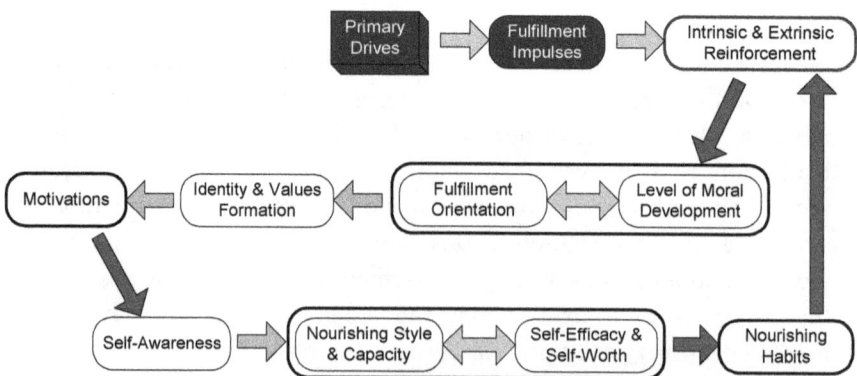

To begin, it is helpful to distinguish motivations from primary drives. A primary drive is a fundamental imperative that everyone shares, and which facilitates survival of the species. A motivation results from a series of complex events and interactions (note that a "Motivations" element is pretty far along in the diagram), but ultimately serves one or more of these primary drives. It's like having different approaches to achieve the same outcome, and as we have already seen, each approach will be uniquely suited to each situation, and each person has a unique way of creating and expressing their own approach. But let's dig into this a little. First, here are the four basic survival drives as they are defined in *Integral Lifework*:

- To Exist
- To Experience
- To Adapt
- To Affect

These fundamental drives govern everything we do and relate to every aspect of our existence. The focus of each drive – the processing space within which it is most operant – shifts constantly, but the drive is ever-present. For example, in one moment I am concerned only with myself in the now: how I exist in this instant; how I experience this instant; how I adapt to this experience; and how I have an effect on my own experience. In the next moment I am concerned with someone or something else, perhaps in a more expanded time-space: how some event in history perpetuates its existence; how others may share my experience of joy; how my elderly neighbors will adapt to the impending road construction; how a child will affect the life of their canine companion. The concept of widening circles of interaction will also become important in understanding our own evolution of being. But regardless of where we are along the arc of an ever-expanding self-concept, we cannot escape our primary drives.

We do, however, have a great deal of choice in how those drives are satisfied. Layered on top of primary drives are sixteen different fulfillment impulses. These fulfillment impulses contribute to how our motivations are defined and reinforced, and are instrumental in corralling all our efforts to serve primary drives. They also help us understand what constitutes full-spectrum nourishment, because every type of nourishment ultimately satisfies one or more fulfillment impulses. So primary drives generate fulfillment impulses, which in turn lead to motivations that are satisfied by essential nourishment. Simple, right? It will become clearer in a moment, but here is why this process of motivation synthesis is relevant: once we understand how motivations are formed and how they contributed to our day-to-day well-being, we can begin to consciously shape that process. And once we shape that process, we can resist the pitfalls of externalized or habit-based motivation. We can then be set free from attachment to past patterns of survival and reliance on external structures to nurture ourselves. We can live fully in this moment for a clear and empowering purpose we choose in accordance with the values we cherish. And we can allow true love its prominent role in this process. In other words, we can ultimately become more effective in fulfilling our primary drives. This is what it means to thrive.

Okay, so let's take a look at the diverse menu of fulfillment impulses available to us. In the following chart, each impulse is defined by its most common expression in our volition and behavior (active expression), and by the emotional responses we frequently associate with it (felt sense). Take a gander at the chart and see what you think.

FULFILLMENT IMPULSE	ACTIVE EXPRESSION	FELT SENSE
Discovery	Observe/Explore/Expand/Experiment	Sense of adventure, risk, opportunity
Understanding	Contextualize/Evaluate/Identify/Interpret	Sense of purpose, meaning, context, structure
Effectiveness	Impact/Shape/Actuate/Realize	Sense of activity, success, achievement, accomplishment
Perpetuation	Stabilize/Maintain/Secure/Contain	Sense of safety, family, security, "home"
Reproduction	Sexualize/Gratify/Stimulate/Attract	Sense of attraction, arousal, satisfaction, release, pleasure
Maturation	Nurture/Support/Grow/Thrive	Sense of caring, supporting, growing, maturing

Fulfillment	Complete/Transform/Transcend/Become	Sense of wonder, awe, fulfillment, transcendence, self-transformation
Sustenance	Taste/Consume/Quench/Savor	Sense of fullness, enjoyment, contentment, satiation
Avoidance	Escape/Evade/Deny/Reject	Sense of fearfulness, self-protectiveness, wariness, stubbornness
Union	Accept/Embrace/Incorporate/Combine	Sense of "being," union, interdependence, continuity
Autonomy	Differentiate/Individuate/Rebel/Isolate	Sense of distinct self, uniqueness, freedom, personal potential
Belonging	Cooperate/Conform/Commit/Submit	Sense of belonging, trust, community, acceptance
Affirmation	Appreciate/Enjoy/Celebrate/Create	Sense of "I am," play, gratitude, aesthetics, inspiration
Mastery	Empower/Compete/Dominate/Destroy	Sense of strength, power, control, skill, competence
Imagination	Hypothesize/Consider/Extrapolate/Project	Sense of limitlessness, possibility, inventiveness, "aha"
Exchange	Communicate/Engage/Share/Interact	Sense of connection, intimacy, sharing, expression

One quick way to put this into context is to think about people you know who exhibit some of these fulfillment impulses as a pronounced part of their values, personality or identity. For instance, a relative who is compelled to win every argument, or to achieve more than anyone else in the family, or to always be stronger, more knowledgeable or more capable than everyone else. For this person, it may be that Mastery has taken a prominent role in their approach to fulfilling primary needs. Or how about the friend who can't stand conflict or competition, who strives to be absent from any argument or confrontation, or who avoids challenging situations and difficult people altogether? For this person, perhaps Avoidance has become their default method of primary drive fulfillment. Or what about the coworker who joyfully supports the corporate mission statement, who relishes everyone getting along well and participating in each project, who believes fervently in the benefits of cooperative effort? Perhaps they have embraced Belonging as the most effective approach to survival. Of course, in reality, all of these impulses are jumbled together in a complex, dynamically changing amalgam within us, but when we reflect carefully on the nature of our actions, we will see one or more of these fulfillment impulses shine through as prominent contributions to every choice we make.

> **Exercise: What Fulfills You?** Using the *active expression* and *felt sense* columns in the chart as a guide, take a moment to reflect on the fulfillment impulses that infuse your daily life. What impulses do you think are behind many of your actions and reactions from moment to moment? Which ones seldom seem to prompt you at all? Why do think either pattern exists in your life? Are there events in your past that have influenced which impulses you've relied up on over time? Can you see how these impulses tie into your primary drives? I encourage you to capture your thoughts in your journal.

What often happens over time is that a particular combination of fulfillment impulses becomes our habitual survival mechanism – our unique set of integrated motivations – and we lose the flexibility necessary to shift our fulfillment patterns in new situations. In other words, one or more fulfillment impulses are reinforced by our life experience, and so we come to rely on the motivational patterns and external structures created by those successes. We continue to generate empty habits and reflexive reactions that indulge cycles of reinforcement, until this whole process begins to feel familiar, safe and self-protective. As these experiences are integrated into our moral valuations, our sense of identity, our worldview and our prioritizations of thought and action are funneled into each choice and interaction, and, in turn, each choice and interaction sustains and supports those same facets of our being. Once this pattern is set, we become the happy hamster on a wheel – satisfied and certain we are making progress, but really going nowhere.

An almost universal consequence is that we then cease evaluating the current moment, cease believing that we have other internal resources, capacity or flexibility – we have already unconsciously integrated an arbitrary set of values defined by our most formative experiences and, by golly, we're going to stick to what we know. For some people, the resulting mode of being serves them well in most situations, facilitating nourishment in healthy ways. For others, self-nourishment is less successful and their suffering is more extreme. But for all of us, there will come a time in our lives when our ingrained habits and set motivational patterns will fail to work well for us in some new situation, relationship or level of exchange. We will inevitably fall off our wheel. At that point, we can either choose to avoid or escape the new challenge, or embrace a new mode of being that helps us thrive.

What *Integral Lifework* seeks to accomplish is a way to meet such challenges head-on. How? Through deliberate diversification of self-nourishment, so that all fulfillment impulses are being satisfied regardless of our habitual modes of operation and our unconscious, reflexive motivations. Once that diverse nourishment floods through us, the dominance of any individual or select group of fulfillment impulses tends to subside. Once we experience reliable full-spectrum nourishment, we can relax those rigid patterns of gratification and allow energy to flow through all the circuits of our being. At the same time, we can begin to evaluate our motivations and consciously restructure them. As the energy shift and restructuring occur, the efficiency with which integral practice satisfies our primary drives amplifies the positive cycles of holistic self-care and conscious self-motivation. Instead of operating from an arbitrary set of values, our focus becomes more conscious and directed. All at once, new vistas of actualization open up before us.

Motivating Change: From Downward Spiral to Upward Spiral

How can we discover motivations that help us migrate away from unhealthy habits into healthy ones? And how can we sustain a healthy and self-supportive motivation over time? These are central questions in transformative practice and deserve careful reflection and exploration. Why? Because there two of the most powerful forces within us are working at odds: a desire to grow and thrive that actively seeks change (corresponding mainly to the *experience* and *adapt* primary drives), and a desire for safety and stability that is ambivalent about or resistant to change (corresponding mainly to the *exist* and *affect* primary drives). If either of these forces ever dominated us completely, our quality of life would quickly degrade. For we can neither remain in stasis, nor constantly cast aside established patterns in favor of new ones. One condition would lead to stagnation and depletion, and the other to chaos and overstimulation; once again, we must find the middle ground, the optimal range of effective effort. First let's cover some common methods and principles that have been utilized over time to confer new modes of being. For simplicity we will describe each as a relationship between student and teacher, but these could just as easily describe the relational qualities between a child and parent, an employee and manager, a client and therapist, a patient and healthcare provider, or our ego and our higher Self.

- **Discipleship.** The concept here is very straightforward: when someone submits to this particular mode of training, they willingly accept that they cannot always understand the benefit or even anticipate the outcome of certain patterns of thought, action and interaction. As a result, they either receive specific direction in various areas from their teacher, or are given the more general instruction to imitate their mentor. Explanation of the rationale for the instruction is seldom provided, often because it is assumed (often with reasonably supportive evidence) that such elucidation will only distract the student's learning process. As they dutifully imitate or comply with direction, the student begins to experience the benefits of that instruction. Once the benefits become clear, then the student can integrate the new information, shifting their motivation from willing submission to external conditioning to an intrinsic appreciation of the outcome and a desire to perpetuate that outcome. So extrinsic discipline becomes intrinsic motivation. This approach has been used for centuries with much success, and relies on the willingness of the student to submit to this type of training – whether that submission is a result of cultural expectations and pressures, an intrinsic yearning for betterment, or some fearful compulsion is less important than the act of submission and its eventual benefits.

- **Socratic dialogue.** At the other end of the spectrum, this approach relies on a series of questions from teacher to student that help the student reason out their own conclusions on a particular topic. Once these conclusions have been reached, the student can then apply the new concepts and convictions to their lives, making better decisions through their revised understanding. Here again, as with discipleship, the assumption is that the student will follow through with transformative action because of their willingness to submit to instruction. That is, because of their curiosity and desire for understanding, the student will be compelled to apply what they learn. So this method tends to rely on an intrinsic motivation to learn and grow.

- **Empathic connection.** When a teacher has genuine empathy for a student, they not only better understand the student's current state of being but also build a trust relationship. Why should a student care what a teacher thinks if the teacher doesn't demonstrate that they care, appreciating the student's perspective in a felt way? This is of course differentiated from sympathy in that a teacher does not merely feel sorry for a student's situation, but rather tries to step into the student's shoes and feel what they are feeling. This invites a more comprehensive mutual understanding through the common ground of shared emotional experience.

- **Enforced independence.** There is a rich vernacular for this approach: tough love, being thrown to the sharks, getting kicked out of the nest, learning to adapt or perish, an Outward Bound experience and so on. The idea here is that the teacher sees a capacity in the student that the student hasn't experienced or doesn't believe to be present in themselves. So the teacher seemingly abandons the student to an environment where they will either learn self-sufficiency or fail, and in either case be responsible for the outcome. Often the teacher remains within reach if a crisis develops, but resist being drawn into the student's process of self-discovery. This approach is often utilized when someone has established a deep rut of dependence on externals and is terrified of letting that dependence go. One advantage of this approach is that the student does not need to demonstrate willingness to enter the learning process.

- **Cathartic experience.** The idea here is to evoke an internal break-through of awareness by introducing the student to intense emotional, spiritual or intuitive material, usually through a guided therapeutic mechanism. Because that material is internal, the subjective perception is that the epiphany is self-generated and carries profound or conclusive weight in subsequent decisions. This has become a stock tool for self-improvement teachers, especially in group instruction where there may be a compressed timeline, and it relies on students' active participation.

- **Physiological amenity.** Altering physiology can have sweeping short-term benefits. Drugs, fasting, therapeutic bodywork and acupuncture could be grouped into this category. As external agents supplied by the teacher to act on the student's physiology, these mitigate barriers to healthy function, relieve discomfort and pain, or stimulate new avenues of interior processing. In most cases, this approach expects students to remain passive and receptive, rather than actively participate. Because of this, sustained, long-term benefits of this approach are limited.

- **Cultural conformance.** As a didactic tool and motivational force, cultural conformance is always present, nudging us towards one communally approved set of choices. Even when student and teacher are unaware of it, this influence works itself into the instructional relationship. Perhaps someone attends a seminar because their friends or loved ones pressured them to do so, or because they identify with a particular group or belief system that holds a particular status in their culture. Perhaps someone teaches a class because their culture has corralled them into a teaching role, or because their culture places value on what they teach. If there is a cultural stigma associated with being single and childless, then a person in that situation might be motivated to consult a mentor or read books on how to find the perfect mate. If a culture promulgates the idea that happiness is a commodity that is easy to purchase, then students and teachers alike may be compelled to engage in instruction on that topic. And so on.

- **Deceptive manipulation.** Here the teacher deliberately misleads the student to achieve a specific outcome. Sometimes this is a conscious deception, and sometimes the teacher themselves has become deluded by the manipulative content of what they teach. This approach is used when students are unreceptive, passive or resistant, or when students are willing but the teacher lacks confidence.

- **Consequence inducement.** This is all about rewards and punishments. If the student jumps through a given hoop, the teacher will reward them. If the student trips and falls, the reward is withdrawn or students may be subjected to a harsher punishment. This can be an efficient short-term control, but it seldom encourages the self-sufficiency necessary to advance to more mature stages of being. This approach can be used with passive, resistant and actively engaged students.

- **Values alignment.** If the student has deeply internalized values that do not align with their current beliefs, assumptions or behaviors, the teacher first helps the student recognize this disconnect. Once this is achieved, the teacher invites the student to begin aligning their thoughts, emotions and actions with professed values, providing tools and resources to evaluate and maintain that alignment. A variant of this approach is for the teacher to explore a student's values and judgments that unwittingly support self-defeating beliefs and assumptions, and then to help the student consider the ultimate consequences of such a pattern. The final step in this process is assisting the student in first considering, then envisioning and actualizing new values, goals and outcomes that are more self-supportive. Student willingness and openness are not a prerequisite to this approach, but of course accelerate positive results.

- **Influencing the unconscious directly.** Here the student is subjected to techniques that directly access their unconscious mind. Sometimes the student contributes active components to this process, and sometimes they remain passive; their willingness can assist but it is not necessary. Techniques to access the unconscious include hypnotherapy, induced relaxation, body-centered psychotherapy, verbal probing techniques, music and art therapy, guided visualization and imagination, certain types of meditation, affirmation or other self-talk, and many others. As methods for the student to achieve new awareness about their inner workings or to intervene in a self-destructive crisis, these can be extremely beneficial. As methods of ongoing learning, healing and self-actualization, they may be of less value when they encourage the student to remain passive. This tends to bypass active self-governance and medicate difficult internal material in much the same way that physiological amenities do.

- **Non-judgmental introspection.** This includes techniques the student learns from their teacher and applies willingly and independently. These include things like meditation, heightened intuition and somatic awareness. The central theme is that whatever the student encounters during introspective practice is observed and accepted without reaction or judgment. As a long-term tool for continued self-discovery and motivational transition, this approach is indispensable.

- **Faith reliance.** To believe in a power greater than ourselves is the basis of nearly all faith traditions. When a teacher-student relationship centers around reliance on such faith, both parties are encouraged to let go of volitional control over outcomes and trust in the benevolence of a higher power. This is an important tool for many reasons, mainly because it disengages ego from the transformation process. This in turn frees up internal resources (i.e. the energy behind each fulfillment impulse) so that they can be focused on change rather than ego's main function, which is generally maintaining the status quo of previous mental, emotional and behavioral patterns. In other words, faith reliance is intended to foster humility and letting go. And once an ability to acquiesce is conditioned into the student's psyche, other barriers to growth and transformation can also be eliminated with more ease. This method has been effective for both short-term intervention and longer-term healing.

- **Collaboration.** Working together toward a mutually beneficial outcome provides many opportunities for learning and growth. The synergy created through collaboration is in itself a motivating factor, empowering the student to contribute to the learning agenda and process, and encouraging self-reliance. Collaboration also benefits the teacher by reinforcing humility and exposing them to higher accountability. Although this process often requires more time than other methods, the outcome is almost always beneficial to everyone involved over the long term.

•   **Getting out of the way.** In this method the teacher establishes a safe and supportive atmosphere for the student to explore new material, but otherwise does not interfere with the process of discovery and learning. Here the teacher trusts the student to find their own way, withdrawing to a non-directive distance in terms of their own role, while modeling a truly caring relationship. In this approach, the teacher's way of being exemplifies positive outcomes for the student, and gently places the responsibility for those outcomes in the student's hands.

In order to be productive, all of these methods rely on our fundamental drives – to exist, adapt, experience or affect – and their subsequent fulfillment impulses to sustain forward momentum. The motivation to change is therefore directly linked to the fulfillment we receive in each of those areas. In *Integral Lifework,* that fulfillment is framed as essential nourishment of our twelve dimensions of self, which in turn satisfies our basic drives. If we lose our ability to self-nourish, to satisfy all of those fulfillment impulses, then our intrinsic motivation is increasingly undermined. As a result, our ability to adapt effectively, experience fully, affect capably or even exist safely is also compromised. So it follows that, unless and until we fully nurture ourselves holistically across all dimensions, we will sabotage intrinsic motivations. Those basic drives will still exist, still pull us forward through each day, because they are the building blocks of our volition and the irreducible fundaments of who, what and how we are. But our capacity to act on those drives, to translate them into meaningful, self-sustaining patterns will be greatly curtailed. So the first step in energizing our motivational orientation is to take advantage of the motivational approaches listed here to ensure we have full-spectrum nourishment; that is, to make certain we are satisfying all of our fulfillment impulses as part of a daily integral practice.

So which of these mode-shifting methods works best? Interestingly, in terms of conveying healthy or corrective modes of being, they all work well in certain situations, with each method appealing more strongly to the unique combination of aptitudes, skill sets and barriers each individual possesses at a given time. For one person, the most effective way to jump start learning is through body-centered treatment. Another person thrives in a discipleship relationship. Others will not be able to integrate new information without a strong, empathic connection. Moreover, many different methods may need to be combined…and then, over time, people change and respond differently.   As an *Integral Lifework Practitioner* and instructor of mystical practice, I have experimented with many of these approaches. What I have found is that no single method appears to be superior to any other in the short run, but there are a few that provide enduring results over the longer term. In particular, approaches that incorporate non-judgmental introspection, empathic connection, Socratic dialogue, discipleship, values alignment and enforced independence seem to have the greatest long-term success for all but the most difficult situations. These have a built-in cycle of reinforcement that empowers people to continue with courage, hope and self-reliance. This is why you will encounter many of those methods in some form among the following pages.

Are there any methods that tend to be less productive?   Clearly, deceptive manipulation is disempowering at best and unethical at worst. Beyond that, many practitioners of traditional and alternative healing gravitate toward modalities that resonate with their own experiences and preferred mode of being, but exclude other approaches. By doing this, they are sometimes unable to find common ground with clients or patients; I have experienced this myself.   We are also influenced by culture.   Quick, externally oriented fixes are the cultural norm in the West, and therapeutic environments are often subject to a rushed, assembly-line, profit-driven ethos.   Certain approaches adapt more easily to such environments.   In particular, cathartic experiences, physiological amenity, deceptive manipulation and direct influence on the unconscious are widely embraced in Western healing.   All but deceptive manipulation can retain an important place in the healing, growth and transformation process. I see them as intervention tools for short term barrier reduction and illuminating self-discovery. However, although they can be helpful in the short run, they may become impedances to self-sufficiency as people regain their motivational compass. Why? Because they tend to be externally-oriented, incurring ongoing dependence rather than inspiring self-directed effort. In other words, they tend to provide rapid relief and escape from the more difficult – but necessary – phases of our interior journey. So to accelerate initial intervention and awakening, these methods can be miraculous, but for longer term maintenance and maturation they are not.

There are, of course, always exceptions to the rule. Sometimes doors open or close of their own accord, regardless of our quality of effort or the tools at our disposal. In fact, I believe successful outcomes have more to do with a certain magic ingredient than any particular method of self-transformation. This one ingredient will have the greatest impact on our ability to convert a downward spiral of suffering and despair into an upward spiral of effective, hopeful living. And that special magic is what we will discuss in a moment.

Useful Combinations

How to motivate and sustain personal change is a critical question in all healing, growth and transformative practice, and no less so in *Integral Lifework*. So I will focus special attention on techniques that have been successful in my own development, teaching and integral approaches. A main emphasis in *Integral Lifework* is self-empowerment and intrinsic reinforcement, so is there a combination of mode-shifting methods that lends itself most readily to this? Unfortunately, an inflexible approach is seldom effective for every person; instead, as an ILP I must rely on careful assessment, probing, intuition and feedback to discover what works best for each client. The key is finding that first spark of interest, that initial resonance with motivations that are already close to the surface. Sure, motivations will change over time, but that first foothold is critical. This is equally true when we are self-selecting options for personal growth. Thankfully there are several methods to choose from, and a manageable enough number that we can experiment to see what dovetails with temperament, learning style and initial motivations. So the following are combinations of mode-shifting motivational methods that have had the broadest, most consistent impact on positive upward spirals for my own evolution, and in my sessions with *Integral Lifework* clients.

Values Alignment with Empathy, Non-Judgmental Introspection
& Getting Out of the Way

When we recognize the benefits of a change and how those benefits align
with our core values, is strengthens our motivation to change. The more
we explore and discuss those benefits and values, the clearer our vision
of change becomes, the deeper our conviction about its necessity, and the
easier our first steps toward meaningful action. For instance, if my core
values include having close and rewarding relationships and being a
caring and skillful teacher, then once I realize how improving my
communication skills will facilitate these values, I will be more
motivated to learn about effective communication. When presented with
an opportunity to take a class or put the ideas I have just read about into
practice, I will have more enthusiasm and less ambivalence. For change
to happen, I have to be able to connect the dots. There must a context for
what I am doing or learning that makes it meaningful, and if the
potential outcome of that education or action is to actualize what I
already believe is important, then absorbing the information and using it
to improve my life are much easier. The motivation to follow through is
intrinsic.

This is why we constantly ask "Why?" Why am I doing this? Why is it
important to me? How does it connect with my core values? How is it
facilitating the outcomes I hope for? If we can't answer these questions
with confidence, our motivation to continue will be undermined. If we
know that our primary drives are to exist, experience, adapt and affect,
we should be able to plug every component of our life into that
framework – every goal, every hope, every impulse, every action. And if
we also know that our fulfillment impulses also serve those underlying
drives, we have a way to interpret our motivations in that context. Am I
trying to feel safe? Do I want to belong? Am I avoiding something
painful? All of these are normal responses that serve our primary drives.
What tends to confuse us, get us off track and even injure our well-being
is when we begin overemphasizing one type of fulfillment and
neglecting others. All those fulfillment impulses are part of us for a
reason. They allow us to achieve balance, harmony and growth. When
our motivations become so single-minded, so focused on one thing that
we choke off the full array of additional fulfillment available to us, then
we are really choking off our ability to thrive. A part that we need to be

whole is forgotten; a part that was designed to help us exist, to be effective in realizing our day-to-day choices, to enliven and enrich our experiences, and to provide us the flexibility we need to adapt to new situations.

So, understandably, even if we align beneficial actions with our core values, if we have forgotten to nourish every dimension of our being, our ability to create or maintain positive change in our lives will be greatly curtailed. And that is one of the reasons *Integral Lifework* came into being. When we provide ourselves with balanced, multidimensional nourishment we are propelled and sustained through the highs and lows of our achievements and failures, because our goals and vision are moderated to include fulfillment for every aspect of our being. In essence, through integral practice we avoid putting all of our volitional eggs in one basket, and honor our whole self rather than just one portion. To illustrate through the starkest of contrasts: what if the only thing that motivated me to get out of bed in the morning was the promise of capturing a beautiful image with my camera? It might be satisfying to have such a clear and easily gratified purpose. But what if I then lost my sight? What would inspire me to get out of bed? If I had focused my entire life in just this one area, my other talents and skills would be underdeveloped, and any path out of my grief and devastation would be that much more difficult. Although this is in many ways an oversimplification, it is a principle we see reflected in everyday life. Consider the increased risk of heart attack or stroke within six months of retirement. Or the many partnerships and families that end up in crisis when one person is so driven they disconnect from their loved ones. Or the depression and emptiness many people experience after the initial excitement of achieving a long sought-after goal. These are all manifestations of the same pattern: imbalanced and exclusionary nourishment.

For any values-alignment process to be productive, the characteristics of empathy and non-judgmental introspection must be present. The more we are able to feel our way through each introspective question without being compelled to exonerate or condemn ourselves over what we find, the more accurate our assessment will be and the freer we will be to act on our discoveries. If we can't navigate our values with emotional sensitivity – if we can't feel the importance of each value we uncover – it will be difficult to answer the question of "why?" as well as discover a clear prioritization within. In other words, there must be an empathic connection with each of our values for them to hold importance for us. What is empathy? Empathy allows us to recognize, honor and validate whatever we encounter on a felt level. Empathy encourages us to say "Yes, I can feel that this is part of me and is important to me." At the same time, if we can hold what we discover in a neutral, non-judgmental space, we will be able to actuate those values with minimal effort. If self-degrading reactions enter into the process (i.e. guilt, shame, fear, anxiety, dismissal, avoidance, etc.) our ability to put our core values into practice will be short-circuited. So non-judgmental introspection allows us to say "Yes, this is part of me...and, for now, that's okay. It just is. I can accept this about myself."

In many ways our level of empathy and neutrality of judgment reflect our current stage of moral development. Why? Because what we are really doing here is entertaining a contradiction: we are examining how we evaluate the world while suspending valuation of that process. As a brief peak experience, anyone can achieve this perspective whatever strata they inhabit. But as a sustained self-examination it requires a fairly advanced level of moral navigation. Therefore our goal shouldn't be perfection in this process, but a best effort that helps us glimpse a facet of our True Self. And that is where *getting out of the way* comes in. Once we get the transformational ball rolling, any attempts to constrain, control or grab hold of its bounding elation are inherently dampening. To let go, to let things be, to let our natural inclination to thrive take over and take off is just as important as setting the stage for transformative experiences or fueling their progress with holistic energy exchanges.

All of these principles originate from the observed dynamics of successful teacher-student relationships, all we are doing here is making you both the teacher and the student. With this in mind, spend a few minutes with the exercise below and see what you can discover.

Exercise: Values Alignment   Take a moment to review some changes you would like to make in your life by envisioning some specific outcomes. Put today's date at the top of three blank pages in your journal. On the first page, write five specific goal statements and their benefits using the following format: "I would like to _____ starting/by [specific date], because I want _____." For example, "I would like to learn basic phrases in Italian starting next Monday, because I want to have some proficiency before I travel to Italy." Or ""I would like to lose ten pounds by the first of next month, because I want to have more energy throughout each day." In these statements, try to use language that is both positive and concrete. For instance, I could have said "I would like to be less fat," but that is neither as positive nor as concrete as "I would like to lose ten pounds."

On the second page, write down as many contrast statements you can think of that amplify benefits for each goal. The question you are answering here is the deeper justification or desire behind each goal. Why is each goal important to you? Try using this format: "Right now, I _____. But when I _____, I will feel _____." For example, "Right now, I don't know much Italian. But when I learn some phrases, I will feel more confident while I'm traveling." Or "Right now, I seem overweight and tired. But when I lose ten pounds, I will feel more positive about my body." Notice the shift to underlying justifications for these goals. Keep writing statements until you run out of room.

On the last page, explore some core values that align with your goals. This may take a bit longer to think through, so try not to rush. Using the following format, see what comes to the surface for you. List all of the last phrases from the second page down the left side of the third page. On the right side of the page, keep answering the question "Why is this important to me?" after each successive answer...until you burrow down to the core value that supports your desires. For example:

> **Feel more confident while I'm traveling** – (Why is this important to me?) So the trip goes more smoothly. (Why is this important to me?) So that I will have a more enjoyable trip. (Why is this important to me?) I want to have more fun in life! *Thus a core value uncovered through this examination is "having fun in life."*

Feel more positive about my body – (Why is this important to me?) Because I want to feel better about myself overall. (Why is this important to me?) Because if I feel better about myself, I'll be more confident and assertive. (Why is this important to me?) Because I want to be more empowered, and to have more control over my life. (Why is this important to me?) Because if I have more control, I will feel more safe. And if I am more empowered, I'll get more things done. (Why is this important to me?) Because feeling safe is important to me! And getting things done is important to me...it helps me feel satisfied and productive. *Here the core values revealed are "feeling safe," "being productive" and "experiencing satisfaction."*

Spend a few minutes more reflecting on what you uncovered here. Notice how the last of your answers on page three relate to your desired outcomes on page one. In the example above, my desired outcome of losing ten pounds is so I can feel safe, satisfied and productive. And my learning phrases in Italian is so I can have more fun in life. When I see the connection between my underlying values and those outcomes, I can remain committed to them more easily. It can also be enlightening to decipher how those core values align with the fulfillment impulses in that chart, so I encourage you to try that as well. Take a moment to consider the following questions while reviewing the fulfillment impulse chart:

- What impulses keep surfacing for you?
- Which ones seem to be neglected?
- Which ones seem to align with some of your core values?
- Which ones do you think would aid you in achieving your desired goals?

If you'd like you could also think about other areas of your life you would like to change to align with your core values, and see where that leads you. Just return to the first page you recorded as part of this exercise, and write down the new areas you wish to focus on, repeating the same steps. This may uncover still more values that are important to you, and both help you align your goals with those values and actuate a specific action plan.

Discipleship with Empathy, Collaboration and Enforced Independence

In certain areas, especially those where we have experienced little success in the past or have a particularly steep learning curve, a discipleship relationship can be extremely beneficial. But let's clarify some of the parameters of such an involvement. A number of my therapeutic and teaching relationships have begun with a client or student assuming there is a power relationship present that must be respected. This is, I believe, the result of cultural programming regarding societal and situational roles. However, this assumption of positional power can become a disempowering trap for both parties, shifting genuine, intrinsic motivations into external and artificial ones, and creating an unhealthy dependence that stifles growth. To redefine this dynamic can be challenging, but it has to be done. The healthy responsibility of the teacher is one of sharing their knowledge, insight and experience in the context of collaborative problem-solving; they are facilitating a joint inward exploration of past, present and future phenomena. There is no hierarchy inherent to this role, only a difference of learning based on skills the teacher also had to acquire. The student's responsibility is then to take utmost advantage of the teacher's experience, insight and skills without annihilating their sense of self, their willpower or their intrinsic dignity and sovereignty. The tendency for each party to gravitate towards a more hierarchical, one-up to one-down relationship instead of shared discovery and cooperation is understandable but always counterproductive.

A learning gap will eventually present itself that requires a blind leap of faith, when the student can't comprehend one or more taught principles in a direct, felt way. At this point the teacher asks the student to follow a set of instructions, knowing that the student would otherwise only have a vague comprehension of the process and its outcomes. If the student willingly submits and follows the instructions, they will discover for themselves the value of those instructions. But if they question and challenge, trying to gain an intellectual handle on the process or its outcomes, this may make them feel better about moving forward, but it won't encourage same depth of instruction as simply following the process. So discipleship requires patience and commitment from both teacher and student. From the teacher's perspective, it may seem easier at this point to use other methods to induce compliance other than trusting in the student's willingness. Cultural conformance, deceptive manipulation, consequence inducement, Socratic dialogue, cathartic experience and faith reliance have all been applied in this context – but really these are often pretexts for the more potent justification, which is basically "just give this a try and you'll experience the benefits firsthand."

In my experience the most supportive and constructive way to bridge this initial learning gap is to enter the entire process in a collaborative and cooperative spirit, and then reinforce that relationship with an empathic connection. Genuine empathy builds trust, and collaboration empowers students to take first steps on the basis of their own reasoning and conclusions. The teacher can then be a less intrusive guide, reminding them, encouraging them and holding them accountable to the tasks and goals they set for themselves. This isn't always as touchy-feely as it sounds, because the process requires honesty that can be difficult to deliver and difficult to hear. It also requires a healthy dose of enforced independence. What this usually means is that the teacher deliberately and repeatedly nudges a student out of their comfort zone – and eventually out of the "nest" of the discipleship relationship entirely. But enforced independence can (and should) originate from both sides, because students also have a responsibility to push back at the teacher whenever the learning process becomes too hurried, too overwhelming with unfamiliar territory, or begins to undermine a student's sense of self or self-direction. Both parties have to be fiercely courageous for discipleship to be effective.

So how can discipleship principles be applied to a book? Well, you'll notice that there are several exercises scattered throughout these pages. Each one is intended to engage the reader in the same way a discipleship relationship does – imparting experiential information through the reader's willingness to experiment and follow a set of instructions. There are concepts we simply won't grasp until we begin to experiment and explore through rote practice. And of course enforced independence is the subtext for all of these exercises, because this particular teacher-student relationship is abstracted through the medium of the written word. Unlike direct interaction, however, neither of us gets to benefit from the same level of collaborative effort. And empathy? Hopefully there is at least some empathic connection between us, perhaps generated by some of my more personal examples, or some shared epiphanies and core values that might be inferred through careful reading, but the empathic element is admittedly attenuated in this medium. On the other hand, you have the advantage of spending as much time as you desire mulling over the concepts laid out here before trying any of the exercises. You get to choose the terms of your engagement in the process. That's one reason I myself like books – I get to digest and relish them at my own pace.

Motivational Breakdown

In the *Integral Lifework* approach, we will always remain sufficiently motivated to change, grow and maintain our progress if we achieve balanced nourishment in all dimensions of our being. That is because, if we satisfy all of our fulfillment impulses in a measured and caring way, we will be able to sustain an upward spiral of transformation. This is an important goal of integral practice. Conversely, when we are not able to nourish ourselves holistically, our motivation to continue will begin to break down. When one or more areas become depleted, our natural tendency will be to compensate by focusing on some unrelated aspect of our lives. We will tend to substitute for undernourished areas rather than addressing them directly. And achieving high levels of fulfillment in one area can seem enriching and exciting over a short span; eventually, however, this can no longer compensate for serious depletions. Even if we are skilled at synthesizing new horizons for ourselves, inventing new and compelling goals to draw us forward through life, the neglected parts of us will end up feeling frustrated, lost and empty. If we continue to ignore them, our existence will become ever more strained and dissonant, until at some point even our most skillful efforts will lose resonance, and our most celebrated accomplishments will seem empty of meaning. At this point, our reliable habits of self-nourishment will begin to fall apart, and the thin veneer of normalcy atop our existence will be ripped away.

For many people, arriving at this place of emptiness and motivational breakdown is the beginning of a quest for balanced nourishment. They recognize the need to adjust their patterns of thought, emotion and action before things get any worse. For others, the spiral must descend further into real depression and despair before they begin to reach for fresh understanding. And for some, the awakening to a new way of being does not arrive until they collide with life-threatening conditions. We all have different tolerances for suffering and different habits for coping, and the great irony of the modern age is that many of the attitudes and behaviors that help us survive and even thrive in Western culture directly contribute to imbalanced nourishment and accelerated depletion. Consider the influence of fast food, stress-filled careers, conspicuous consumption, broken communities and failed relationships on our ability to care for ourselves and our loved ones. It is all too easy to jump onto the fast-moving train of modern conveniences and inadvertently rush past our most fulfilling and multidimensional opportunities for healing and growth.

What happens when one or more fulfillment impulses continue to remain unattended? We begin to lose the joy of life. And when we lose the joy of life, our ability to self-nourish is crippled in many areas at once, and the downward spiral accelerates. Then, once we reach such a dark and foreboding place, it is easy to feel like a victim, to feel disgusted with our situation and sorry for ourselves without any real hope of liberation. We might turn to others in the hope that they will somehow rescue us from our predicament. And that might even provide superficial relief for a time. But the natural progress of motivational breakdown is to destroy our lives even further so that easy recovery becomes impossible. We may even convince ourselves that the downward spiral is bottomless, and that we are powerless to stop it. After all, if we keep resisting or denying accountability for our own well-being, we will never be responsible for what happens to us. Eventually, we can come to fully identify ourselves as *the helpless victim*. In order to arrest this self-disabling momentum, we must discover the kernel of resolve within us that will recharge our motivational battery. We need to flip the switch in our hearts from self-destructive impulses to self-preservation impulses, and take responsibility for our own wellness. How can we best do that?

In the following chapters we will explore in detail how to turn a downward spiral into an upward one, and how to sustain that upward climb to a joyful and productive life. But there is a first critical step that will inform every other step along the way. We need to tap the force that will jump-start our conviction to care for ourselves. It is the force that energizes all positive momentum in our lives. I believe it is also the fundamental causal agent for life itself. In its most authentic form, this magic ingredient is perhaps the most powerful of all mechanisms of change. It answers the "why" of all primary drives confidently and conclusively, shaping values that govern the highest levels of fulfillment and the most nourishing of intentions and actions.

Love: The Magic Ingredient

There are many emotionally felt experiences that can motivate us to adjust our life direction. We might become angry about some situation and from that anger find the strength to change it. Or we might experience a cathartic epiphany about some new direction in our life and translate that into the first steps of constructive progress. Or we might begin to alter our habits out of guilt, or fear, or anxious compulsion. In fact, just about any strong emotion can light a fire in our awareness that illuminates the imperative of new direction. But none of these will keep us going for long – we are simply not wired to continually function that way. Once we experience a little relief from the suffering that initially incited our change-response, or are distracted from our epiphanies by novel insights and experiences, or discover a way to medicate ourselves and numb any uncomfortable feelings, we will inevitably begin drifting away from our newfound path. There is only one felt experience that can energize us both with that initial kick-start spark of inspiration and sustain the positive vision, prodding and enticement that will help us persevere in our journey. And that, of course, is a certain quality of love. When the felt experience of authentic love inhabits us completely, guiding every thought and action, we are both gently invited and strongly compelled to nourish every dimension of our being. And when we then fulfill those needs with authentic love, the cycle amplifies itself. When our efforts are permeated with caring and affection, they are more likely to flourish and we will be much more forgiving of ourselves if we fail. And, as our fulfillment impulses are satisfied, that reinforcement inspires us to continue, and because we are anchored in compassionate understanding we are much less likely to stray into depleting substitutions or excesses.   Through love we discover that ideal moderation – the narrow band of optimal function that strengthens us – with increasing ease.   And because love is as much a product of multidimensional nourishment as it is a facilitator of the process, the upward spiral is never-ending.   Even the natural barriers we encounter along the way become just one more opportunity for love to triumph – in encouraging our patience, in inspiring faith in our own healing, in comforting us when we stumble.   Without the magic ingredient of love, our loftiest goals and most impassioned disciplines will inevitably crumble back into empty, unsatisfying habits.

A stronger way to state this principle is that without the cofactor of love, the nutrients available to different dimensions of our being cannot be properly metabolized.   You could even say that a paucity of love is our greatest barrier to wholeness and well-being.   The felt experience of compassionate affection must develop in parallel with every other aspect of self; it is both a prerequisite and product of nurturing efforts. Returning for a moment to the strata of moral valuation, consider that movement from one stratum to the next cannot occur unless love is firmly seated in our consciousness.   Authentic love, in this context, is the fullest expression possible of our particular level of moral development; it progressively defines what we value and how courageously we act on those valuations.   This leads to one way we can define love-consciousness: love that has become fully conscious within us, producing a sensitivity that is wholly infused with love and grounded in ever-expanding arenas of affection.   Another way to say this is that our moral development reflects the maturation of love within us, and this in turn defines how skillfully we can achieve multidimensional nourishment for ourselves and throughout all of our interactions.   Our energy exchanges become the very currency of love and the evidence of its sovereignty in our life.

With these principles in mind, the following chapters will introduce both the road to wholeness through integral nourishment, and the means to invoke a sustaining force of love throughout that journey.   You could even say that the middle way – the zone of mature and optimal effort – is a direct result of recognizing what balanced nourishment looks like when it is energized by loving intentions. The rest is just learning to rely on innate strengths and acquiring some simple skills to enable our voyage. We all have, in our innermost being, the tools to succeed in this adventure. We just have to remember what those tools feel like, and when and how to use them.

If I feel affection for myself, won't I want to nourish every aspect of my being? And if I can care for myself effectively, won't that help me become more competent in facing new challenges? Thinking, choosing and acting from a place of loving kindness, we have the courage to be flexible and allow appropriate fulfillment impulses to take the upper hand when needed. Then our love can flow forth into the world around us as well. I am sure you can intuit the critical role that compassionate affection plays in the nourishment process – it is the beginning and end of our journey. True love is the kernel of enduring strength at our core, the wind that lifts us, and the distant horizon towards which we fly. It is the cofactor for metabolizing healthy nourishment in every dimension of self and the sunlight that enables growth. It inspires change and supports us as we test our wings. Love then provides the courage to see ourselves and the world around us clearly, and envision a future appropriate to who we really are. In the end, it is only through love that we can grasp the importance of the life we choose to live, or measure the real worth of our triumphs.

BUILDING BLOCKS OF WELL-BEING

Compassion is an endless journey, changing and evolving with each breath. It is at once subtle and elusive and omnipotent and all-pervasive, yet learning how to love is our natural inclination; our desire to love doesn't require any training at all. Does a systematized approach to loving kindness dilute its freshness, spontaneity or miraculous effects? Not at all. Because of its organic nature, the essence of love pervades everything we do, whether we feel it or even choose to recognize it. So learning about love – how to experience it as well as how to express it – is less a synthesis of desirable traits and practices, and more an unfolding discovery of what is already there, right beneath the surface of each moment. And sometimes, especially in a world full of distorted or incomplete reflections of ourselves and the affectionate impulses within us, it is helpful to have support and guidance through this process of discovery. That is in part what I hope to provide here.

Before delving into the full blossoming of authentic love, it is helpful to understand some prerequisites for our own capacity to love fully. That is, there are certain conditions which, if they have not yet been encouraged or sustained, will inhibit our ability to experience the love we already possess and the potential of that love to flourish and grow. We have already touched on the idea of maturity's role in this process, so let's examine some of those key maturity factors. Among the most critical interior structures that support love are our identity and self-awareness, the belief we have in ourselves, and the governing intentions that infuse our daily life. These are the primary building blocks of integral practice, which in turn help us become more receptive to the deep and enduring foundations of love-consciousness. Really, they answer the three basic questions of preparation: Are we ready to love? Are we able to love? Are we willing to love? How accurately and thoroughly we answer these questions will define our ability to share ourselves in loving ways and constructively receive the caring attentions of others.

How can we begin to answer these questions? In part, initiating an integral practice will provide an experiential answer. As we nurture ourselves in every dimension, we will quickly encounter barriers to nourishment that provide some helpful insights, and the sense of expansion and strength in other areas will unveil additional wisdom. Integral practice offers us direct access to new information about ourselves, and rather than a static snapshot of strengths or weaknesses, much more qualitative information will unfold for us as we continue in our personal practice. It's an exciting process – so let's get started.

What is Nourishment?

One way of understanding nourishment is as an exchange of vital substance, an intermingling of essences between one thing and another. As those essences engage, one of them may be consumed so that the other grows stronger. And yet that is not how all nourishment occurs. There are also energy exchanges that are symbiotic, mutual or complimentary, so that every essence involved is reinforced, supported or strengthened through the interaction. For instance, if I smile at someone I pass on the street, I am not expending much energy, but I may receive a great deal of energy in return should they smile back at me. Or perhaps my own reason for smiling generates energy within me that touches everyone I pass by. Regardless, nothing is lost here. In this way, joy is mutually nourishing energy, as is encouragement or any expression of affection. And what is energy? A wave, an excited particle, a continual transmutation of matter from one form to another, and from one spectrum to another. And like all energy, there are different wavelengths and harmonics, resonances and interferences involved in the nourishment process. Each wavelength emanates from a particular dimension, with its own unique resonance in space and time. The spectra of nourishment in *Integral Lifework* include the spiritual, the emotional, the physical, the mental, the social and so on, with each satisfying many different fulfillment impulses at once. We will define twelve nourishment dimensions in a moment, but it's important to remember that the main objective of integral practice is to nourish many areas at once, as fully and as skillfully as possible, so that the broadest band of nourishment energy is both received and expressed in each dimension. That is full-spectrum nourishment.

In order for efficient energy exchange to take place there must be intimate connection. This is very important. Think of an electrical current traveling from one wire to another. If there is a gap in the wire the current will either be unable to continue its journey, or it will arc in a blaze of expended light and heat. If the wires are well-connected, the current travels on without mishap. This simple analogy applies to every form of nourishing energy exchange. If I am intimately connected to something from which I receive nourishment, that nourishment will flow efficiently into the appropriate parts of my being, without meandering off into some other place, and I will be able to reciprocate in kind. So for there to be satisfying spiritual nourishment, there must be an intimate spiritual connection involved. For effective emotional nourishment there must be an intimate emotional connection. And so on for the physical, the social, the mental and all the other dimensions or wavelengths of nourishment.

Another way of understanding nourishment is through relationship, and at the center of relationship is reciprocation. The more supportive, fluid, open and balanced that reciprocation becomes, the more intimate the relationship can become. One-sided love affairs are not very satisfying, but when affection is mutually recognized then sharing can deepen. With mutual love comes an intermingling of essences, an unguarded sharing of meaningful experiences, and – if the match is well-suited – a broadening foundation of supportive values and beliefs. As we apply this to different arenas of affection and various nourishment centers, you will see that full spectrum nourishment cannot occur without this openness and interaction. In fact, without falling in love with every aspect of ourselves and every aspect of our lives, we can never be fully nurtured. Like a friendless soul lost in loneliness, we will forever be trying to connect with something or someone – forever trying to generate relationship – without being able to support the exchange.

High Quality Relationship

So how do we make an enduring connection and deepening relationship possible? In this context, all the principles and guidelines that facilitate open, high quality communication and intimately satisfying relationships also allow effective connection and energy exchange – and thus efficient nourishment. As an example, here is a quick overview of some key factors that contribute to the kind of connections and relationships that support *Integral Lifework*. If all of these factors are present in some form throughout our energy exchanges with each facet of self, then we have created high quality relationship.

- **Connectedness.** A presumption and mutual acknowledgement of connectedness, interdependence and equivalent fundamental value.

- **Validation.** Authentic desire to understand, appreciate and support each other's perspective, individual journey and unique contributions.

- **Compassion.** Recognizing the circle of intimacy and arena of affection within which the exchange is occurring, and consciously honoring that with appropriate empathy and love-in-action.

- **Clear priority, balance & boundaries.** Seeking first to understand, and then to be understood; to appreciate before expecting appreciation; to listen before expecting to be heard. At the same time creating an intentional, mutually beneficial balance in the flow of expressing and listening, empathy and expectation of empathy, and giving and receiving. This is accomplished by mutually respected boundaries of action and interaction.

- **Insight.** Discerning what strengths and limitations factor into the exchange, while remaining neutral and open to the outcome regardless of those insights.

- **Tension.** Allowing conflict, counterforce, ambiguity and dialectic tension to exist in order to encourage growth; accepting these without trying to resolve them.

- **Acknowledged genius.** Celebrating the truly exceptional whenever and wherever we encounter it.

- **Authenticity.** Presenting only a genuine face of ourselves in our interactions and harmonizing our thoughts, words and deeds so that they reflect that genuine self. This implies acting out of intrinsic vision rather than in reaction to extrinsic pressures.

- **Spaciousness.** Creating interior and exterior space for new possibilities to occur. This allows us to engage in many connections at once, or shift rapidly from one mode of exchange to another, or be flexible in how exchanges occur.

- **Sovereignty.** Mutual recognition of the innate right to think, feel and act independently from a place of self-governed will and responsibility for outcomes.

- **Quality input.** Paying attention to the quality of our interactions is paramount. Is this exchange mutually supportive? Does it evoke new spectra of emotion, or expose us to new information and experiences that stimulate and inspire? Does it challenge us?

- **Integration.** Incorporating the synthesis that results from all high quality interactions into our own being.

Let's consider some practical examples. If I eat a little spinach, it may not seem like spinach is getting much out of the deal. But let's look a little more closely at this simple act. Did I grow the spinach myself? Well, then I was involved in providing some of the energy it contains – I prepared the earth for it, I watered it, I kept the weeds from choking it and so on. I contributed – along with the sun, the earth worms, the favorable weather and countless other factors – to its existence. So there was communication. In fact, there was more than that, as most gardeners will tell you, because the communication occurred within the context of a relationship. Those who really enjoy gardening feel for their plants; they care for them and, on occasion, can even be heard talking to them in conversational tones. So if I grow the spinach myself, well, there is likely a great deal of energy involved, and so the exchange – the communication – is mutual. It may seem less the case if I buy the spinach in a store, and the communication is perhaps further removed, but it is still occurring. After all, the money I use to buy the spinach was earned with my own energy, and some portion of it will eventually arrive at the place where the spinach was grown. But as any spinach connoisseur knows, most spinach purchased in a store doesn't taste nearly as good as spinach grown in your own garden.

And so we come to another overarching principle in nourishment: the highest quality communication, and thus the highest quality nourishment, occurs when there is a high quality relationship. And the more that relationship flourishes, the greater the nourishment it contains; and the greater the nourishment, the more the relationship flourishes. Ever upward in a pleasant, satisfying spiral. Where there is a deep and enduring connection, the energy exchange is both easier and more nourishing on many levels. As an example, when I spend time with good friends I have known for years, I am always deeply gratified by the exchanges that occur. The food we share tastes better, the conversation feels more satisfying, and the sharing is more substantive – that is, as compared to eating a sandwich alone as I drive somewhere, or discussing a computer problem with an automated tech support line, or commenting on politics with a stranger at a bus stop. Not that these other exchanges don't have their place, but I am sure you see my point. When a mutually beneficial relationship has already been established, and there is trust on both sides that the relationship exists to support and invigorate each other, then the pump is primed for full-spectrum energy of the highest order.

So now we are getting down to some really interesting stuff: what constitutes a high quality relationship? Well, we have heard for years that satisfying relationships of all kinds are founded on and sustained with effective communication, but in the context of integral nourishment that advice has a whole new meaning. Because in all relationships, and all interactions with everything and everyone in our lives, communication and energy exchange is occurring in countless ways. The question is, is that exchange building us up, or tearing us down? Is it enriching our lives, or impoverishing our lives? Is it completing us or depleting us? Understanding high quality relationships from some different angles will help answer that question.

Returning for a moment to the cycle of motivation, we can observe another series of interactions that facilitate nourishment. When we satisfy our primary drives and fulfillment impulses, we nourish ourselves. And a brief consideration of those impulses reveals that nearly all of them manifest in our communication and relationship. In fact, as a species we have become extraordinarily efficient at nourishing ourselves through almost any conceivable interaction, and the success of humanity over the past few millennia is likely the result. We have developed a broad spectrum of energy exchanges and also gradations of sustenance within it. That is, some nourishment only supports existence in barest sense, while other levels help us soar to the heights of new experiences and growth. At the pinnacle of finely tuned nurturing is transformative practice, which fulfills many dimensions if our being at once in the fullest ways possible. How does all this go together? What do these levels and dimensions of nourishment look like, and how do we engage them? That's what we will examine next.

The Twelve Essential Dimensions of Nourishment

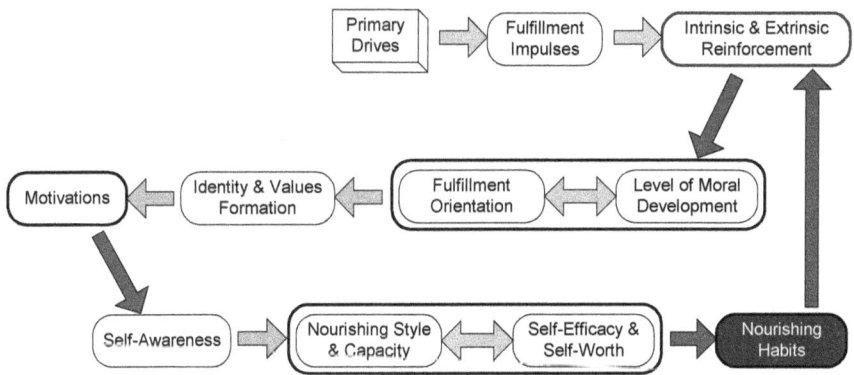

The twelve dimensions of nourishment in *Integral Lifework* are derived from the complex interaction of all primary drives and fulfillment impulses that inhabit our being. If you examine each of the twelve nourishment centers closely, you can perceive all of the sixteen fulfillment impulses percolating to the surface through them. In fact, all of our nourishment centers facilitate fulfillment impulses in much the same way our senses facilitate a dynamic perception of the world around us. Those senses – touch, taste, smell, sight, hearing, etc. – interact through our consciousness to create composite impressions, representations of all the various relationships of matter. As our eyes see and skin feels, we comprehend sunlight as warmth. As our tongue tastes and our nose smells, we experience a savory flavor of food. And likewise each nourishment center combines with others to satiate the diverse interplay of needs that constantly course through us; needs that are inspired by fulfillment impulses, which in turn serve our primary drives.

As a whole, supporting these twelve dimensions creates the solid, reliable formula for both strengthening our capacity to love and growing our being. If any of these essentials are neglected, that formula begins to weaken and crumble, and our progress will be interrupted, the quality of our experience will degrade, or we will begin sliding back into unhealthy and ineffective modes of being. Without holistic nourishment, daily existence begins to feel strained and empty, and we may become depressed, anxious or even physically ill. That is the natural consequence of interruptions to any communication or relationship. And no matter how we compensate for the neglected exchange, we will continue to feel incomplete, fragmented and depleted if we lack full-spectrum nourishment. Later on we will discuss each of these essential dimensions in more depth, but to begin here is a brief overview of each one:

- **Healthy Body.** Sustaining and strengthening our physical being through conscious patterns of diet, exercise, sleep and other key factors uniquely suited to who we are.

- **Playful Heart**. Maintaining healthy emotional expression and connection with our inner life, and engaging in regular playfulness and creative self-expression from day to day.

- **Supportive Community**. Inviting love and acceptance into our lives, both in what we receive from others, how loving and accepting we are of others, and how actively we participate in our community.

- **Expanding Mind**. Building, broadening and routinely stimulating our knowledge, understanding and mental capacities and abilities.

- **Fulfilling Purpose**. Discovering and actuating a satisfying life-purpose that is perfectly matched to our authentic self, and which supports the focus, strength and healthy expression of our personal will.

- **Authentic Spirit**. Establishing and increasing our connection and interaction with the ground of being – described in different traditions as the fundamental essence, spiritual energy, universal soul or divine nature of reality – and translating that deepening connection into a spiritually authentic life.

- **Restorative History**. Acknowledging, honoring and, when necessary, reprocessing all the experiences of our lives – whether remembered or forgotten, integrated or rejected – that have contributed to our current state of being; every significant relationship, trauma, milestone, accomplishment, perception or influence that has led us to the present moment.

- **Pleasurable Legacy**. Creating and sustaining new life, pleasurable experiences that are shared, and an enduring and positive impression on our world, while at the same time maintaining a sense of safety and stability for ourselves and those we love.

- **Flexible Processing Space**. Being able to regularly and effortlessly transition through different modes of processing, with each centered in different facets of our being -- the heart, mind, body, spirit and soul – so that we fully nourish those facets and create transparent access to the insights, wisdom and discernment each has to offer.

- **Empowered Self-Concept**. Tuning our self-awareness, self-worth and self-efficacy the most realistic, compassionate and supportive range of function, so that we both strengthen our nurturing capacity in all other nourishment centers, and continually address any barriers that arise.

- **Satisfying Sexuality.** Exploring the nature of our own sexuality – through the dynamics of our sexual relationships and our expectations of intimacy – in order to clarify and communicate our needs and desires and arrive at fulfilling nourishment for ourselves and those we sexually engage.

- **Affirming Integrity.** Consciously aligning the unfolding essence of our being with our thoughts, feelings, words and actions, so that *how* we are from moment to moment authentically reflects *who* we are in our innermost depths.

These nourishment dimensions are listed in no particular order, because they are all equally essential; none of them can be neglected for long without antagonizing our well-being. In reading over the list you may find yourself checking many of them off as part of your personal routines – perhaps even all of them. If so, that's really fantastic. However, because of unique barriers each of us will face throughout our lives, one dimension may be particularly difficult for us to recognize or access at particular times, even when we have been diligent and successful in the past. In fact, the one dimension we feel is our greatest strength may become a barrier to other dimensions of nourishment. It is also very easy to misinterpret one form of energy exchange for another, which is why advanced modes of self-awareness are so important when evaluating self-care. Adding to these challenges, our surrounding culture can also be quick to gloss over one type of nourishment in favor of other, more readily accessible ones. In the same way, many conventional approaches to wellness and personal growth tend to overemphasize one type of nurturing over everything else. As we explore each of these dimensions in depth, it will be helpful to keep these caveats in mind.

Consider the example of Michelle. She lives in a rural area, far away from the city culture and amenities she grew up with or a supportive community of friends, and she longs to spend more time at the theatre, at music concerts or perusing art galleries and to share those experiences with friends. Likely as a result of a recent onset of menopause, she is also having trouble sleeping and, because of the resulting fatigue, is not motivated to exercise during the day. Adding to her unhappiness, she no longer has a meaningful relationship with her only son and is struggling to connect emotionally with her husband. Although she takes a number of supplements and is aware of proper nutrition, she is extremely weight conscious and tends to eat lightly or even skip meals. In fact, when she and I discuss each dimension of nourishment, it quickly becomes clear that in nearly every area of her life, Michelle is not adequately nourishing herself. She has become severely depleted in so many ways that it is hard for her to see any hope for herself.

How did this happen? In today's world, even in the health-conscious culture of southern California where I live and practice, a downward spiral of depletion in multiple dimensions is exceedingly common. In Michelle's case, a series of decisions which initially held the appearance of self-nourishment led her down this path. Her choice of husband and their relationship style, the social status and lifestyle that she desired, her unconscious parenting choices and a few self-limiting beliefs all contributed to a landscape where one nourishment avenue after another was closed to her. It did not take long for us to identify the barriers she had accumulated over the years, as well as their possible remedies, but at the point Michelle contacted me she had little to no energy to begin moving in a more positive, self-nurturing direction. She had bottomed out, and was feeling an intensity of darkness and despair never encountered before. On many levels at once, she was starving to death. Over the subsequent months Michelle created a door for herself out of that darkness – through small changes that helped her rediscover what real nourishment felt like in each of the twelve dimensions. She also disrupted some persisting barriers and refreshed her self-concept. From there, she could test her wings a bit and at least fly around the yard. But imagine how many people spend decades trapped in a self-depleting situation like Michelle's? Taken in small steps, it is relatively easy to free ourselves from these unhealthy patterns, but finding that first glimpse of light in the darkness can often be the hardest.

In order to asses your own nourishment, try spending a few moments with the following exercise:

> **Exercise: Nourishment Levels**   In your journal, list all the dimensions of nourishment down the left side of a page, equally spaced. On the right side, reflect how you have nourished each dimension in the last three days in targeted ways. In other

words, what did you do that actually provided immediate nourishment in specific areas? How did you fulfill your purpose, exercise your creativity, add to your legacy, connect with the ground of being...and so forth? There may be one or two activities you regularly perform that nourish you in multiple dimensions, so you can certainly write the same activity down for more than one nourishment center. Take your time with this. In *Integral Lifework* classes, some people fill up the page quickly and move on to fill up a second, while others write down just a few brief notes. Regardless, after you make your list, spend some time reflecting on why certain of your dimensions may receive more nourishment than others. What is filling up your time or demanding your energy, and why?

As we initially identify where we are and what areas need to be addressed, there can be strong resistance to holistic self-nourishment; this is not always a simple or easy path. There is often both internal resistance from years of self-depleting habits, and external resistance because our current relationships and environment do not allow us sufficient time or volitional space for integral exchanges. Consider also that one narrowly focused solution simply cannot work for everyone, and the same mode of being will not remain effective for us over time. Not only is each of us unique to begin with, but we constantly change and grow. That is why an integral approach customized to our aptitudes, abilities and barriers in the present moment is so important, followed by ongoing self-examination and adjustment. Without carefully evaluating our self-nurturing routines, it is unfeasible to appreciate where we have become depleted and why. And when we take all of our cultural, historical and personal factors into account, we often believe we must learn to live with sub-optimal sustenance in crucial areas. I have concluded that this mistaken belief is what leads to many chronically debilitating conditions of mind, heart, body and spirit. In fact, one way we can define all illness, unhappiness, pain and suffering is to identify what nourishment is being blocked. Even death itself can be defined simply as the interruption of nourishment to many areas at once. The good news is that we all have the capacity to untangle these obstacles and achieve fulfilling, multidimensional self-care.

Why Twelve?

Why are there only twelve centers of nourishment? For that matter, why are there sixteen fulfillment impulses or four primary drives? In reality these are pragmatic placeholders for umbrella concepts, and could just as easily have been grouped differently, using other numbers and with different names. It would also be quite easy to break them down further or add to the list. But what I have found over time is that these labels and groupings have a practical relevance when trying to convey an integral nourishment framework, especially when working with *Integral Lifework* clients on the specific challenges they face. Clustering these ideas in such a fashion softens the learning curve and allows us to more quickly map them to the details of our daily life. Additionally, the way each dimension combines certain elements of nourishment appears to track with how many people naturally differentiate or relate to them. In essence, the twelve dimensions are manageable concepts that capture the gist of underlying factors – factors that undeniably contribute to human motivation and well-being. The exactitude with which we divide, combine, name or describe those factors is important in a theoretical sense, but in a practical sense what is most important is having some handles – and some sort of pragmatic process – for sorting them out as nourishment. It is human nature to delve deeper and deeper into specificity until, at some point, the relevant context is lost. So I have settled on these groupings because they seem to stop just short of fracturing context and meaning, while still providing a convenient, working model for the nitty-gritty necessities of life.

Over the course of theorizing and applying those theories, I have encountered new components of nourishment that weren't addressed in earlier models, and I expect that this will continue to be the case. The first few times this happened, I was certain I had uncovered a nourishment channel that was unique enough to deserve its own separate category – a fresh dimension to be explored. Sometimes this was indeed the case, but through my own integral practice and my work with clients, I concluded much of the time that the new facet nestled neatly into one of the previously defined dimensions. There is almost always a natural fit. As we investigate them in more detail, I expect you will discover how different channels in one dimension harmonize with each other; this is especially true when those concepts become practice.

That said, this arrangement of twelve distinct but equal nourishment centers is intuitive in nature – it can be sensed and experienced, but is sometimes challenging to intellectualize. Perhaps in the fullness of time a correlation with neurological structures in the brain, physiological sympathies in the body or even patterns of energy or matter in the Universe will someday hint at the appropriateness of this model or suggest some other. For now, this provides us with a working vocabulary to manage some important concepts.

Of course, no matter how grandiose and all-inclusive an initial vision intends to be, there will always be room for improvement. In fact, I will throw one final wrench into the works before leaving this topic: in the last months before this book went to print, I explored what I believe may be an additional dimension of nourishment that doesn't fit into any of the existing twelve. It may in fact require a new, thirteenth dimension to accommodate it. However, my ideas about this frequency of energy and how its nurturing patterns are structured and facilitated have not fermented long enough to be included here, and will undoubtedly be the subject of future writings. So there you go…the only constant is change.

Prerequisites for Full-Spectrum Nourishment

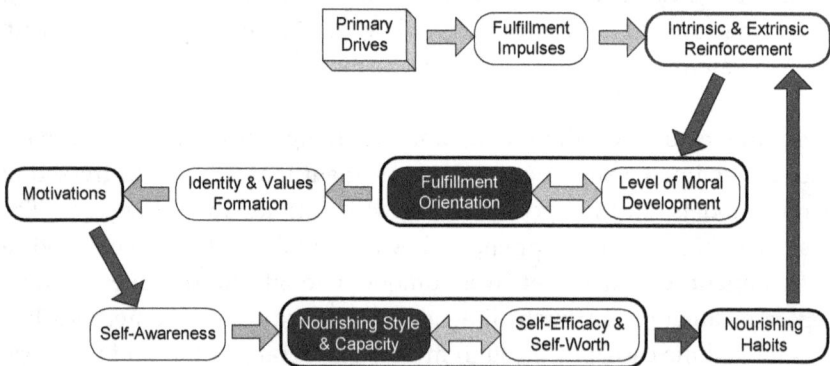

In some ways, we can never fully prepare ourselves for any relationship. We venture forth with what little we have observed or believe about how successful relationships function, and we do our best. We take each step forward with hope that we can sustain a meaningful connection.

And, often, we fail, stumbling over hitherto unperceived obstacles or the inevitable twists and turns any growing relationship will take. But we don't have to stumble in the dark. If we understand what we bring to the relationship and how we can share it, then we can garner a bit more confidence as we begin, and the journey need not be quite so unpredictable. To that end, I have provided some of the prerequisites for full-spectrum nourishment. Understanding our current states and modes of operation in these areas will unlock new potential for effective self-care in any dimension. They also define some of the more common barriers to our innate nourishing capacity.

Fulfillment Orientation

We have already touched on one important differentiator in the quality of our motivations: externally dependent vs. internally generated. This is an important component of the broader topic of our *fulfillment orientation*. That is, what do we believe is the most effective way for us to satisfy our fulfillment impulses and become fully nourished? Are we relying on external resources or ourselves? Are we willing to engage in mutual exchanges that benefit everyone, or do we mistrust that level of connection and confine our efforts to actions that clearly benefit us alone? Have we individuated from our family of origin or other group identifications, or are we still overly dependent on others – and perhaps on our identity in that larger group – to nourish ourselves? As we will see, having self-awareness in this area is vital, as it has a direct impact on our well-being.

Here then are some of the more common patterns of fulfillment orientation as framed by the maturity model described earlier:

DEPLETION ←	OPTIMAL RANGE	→ EXCESS
Protective → Fixated	Self-Reliant → Love-Consciousness	Dependent → Codependent

- **Protective** – Here we isolate ourselves from external influences on our well-being and persistently reject mutual exchanges. A protective orientation constraining all effort to purely self-referential nourishment. In other words, instead of having healthy interactions with our friends, family or society at large, we isolate ourselves in some way – physically, emotionally, psychologically, spiritually, etc. This often involves a forceful rejection of any perceived dependence on anyone or anything; we want to be in complete control of our own fulfillment in one or more areas. Unfortunately, this eventually leads to depletion in whatever dimensions are being protected.

  → **Fixated** – Narrow focus on one or two fulfillment impulses to the exclusion of all others. The emphasis here is tight control over specific exchanges or certain arenas of affection, much the same way as in the protective isolation just described. For example, what if all of my energy were constrained to satisfying my Understanding fulfillment impulse? What if I spent an excessive amount of time evaluating the new information I have just encountered. As I tried to interpret and contextualize this new information, my health would fail, my relationships would unravel and my ability to nourish myself in other areas would be undermined. I am chronically substituting one form of nourishment for all others. In a way, this is a sort of overly aggressive protective orientation, because it most often stems from a compensatory need to fulfill one or more areas that we abused or neglected in the past. As a result, it often manifests as behaviors that are abusive or destructive.

- **Self-Reliant** – We are able to fully nourish ourselves in all dimensions, with a careful balance of internal and external exchanges, but not always with much interest in widening arenas of affection. We trust both our abilities to self-nurture and our discernment to allow others into that process. We know how to be safe and stay safe, while at the same time being open and vulnerable to all levels of relationship. This is a "steady state" fulfillment orientation, where maintenance and gradual healing are common, but multidimensional growth is less so. Self-reliant exchanges do mutually nourish, however, so the more arenas of relationship into which we allow ourselves to expand, the richer and more complex those exchanges will become.

→ **Love-Consciousness** – Through authentic love-consciousness, we have fully integrated an affectionate motivation to nourish ourselves and everything around us as a natural outpouring of our way of being. Exchanges in multiple dimensions tend to be both frequent and effortless, and result in more accelerated healing and growth, ultimately exciting new and unexpected transformations. This is the next phase beyond self-reliance and expands interdependence into new types of relationship. For instance, my relationship with my community, with society as a whole, with the Earth, and so on.

• **Dependent** – As a dependent, we are not yet fully individuated from our parents, our family of origin, our peers, our tribe or some other perceived group with whom we strongly identify. As a result, we tend to rely on that group or self-identification for all nourishment as well as our overall sense of well-being. A dependent is almost completely defined by externals. This is the logical and necessary place for an infant to begin, but we often hold onto some patterns of dependency well into adulthood. For instance, when someone cannot confidently make a decision or initiate a course of action without first consulting a parent, spouse, friend, etc. this indicates residual dependency.

→ **Codependent** – As an exaggerated form of mutual dependence, here we not only rely on perceived satisfaction of other people's wants and needs for our own sense of well-being, but we engineer enmeshments with them that cause their well-being to become dependent on us as well. As might be expected, this coincides with little understanding or consistent satisfaction of either party's nourishment centers. Where the dependent person might require someone else's approval to feel confident about their choice, the codependent person cannot feel safe or certain without first confirming their decision garners approval, then ensuring that they have power or control over another's nurturing. This is hardly ever a conscious act – it is the consequence of an unconscious belief that distort the nature of love. This belief sounds something like this: "You can't be nourished, safe, loved or whole without me, and I can't be nourished, safe, loved or whole without you, so let's make sure we stick together...even if we are hurting each other." A codependent orientation thus substitutes the perceived well-being of another for authentic self-nourishment in both directions, conditioning all parties to become dependent on external relationships and environments. This eventually leads to serious depletion across multiple dimensions for everyone involved. In nearly all cases, the codependent orientation results in difficulties both in taking responsibility for one's own well-being, maintaining clear boundaries between ourselves and other people, and respecting the sovereignty of anyone else to care for themselves.

The outcome of all fulfillment orientations that are not grounded in self-reliance and love-consciousness is nearly always the same: depletion in one or more dimensions of nourishment. Self-reliant fulfillment can stave off depletion, but it still limits our ability to grow. Only one orientation, love-consciousness, greatly enhances healing and growth, then leads us into enduring evolutions of being. And what is the main difference between this transformative mode of fulfillment and all the others? The infusion of authentic love. And that will continue to be a common motif in our exploration of nourishment: when we add sincere, discerning and all-encompassing love to the equation, our capacity for and skillfulness in all dimensions of nourishment will increase in many directions at once. Of course, it is important to recognize that we will rarely operate from one fulfillment orientation for any length of time. In nearly all cases, we will cycle through all of these modes of fulfillment over and over again. That is part of our humanity. So in *Integral Lifework*, our objective is simply to dwell most often in the self-reliant and love-consciousness orientations, and to heal from experiences and habits that cause us to gravitate towards less nourishing modes of being.

Some real world examples of fulfillment orientation seem in order. Consider Judy, a fifty-year old woman who operates in a fixated, protective mode. Although on the surface she appears happy, jovial and confident, she is extremely insecure about all of the relationships in her professional and private life. This is because she has never really allowed honest, intimate exchanges to take place. She has carefully controlled each interaction so that they are always on her terms, serving her agendas and obscuring or excusing what might be perceived as weaknesses or vulnerability. To reveal her true needs or allow herself to rely on someone else to fulfill any of her needs is out of the question. Like many such patterns, this was a lesson painfully learned in her childhood. Judy's mother was both emotionally and physically absent for much of the time, and when she was present she was the harsh, authoritarian matron of their home. Judy's father was both disempowered by her mother and relatively disinterested in Judy, preferring to invest his time in his son. It was only natural for Judy to conclude that she herself was the only person she could rely upon; all she had to do was decide what she really wanted, and chase after that. So Judy set up a series of life goals for herself – some professional, some having to do with starting her own family – which she pursued with laser-like focus. Every relationship in her life then became a means to those ends, or was left to languish in a junkyard of ever-enlarging emotional wreckage. Denial about those failures and abandonments – which were in fact echoes of how she herself had been treated as a child – became second nature, until all Judy had to offer the world was a cajoling laugh, a recitation of her most recent accomplishments, and other rapid redirects away from her darkened and deeply detested interior.

Now let's consider Rob, a man in his forties who operates primarily in a codependent mode. For Rob, nearly every conversation is a stressful test in which he must discover precisely what the other person wants from him, and then quickly decipher how he will respond to their request. His own needs, buried beneath layer upon layer of reflexive tension, seldom rise to the surface in daily life. At the same time, he is absolutely certain that he is responsible for the well-being of others, and sees his own overbearing devotion as kindness. For Rob, maintaining healthy boundaries is extremely difficult; that is, on an emotional level it is inconceivable for him to not become involved in someone else's crisis or pain.   He is affable, intelligent, well-educated and has a wealth of personal skills to draw upon, but he has spent his entire life walking on eggshells around people who either were so unhappy they didn't realize they were being abusive, or whose personalities were so strong that Rob reflexively fell into a submissive, pleasing role. As a result, he now does not believe he is capable of nurturing himself other than vicariously through the satisfaction of others, nor that others should be allowed to nurture themselves without his involvement. In Rob's case, this strong desire to please and appease resulted from years of living in an alcoholic household – that was how he survived in that environment. Now every interaction has come to rely on the survival lessons he learned when he was young, which have been reinforced again and again as he unconsciously chose abusive or domineering people to associate with – or unconsciously became a controller himself.   So he masks his discomfort with an elaborate act, a persona that seems to offer up his every asset as a resource for those he loves, while he secretly suffers from exhaustion, resentment and a strong sense of inadequacy. So this is what one form of codependence looks like.

And lastly let's consider Gustavo, who has worked hard to maintain a self-reliant orientation.   Through years of interior work, Gustavo has come to realize both what drives him and derails him. Most of the time, he is able to remember how to nourish himself and avoid those derailing habits. The key to his own well-being, he has found, is to open himself up wide to those around him while at the same time remembering his own purpose, strengths and resources so that he knows which exchanges are appropriate and which are not.   For example, he will not engage anyone in a political debate, because he does not feel that is constructive; for Gustavo, political views are so closely tied to personal convictions and core values that debate is seldom fruitful. On the other hand, if you wish to discuss healthy diets with Gustavo, he'll dive right in. Gustavo also has no problem sharing the secrets of his own profession, to the extent that others have brazenly taken his ideas and duplicated them for their own profit. This doesn't bother Gustavo – at least not much; he'll just shrug and say: "I guess that's on their conscience. It's their karma." He is likewise ready to share just about any part of himself or his life…as long as it doesn't interfere with his purpose or subtract resources that would potentially fulfill his purpose. He's very clear about that. So he is able to nourish and be nourished without losing himself or his focus –

and without closing himself off to the world. This, then, is an example of a truly self-reliant individual.

Governing Intention: The Good of All

Energy exchanges within a broader context tend to be much more fulfilling. A meal lovingly prepared for us by a friend is a lot more satisfying than a quick snack alone. Adorn that meal with a special occasion – a favorite holiday, a birthday, an anniversary – and it becomes memorable as well, nourishing our heart and spirit. In the same way, when we approach nourishment with a consistent, guiding intentionality behind our actions, we add value and energy to our experiences. If we care about what we are doing because it supports a deeper conviction about why we should act, then we can make choices with more confidence and execute them with more zeal and perseverance. This is how intentions affect our nourishing style and capacity. In one way, love itself performs this supportive function, and when we are immersed in love-consciousness we tend to act from that state of being without calling upon anything greater. Love justifies itself. But what supports love? What is the governing intention behind the will to be caring and compassionate? Often we will find that the life purpose we identify for ourselves fulfills that function, acting as a backdrop against which all decisions can be measured. But what is the backdrop for our backdrop? What supports us when we temporarily lose our personal vision, or fall out of love for a while, or stumble across new barriers that seem intimidating or insurmountable?

One answer that spiritual traditions offer us is an overarching desire for the good of All. That is, what benefits everyone, including ourselves, to the greatest degree. Before making any major decision, if I ask myself "is this for the good of All?" I can begin aligning my intention with that higher stratum of moral valuation and a broader, more inclusive purpose. I may not always know for a certainty the answer to that question, but if I ask it, I am at least examining my own heart for any signs of willfulness. And creating that softness of heart, that willingness to align myself with a greater good, opens a channel to wisdom and insight. You might be asking: "Wait a minute, how can we ever know for certain what the good of All really is? Isn't that kind of bigheaded?"

And of course that is one of the dangers. If we assert that we have been granted some special dispensation to stand for good in the world, and that therefore whatever we desire is for the good of All, then we can fall into a classic trap of willful ignorance amplified by unrepentant arrogance, and lose ourselves in megalomaniacal delusion. At the other extreme, if we deny our innate capacity for wisdom and discernment, submitting instead to a sense of helpless inevitability, we can annihilate our potential contribution to all-inclusive beneficial outcomes. So this practice requires just the right balance of courage and humility, relying on an inner conviction, a certainty of faith, that the good of All is possible – perhaps even inevitable – and that we can and will contribute to it. We are confident not in our having the perfect solution, but in our willingness and eagerness to be part of a solution. Our fundamental belief that the good of All deserves to be manifested and indeed cries out to be manifested is what calls us forth and draws us onward. I call this the golden intention.

The skeptic might argue: "How can I trust in something if I don't know where it comes from or where it is taking me?" Because it is precisely our not knowing that entreats our faith. Even if we have a pretty solid idea of what is the most beneficial and skillful for everyone in a given circumstance, any failure to actualize that vision – or just the inevitable twists and turns in the road that obscure any outcome – can sap our momentum. And the exact details of that bigger picture are almost always hidden from us. We may catch glimpses every now and then, but it is difficult to differentiate the illusion of our own desires or the realism of our imagination from what is actually happening. So we must trust that our governing intentionality will contribute to a bigger picture, that our will aligns and harmonizes with the good of All simply because we choose this as our destination. As an additional benefit, as we integrate this intention into our modes of being, we will begin operating within higher and higher strata of moral valuation. That is, we will begin to view our choices and the events around us through a more refined filter of spiritual understanding. And this will not only enwisen our insights, but sustain us through great difficulties.

Perhaps you are familiar with the story of the wise farmer. He was out plowing one day when he saw that his horse was just plain worn out from plowing. So he unhitched the horse and set it loose to recuperate on its own. It quickly trotted off out of sight. His friends declared "What bad luck about your horse!" But the farmer replied, "We shall see." A few weeks later, the horse returned to the farmer, fully recovered and with a whole herd of wild horses in tow. "What great luck!" cried the farmer's friends. "We shall see," said the farmer. A few days later, the farmer's son went to break in one of the mustangs, and ended up breaking his own leg in the process. "What bad luck" declared the rest of the village. "We shall see," said the farmer. In less than a month a war broke out, and all the sons of the village were quickly conscripted – except for the farmer's son, because of his broken leg. "What great luck!" cried his friends, though they really weren't very enthusiastic. "We shall see," the farmer replied. And so on, illustrating that the more we hitch our efforts to specific outcomes or the certainty of our assessments, the more likely our lives will become a rollercoaster of elation and despair. We can pretend we have certainty about the outcome of every one of our actions, but that is a brittle faith, easily broken by repeated failures. So instead of depending on immediate results, we can invest in a steady haven of hope amid the unpredictable storms of life. If we trust in the good of All, our confidence does not rest in control of the moment, but in letting go of that illusion and expecting that each surprise serves a greater purpose.

This can be applied quite practically in almost any situation. If my friend decides to try out a new, better paying job in a different city, I can resist concluding that this is either a great opportunity or a foolish risk, and instead trust that the governing intention of everyone involved will create the best possible outcome. And that includes my own, because then whatever help or advice I offer will trickle into the most beneficial eventuality, regardless of whether I know concretely what that eventuality is. This allows me to avoid black-and-white thinking, increasing my tolerance for unknowns and ambiguity, and remain more flexible and better prepared for whatever comes. As I inform myself the best I can, as I listen to the sharing of the people in my life, as I process my own insights and reactions from day to day, I can filter everything through the golden intention. In this way I can welcome unexpected events as nourishment, and become more skillful in how I approach all of my thoughts, feelings, habits and experiences.

This deliberate intentionality is of course really about love. It trusts that love exists as a governing force in the Universe, and that love has primacy over all other forces in the greater arc of time. Even where there is suffering and loss, love is trusted to heal all wounds, to mitigate the negative fallout from our missteps and overreaching, and to transform the bitterest cold and darkness into warming light. More than anything else, this is a spiritual conviction, but it is not dependent on any broader belief system or religious proclamation. As a mystic, I would offer that direct encounters with the governing force and pervasive substance of love are readily available to anyone who engages in the full-spectrum nourishment of integral practice. As part of any regular spiritual self-nourishment, an ongoing connection with the ground of being, however it is achieved, will confirm and promote this reality. The experience of infinite love in the context of spiritual practice is, I believe, the kernel from which most faith traditions have grown, but it is the individual encounter with that Light, rather than agreement with religious dogma, that validates our faith. As Sri Aurobindo wrote in *The Integral Yoga*: "We must find the Self, the Divine, only then can we know what work the Self or Divine demands of us."

What if we drift away from the golden intention? Well, it is highly likely that, regardless of our fervor, at some point we will. There is something akin to the law of entropy in the inevitability of side trips, regressions and confused muddling in the midst of crisis and stress. What comes of these is another sort of substitution – the substitution of self-limiting intention for that which is constructive. Narcissism, egoism and willfulness burst like flies from the midden heap of our inattention, replacing a calm, clear focus of transcendent purpose with aimless, chaotic busyness and confusion. This can happen even if we operate at the highest levels of moral development. And by forsaking the real and lasting importance of the good of All, we cling to temporary illusions that inflate the urgency and criticality of our own desires and the pressing necessity of our immediate contributions. When we forsake the broader vision of a governing intention, we allow the hurried details of our existence to obscure the shared essence of all things, the innate power of our being and the clarity of our discerning insights. And so we become lost in a maze of our own making, and can neither fully self-actualize nor maintain dynamic harmony with the world around us. In other words, we tend to interrupt our own nourishment and the nourishment of everything around us.

To guide our way through that maze, here are three questions we can ask of any situation:

1) Is it nourishment?
2) Does it benefit the good of All?
3) Have I exercised discernment in my choices?

If we can answer these three questions with insight, honesty and humble confidence, then we know we can do no better. But that leads us to another question: What exactly is "discernment," and how can we achieve it?

Discernment

Discernment is a critical contributor to our nourishing style and capacity. As a prerequisite to balanced nourishment and compassionate affection, it is also a result of these things – so the more we exercise discernment, the more discerning we become. Like all the other components of a solid foundation, discernment can be learned through practice. How does it work? In one way, we can view the discernment process as a conscious navigation of energy exchanges. If I can find my way to a healthy diet that is well-suited to my lifestyle and physique, that could be called discernment. The same is true if I engage just the right group of folks as my community of support, or reinforce my individual life purpose with appropriate actions, or celebrate my spiritual connection with the ground of being while still managing to function well in a material sense – all of these involve discerning choices in different dimensions of nourishment. Perhaps we initially arrive at these insights through trial and error, or through the timely insight of a friend, or as a result of listening carefully to intuitive promptings – or a combination of all three. But because we also come to recognize the beneficial consequences of such balance-inducing choices in our lives, we are not operating out of a purely theoretical orientation or rote discipline. We are reinforcing high quality decisions by receiving high quality nourishment. Our choices make healthy sense.

So, by its nature, discernment involves dynamic and flexible perception. We learn as we go along, adjusting to new situations and new types of information. Most importantly, though, this is an internal compass. It does not rely solely on external data. In a world where we are bombarded with overwhelming information, with the themes of mass media and the sells of advertising, with contradictory advice from friends, teachers, experts and Internet searches...we must learn to rely on our own, internally generated insights to govern our lives. Of course we allow external sources a place in the process, but they become only one of many input streams into our discernment engine. Over time, we can learn to suspend the stronger influence of one source and shore up the less persuasive murmurings of another, so that the resulting synthesis can be more balanced and accurate. In *Integral Lifework* we call *this the art of suspension* – that is, balancing all input streams equally within a neutral consciousness. In this way, discernment becomes a central tenet in our overall self-confidence and self-reliance.

How do we cultivate a neutral consciousness, the art of suspension where all information is given fair an equal weight? Much of this has to do with letting go. Letting go of our prejudices, of fears and mistrust of our own weaknesses, of any exclusive reliance on external sources that may have helped us in the past, and so on. Instead of depending on just one or two of our past decision-making methods, we allow as many input streams as possible to co-exist, and depend on a process that aggregates as much information as possible into a neutral interior space before synthesizing a decision. This may sound complicated, but it is really surprisingly simple. It just requires some practice. To that end, the *mystic activator* exercise in the following section introduces one type of interior discipline that will aid in developing neutral consciousness and the art of suspension.

One of the chief characteristics of discernment is our knack for knowing when to employ it. In the context of nourishment, take the example of fasting. Fasting can be a useful tool to clarify the mind, cleanse the body and fortify the spirit. But how do we differentiate fasting from less healthy choices? For instance, I once had a friend, David, who decided to fast for forty days. He had fasted for short periods before and found it extremely helpful in his spiritual and mental disciplines, and he considered this longer fast a logical next step. So, without telling me or any of this other friends, he gave notice at his job, stocked his room with water and bottled juice, and began his adventure. Unfortunately, other than almost dying, he did not come any closer to the Divine or encounter any epiphany other than that he should never, ever attempt such a feat again. In fact, after the first three weeks, all he remembered from the experience were vague hallucinations, physically wretched symptoms and occasional terror when he realized just how weak he had become. At the end, this was not a fast but something closer to an unintentional suicide attempt. In one way, we see the principle of the narrow band of optimal function illustrated here, but more than that we see the clear evidence of action without discernment. If David had been better prepared, if he had let his friends know what he was doing, if he hadn't been significantly underweight and in poor physical condition to begin with...all these *ifs* indicate there could have been a different outcome from a basically fruitless near-death experience.

For someone who forgets to apply their native discernment, "if only" is usually evident in hindsight. For those who reject the need for discernment or who have not yet developed their discerning faculties, even hindsight may not provide any lessons. So how could David have engaged his discernment? First, he could have called upon some readily available external input streams – the advice of doctors and nutritionists, the experiences of other people who had become experts at deliberate fasting, the support of friends, and so on. Then he could have carefully engaged his internal resources. For instance, tuning in to his body's physical condition and readiness, even asking his physical being for permission to undergo such deprivation. He could also have explored what was driving this decision. What were his motivations for taking such a radical step? Was his ego involved? Was his heart longing for some form of connection he had not yet experienced? Was his neglect of other areas of nourishment leading him to compensate through such an act? As you can see, discernment is really a quest, a series of difficult tests that answer difficult questions. Once those questions are answered, we can move forward with confidence. Not that the outcome is therefore guaranteed, but at least we can know we are proceeding in the most informed, considered fashion possible.

How can we know when we have been discerning? That is one of the benefits of making discerning choices: they reinforce themselves. If the outcome clearly benefits the good of All, then it was a wise choice. And discernment always anticipates our governing intention. Feeling compassion and acting from that compassion is not the same as discernment – after all, that is only one input stream. But if compassion went into the decision and the results successfully enhance the well-being of the object of our affection, then we know we have done well. Of course, we should concurrently develop discernment about what well-being looks and feels like, or we won't be able to accurately evaluate results. In David's case, at the peak of his hallucinations some part of him knew that they were just that, just as some part of him knew that his tongue turning black was not a celestial sign or blessing; these were purely physiological consequences of starving himself. And that part – the part that knows – is what we are growing when we enlarge our discernment. It is not just knowledge, not just intuition, not just spiritual understanding or felt sense, but all of these elements combined together with equal emphasis into an amalgam of practical wisdom.

Ultimately, with practice, discernment becomes less a series of explorations, correlations and considerations and more a state of consciousness. By creating a neutral interior space and allowing all these disparate input streams to coalesce there, we can intuit a wise, healthy and supportive conclusion relatively quickly. Shortly we will discuss the concept of *processing space,* and it will become clear that discernment inhabits several processing spaces at once. The question then becomes what is the best way to train ourselves into that processing mode. And that – among many other things – is what the following integral practice will help you achieve.

Mystic Activation: The Cornerstone of Integral Lifework

As you can see, cultivating a supportive fulfillment orientation, governing intention and discernment is an intensive, far reaching undertaking. On top of that, we also want to experience all the characteristics of high quality relationship that facilitate full-spectrum nourishment. How can we achieve all of this? Is there some integral practice that will help us through this process? Yes, there is. There is one discipline that encompasses and accesses all of these nourishment prerequisites at once; in fact, it is an excellent means of mastering each one to a depth and breadth far beyond what we could ever imagine, while expanding our overall self-awareness at the same time. The shorthand I use for this practice is *mystic activation*. This includes a broad range of techniques to stimulate special consciousness in a focused and reliable way, and need not be exclusively yoked to any religious system. It is not always easy to evoke mystical awareness – especially when we first begin to practice – but the methods you will be harnessing to get there will in themselves nourish several dimensions at once.

What quickly becomes evident as we begin mystical practice is that how we approach our practice will determine the extent of integration and the quality of its outcomes. Our state of mind, our moral orientation, our emotional well-being, our spiritual openness, our current level of understanding – all of these directly influence what occurs as we develop new self-nurturing habits. This seems a little like a chicken-and-egg type conundrum, but there is one distinct overriding factor that will align any number of disparate interior conditions into the greatest potential harmony and receptivity. And that, of course, is love. To whatever degree we allow love to permeate an integral process, we will encourage integral benefits. And how do we set the intention to allow love its proper influence over our efforts? Once again we return to the golden intention, the guiding desire for the good of All, as the anchor that keeps us steady and grounded in love throughout the inevitable storms and tumults of self-discovery.

There is an analogy I find helpful in understanding the effect mystic activation has on our being when it is rooted in love: I like to think of a love-infused mystic continuum as matter – in this case the matter of our consciousness – cooled down to a superconducting quantum state. Let's say our normal mode of being is like helium at room temperature, with atoms bouncing seemingly at random all over the place. But when the helium is cooled down to less than about 2 degrees Kelvin (that's just above Absolute Zero and is really, really cold) something miraculous occurs: the atoms share a superfluid quantum state. They lose their distinctness as separate particles and begin behaving in a unified manner – one becomes all and all become one. I am not a physicist so this is probably a clumsy approximation of what is really happening, but as an analogy for evoking mystical awareness it seems useful. As we cool our consciousness down through levels of successive stillness, we encounter the oneness of all that results in our intuition of the Absolute.

At the Center

At the center
   warm silence
     easy to love
     hard to bear

Sacred space blossoms
   welcoming old ghosts
   forgotten selves
   a fount of passion
   and the deity
     of Now

Remembering stillness
   creates Light
   catapults Consciousness
   reprograms genes
     until we become
       the answers we seek

Once we slip into the mystical continuum, we inevitably recognize it as something we have experienced before. Perhaps in a dream, or during previous spiritually-oriented disciplines, or even spontaneously in situations of extreme stress or elation. In truth, we brush against the mystical all the time, but unless we train ourselves to apprehend it, the moment passes us by with little notice. What is really happening in these experiences is that our apperceptions and assumptions about the current moment are being suspended, and we are catching a glimpse of underlying realities unsullied by memory or belief. Having a structured way to invite this alternative form of perception-cognition into our life will, over time, provide us reliable spiritual nourishment. There is an important distinction between spontaneous mystical insight and regular practice. They both can be nourishing, but regular practice strengthens and fine tunes our consciousness so that we can both pick up increasingly subtle input and withstand the intensity of peak experiences that extend beyond previous thresholds. Would you try to fly a hang glider without any training or practice? Of course not, and when we activate the mystical without a supportive discipline we are taking a similar risk.

There are already many well-known techniques available in the West to evoke mystical consciousness, often carried forward over centuries. Some are more spontaneous, such as Nature mysticism, and some, like hermetic practices, are highly structured and infused with complex ritual. Others, like the contemplative tradition of Christianity, are largely confined to a specific religious system or membership in a religious order. Eastern traditions have also found their way into Western culture. Various forms of Buddhist meditation and Hindu Yoga, for example, have gained much attention in the U.S. at different times. More recently, Qi Gong and Tai Chi have also garnered broader acceptance as ways of achieving one flavor of interior concentration. Over the decades, perhaps the oldest spiritual discipline of all – shamanic trance – has been promoted as an avenue of growth and transformation. In the same vein, the psychedelic movement ushered in a wave of chemically stimulated mystic activation – though not always with adequate attention to accompanying disciplines or constructive contexts from the shamanistic cultures where those practices originated.

In fact, this is a common pattern in consumerist spirituality that is derived from other cultural traditions: there is often a rush to achieve mystical awareness without developing a supportive framework for the experience. This is, I think, a strong indication of the addiction to cathartic sensationalism in American culture and the commoditization of "convenient" quasi-religiosity. But aside from such cyclical fads and entertainments, almost all of the spiritual traditions throughout history offer us some avenue to special consciousness that is easily identified as a "mystical" branch or school. Even among monotheistic religions, we have the Sufis of Islam, the Gnostics of Christianity, the Kabalists of Judaism and so on. Taken together, all of this offers clues to the universal structures underlying mystic activation.

There has been much discussion and debate about the various merits of different systems and approaches to mystical consciousness. It is easy to come to the mistaken conclusion that because one technique works well for one person in one situation, it is somehow superior or better suited for everyone else as well. But in my personal experience, observation and discussions with practitioners of different methods, the effectiveness of one mystic activator over another is more dependent on one's intentionality, self-discipline and openness to spiritual cognizance than on a particular technique or belief system. This doesn't mean the belief system and technique aren't important, but those specifics can distract from the universal accessibility of the experience. Consider the Wicca practitioner who embraces an indwelling Holy Spirit, the Christian who encounters their inner Buddha, the Buddhist who raises their Kundalini, the Neo-Platonist who remembers Allah in every moment, the Sufi who journeys through the Ain Soph, the Hindu who raises the Divine Spark in everything around them.... I do not mean to trivialize distinct beliefs or dilute the rich tapestry of human faith into one homogenous glob. I certainly don't wish to alienate those whose hearts are immersed in their unique forms of faith – or even those who are convinced they require no distinct spiritual beliefs at all. But connection with the ground of being, the Divine, the spiritual essence of things, the soul of existence – this connection is the foundation of all spirituality, no matter how unique the experience or the doctrinal framework within which it occurs. Mystic activation, however it can best be accomplished for each person, pursues as its primary goal the reinforcement of that connection.

So why do we have so many unique approaches? I believe all these systems exist because cultures differ and individual needs differ. Of necessity, there is something for everyone. Each approaches mystic activation through a different door – that is, through different methods that emphasize different processing spaces and different activation principles – but they all ultimately corral us toward the same destination. What is that destination? An adventure through intuitive knowing and spiritual insight; a deepening of wisdom and transformation of identity; an immutable *aha* as we lose ourselves in the passionate embrace of the Absolute. It is beyond words, really, and is more readily experienced than explained. One way to describe this process is an attenuation of established patterns of thought and emotion, a letting go of other senses and physical sensations, so that a subtler form of cognizance can emerge, which in turn can transform our consciousness. In the resulting stillness, with appropriately shaped attention, we can apprehend with our innermost, spiritual ear.

And yet, if all of those differing approaches are designed to meet each individual where they are, how can we determine what will be most suitable for us? How can we discover something that fits perfectly with our particular temperament, the type of interior processing that is most appropriate for us, and the particular phase of our life journey? Well, that is a journey in itself, beginning with carefully cultivated intention, introspection and openness. I encourage you to explore whatever resources are available to you, beginning with your own heart. What does it yearn for? How does it wish to connect with the ground of being? Take a moment to pause in your reading, close your eyes, take a few deep breaths, and look into your heart of hearts for answers to these questions. Don't worry about evaluating what you find within yourself, just let it bubble up to the surface of your thoughts.

....No, really. I mean it. Just stop reading and take a moment to consult your innermost Self. About five minutes of inward searching is a great start.

Okay, what did you discover? Whatever was there – a surprising insight, the sound of your breathing, some piercing doubts, a hint of light, or nothing at all – signals the beginning of the mystic activation process for you. That inward attention combined with receptive, non-judgmental intention is the first step of the journey. And regardless of which approach eventually resonates most for you, finding the courage and humility to begin that journey is what will illuminate your way. This type of discipline is the foundation of all integral practice; it is not something that can be sidestepped or delayed. It will nurture your spirit and develop and strengthen the nourishment prerequisites we have covered in the preceding pages. This, in turn, will allow you to formulate more balanced, all-inclusive multidimensional nourishment. Along the way, you will also encounter the forces and personal truths that underlie every principle discussed in these pages – including the nature of true love itself. Sounds fairly promising, doesn't it? That is why mystic activation is cornerstone of *Integral Lifework*.

Beyond my own assertions and exhortations, how can you know that mystic discipline will provide essential nourishment? Well, there have been a few scientific studies to date, but certainly not enough to draw firm conclusions about the self-nurturing efficacy of mystical practice. A

2005 University of Wisconsin study using MRI brain function mapping suggests that Buddhist mindfulness meditation increases brain activity associated with positive thoughts; the same study also found a strong correlation between regular meditation and enhanced immune response. More recently, in 2008, another University of Wisconsin MRI study found that expert meditators have an increased empathy reaction to external stimuli during meditation. A thirty-year study by the Shanghai Institute of Hypertension showed a marked decrease in overall mortality for daily Qi Gong practitioners who suffered from hypertension, as compared to a control group with hypertension who did not practice. Recent results from an MRI study at Emory University begun in 2004 found that Zen meditation decreased "automatic thinking" (reflexive thought patterns) for those who had been practicing daily for at least three years. Studies at Columbia University and All India Institute of Medical Sciences on the effects of Kriya Yoga found similar immune system, concentration and stress reduction benefits for those who practice that discipline regularly. In short, there appears to be a growing body of evidence that different approaches to mystic activation benefit people mentally, emotionally and physiologically. I encourage you to research this yourself to see what you can uncover.

> **Resources:**   See http://nccam.nih.gov/health/meditation/ and
> http://www.ahrq.gov/clinic/tp/medittp.htm, or search the web
> for "health benefits of meditation" or "psychological effects of
> meditation." You might also explore some of the research at
> www.noetic.org.   Meditation is not the only form of mystic
> activation, but it is the shorthand most frequently used in the
> West for mystically oriented practices.

In a moment, I will introduce you to a sample mystic activator that combines many different approaches into one method. Before we go there, take a look at the following chart. It summarizes an amazing diversity of practices that can, with appropriate intention, attention and follow-through, result in powerful enhancements to spiritual perception-cognition and the persistent indwelling of love-consciousness.

MYSTIC ACTIVATORS

- Sufi muraqaba (watchfulness)
- Buddhist zazen (sitting meditation), vipassana (insight meditation/bare attention), and jhana (concentration meditation)
- Bhakti Yoga
- Kabbalist kavannah (holy intention/concentration)
- Christian theoria/contemplatio (contemplative prayer)
- Buddhist metta bhavana (loving kindness meditation)
- Gyana (jnana) Yoga
- Hermetic visualization and meditation
- Transcendental Meditation
- Other mantra or mandala meditation/Yoga
- Sufi dhikr ("remembering" God)
- Hasidic prayer – hislahavus (bursting into flame) and devekus (clinging to God)
- Invoking certain "spiritual gifts" in Christianity (tongues, prophecy)
- Kundalani, kriya, or other tantra Yoga
- Taoist hsiao chou tien (circulation of Chi meditation)
- Qi Gong
- Tai Chi Chuan
- Chanting, breathing and imagery techniques of ecstatic Kabbalah
- Shamanic trance
- Trance-inducement via controlled breathing, psychedelic drugs or extended fasting
- Sufi "turning" (ecstatic dancing)
- Hermetic initiations and symbolic rituals
- Earth-centered ceremonies such as Wiccan rites of power or polarity
- Angelic incantations and use of gematria (numerology of the Hebrew alphabet) in the magical Kabbalah
- Divination (Tarot, I Ching, Runes, Bibliomancy, etc.)
- Christian rituals, such as adult baptism, "laying on of hands" by elders and the Eucharist
- Energetic healing arts such as Reiki
- Spontaneous Communion (an unintentional state inspired by Nature, during sex, through music, during extreme crisis or pain, in a dream, etc.)

How can we know these practices improve our self-nurturing ability and capacity? How can we be certain they will help us gain clarity about our fulfillment orientation, increase overall self-awareness, inspire a governing intentionality for our lives or enhance our discernment? All we really have are the firsthand accounts of mystics around the world and throughout history who testify to such benefits. For inspiration, I suggest you read some of them; try Plotinus, Krishnamurti, St. Catherine of Siena, Chuang-tzu, Baal Shem Tov, Dogen, Teilhard de Chardin,

Aurobindo or Hafiz; read the Bhagavad Gita, Toa te Ching, Dhammapada, Cloud of Unknowing or Corpus Hermeticum. As with practice itself, the act of beginning matters more than where you begin. But regardless of the actual mechanism of change, I have myself observed countless individuals profit from mystical practice. The secret to success seems to be this formula: an introspective attention or sense that feels a lot like intuition, a devoted intention grounded in affectionate compassion, and diligent follow-through over a period of months and years. In every spiritual tradition, these characteristics are described in different ways, but are always central components of the mystic's way.

And what about love? What does mystic activation or spiritual perception-cognition have to do with compassionate affection? Certainly the great mystics have a lot to say about that. But remember that self-nourishment is the first and foremost act of love. Without caring for ourselves completely, we cannot care for anyone or anything else effectively. And our self-care cannot be complete if we have not developed certain skills and attributes. Integral practices like the one introduced in the following exercise are designed to help you do just that. Also, as you will discover, experiencing an overwhelming, all-pervasive love is one of the many fruits of regular mystic activation. Tuning our mystical awareness is just one of many routes to authentic love, but it is an unswerving and potent one. So whether by expanding our capacity, strengthening our ability or extending our perception, this sort of interior discipline is an extraordinarily effective invitation to the real deal.

If you aren't comfortable taking diving into this right now, there are other exercises later on that will nudge you in a similar direction. There are always alternatives. But if you find yourself avoiding this flavor of internal exploration, it provides a great opportunity to ask yourself: "Why am I not willing to explore this part of myself? What part of me is anxious or fearful about this experience? What part of me is resisting it? What reassurances do I need to include this as part of my daily routine...and why do I need them?" Answering such questions will eventually lead us into that tender inner world that mystic activation helps us explore. And one way or another, that is where we must go to fully appreciate our essence. If you decide to experiment with some of the activators listed in the chart, perhaps you will find one that speaks to your heart, mind and soul more clearly than any other. At a minimum you will make interesting discoveries about yourself, and likely encounter stimulating new relationships as well. Realistically, however, not everyone has the inclination – or the time – to investigate such a broad sampling of opportunities. With that in mind, I have included some tools that provide a sampling of mystical experiences and benefits – beginning with the following exercise.

Exercise: Mystic Activation   As an introduction to one potential avenue of mystic activation, I encourage you to attempt the meditation below. Try this out once each day for a week, and see how you progress. If you find the experience helpful, keep it up for a month. Even if it doesn't evoke special consciousness, the exercise offers the possibility of deep relaxation through consciously shifting your mental focus. After a month or more of practice, you should notice both increased clarity and subtle changes in all of the nourishment prerequisites we have discussed so far, as well as many of the twelve dimensions. Keep a journal to capture the aftereffects of each meditation session, then review those notes after a month of practice. If you don't notice improvement in any of the nourishment prerequisites or dimensions, set this practice aside for now and concentrate on other nourishment disciplines.

1. Objective: Between 15 and 75 minutes of continuous meditation each day. If you can, insulate this with a buffer of five minutes before and after so it never feels rushed, and so you have time to reflect on your experiences.

2. Find a quiet place to sit and relax, and begin your meditation with an inner commitment to the golden intention, i.e. "May this be for the good of All." It will be helpful to be in the same place each time you begin this practice.

3. Relax every part of your body. Start with your hands and feet – perhaps moving them or shaking them a little to release tension – then your arms and legs, then your torso, head and neck.

4. Breathe deeply and evenly deep into your stomach, preferably in through the nose and out through the mouth, so that your shoulders remain still but your stomach "inflates." Purse your lips slightly and allow your cheeks to puff up as you exhale. Practice this until you are comfortable with it in a steady rhythm.

5. With your mind's eye centered in the very middle of your chest, between your backbone and your sternum, silently ask yourself "Where is now?" Search within yourself for a physical locus of the present moment. As words, images, feelings or experiences arise within you, create space for them in your mind and heart without judgment or analysis, and just sit with them for a moment and then let them go. Remember to breathe deeply and evenly. Always return to the question "Where is now?" and, rather than expecting a rational one, search for a sense within yourself of intuitive answers.

6. If you keep practicing and nothing happens, just relax. Resistance to mystic activation is a common occurrence, as are a steady stream of self-distraction, and even a little fear. Keep breathing and keep questioning, perhaps using one or both of the following variations: a) Try changing the emphasis on each word, as in: "*Where* is now?" or "Where *is* now?" or "Where is *now?*" b) Begin to pause in your breathing, at the end of each inhale and exhale – not in a forced way, but enough that your breathing slows substantially to a rhythm of four parts, a "four-fold" breath of in, rest, out, rest.

7. As thoughts, feelings, sensations and images arise, just relax into them for a few moments, then let them go. That is, release any interests or conclusions you might have about internal events, and open the cage of your mind so each event can fly away. You might resist wanting to let go of certain things, and that's okay. Nevertheless, it is important to relax your grip on whatever you're holding onto – try breathing it out with your exhale or flooding it with the interior light of your being. At the same time, avoid forcibly rejecting or denying what you encounter, and allow your

interior to remain spacious and receptive – tenuous and ripe with possibility. Be comfortable in your uncertainty and relinquish your fear.

8. If, even after forty-five minutes of four-fold breathing and interior concentration, your mind still drifts away from the interior spaciousness you are attempting to create, try switching to "Where is now?" as a mantra, repeating it evenly, several times with each breath, either aloud or silently. As in: "whereisnowwhereisnowwhereisnow...." over and over again. Maintain a relaxed rhythm of breathing or the four-fold breath. Remain focused on the rhythm of the words as well as their meaning, and, once again, acknowledge whatever arises without judgment before letting it go.

9. At some point, after a number of practice sessions where you have trained yourself to follow these steps without resistance, you will experience a sense of arrival. The characteristics of this sense are different for everyone, take different amounts of practice for different people, and produce different progressions and intensities of sensation. However, you will recognize on some level that you have encountered "right now." This arrival can occur so suddenly that it jolts us out of our breathing and focus. If this happens, just relax and return to that place of arrival in yourself, resting gently in its light. Immerse yourself in this place for as long as possible, always remembering to breath in and breath out. Know that you are safe, and let go.

10. If any one thing keeps resurfacing during your inner focus, take a break from searching for now and try confronting the resurfacing thought. Challenge it with questions: "What are you? Where are you coming from? What do you want? Why are you here?" And so on. Create space for a response within yourself, and rest in that response just as you sat with your other interior events. Then, whatever answers come, let those go as well. Remember to breath.

11. If you become disquieted, uncomfortable, jittery, or severely disoriented, try to relax through it. If uncomfortable

sensations persist or become extreme, cease all practice for the day, and try again in a day or two.

12. Give yourself time and space after your meditation to process what you have experienced. Open your eyes and just *be* with what has happened without judgment or a sense of conclusion for several minutes. You might consider recording your experiences in a journal as well.

───

Resources: Many contemporary authors offer helpful instruction on mystical practice, either expanding on a particular tradition or reworking shared principles in a conventional context. Try an Internet search on "mystical discipline" to see what's out there. An excellent resource for mystic activation are exercises in the Body and Spirit modules in *Integral Life Practice* by Wilber, Patten, Leonard and Morelli. I also recommend Jack Kornfield's *A Path with Heart* as a superb guide to the Buddhist flavor of mystical discipline. In my books *Essential Mysticism* and *The Vital Mystic*, I define the mystical process more comprehensively than I have here and provide additional exercises to stimulate mystical experience. I've also made an audio CD available, *Deep Relaxation: One*, designed to help those just beginning a meditation practice. One of the best approaches to learning a new interior discipline is to join a local group that both teaches and regularly practices one of the mystic activators listed in the previous chart. This is preferable because, for one, it provides structure and support for ongoing practice; for another, practicing with others tends to expand, enhance and reinforce mystic activation itself. Whatever technique you find works best for you, joining a group will likely be an enriching experience. And remember...if something doesn't work for you after a month or two of regular and thoughtful effort, try something else. All mystic activation techniques are beneficial when practiced in moderation and guided by the golden intention.

This is a good place to stop reading for a while and concentrate on the sample exercises introduced so far. Alternatively, you certainly could power forward through the next chapters to wrap your mind around some of the more advanced concepts. But it likely will only be your mind that you are nourishing. To expand this knowledge into different parts of your being requires operating in different processing modes, and experiencing multidimensional understanding first-hand has a more powerful impact than the written word alone. So give your mind a rest, and let your heart, spirit, body and soul find their own footing in these concepts through integral practice. Then, once you can associate some personally felt experiences with these ideas, you can build on those with the new information and exercises that follow. Remember that the value of your integral practice is founded on appropriate intention, attention and follow-through, and all three of these things spring naturally from the initial seeds of compassionate affection for self. To engage mystic activation creates a personal interface with the immense, unfathomable unknowns of our being. This requires great courage, curiosity and a willingness to suspend beliefs and disbeliefs rooted in previous understanding and experience. To whatever degree true love flourishes within us, these qualities of adventurously being will thrive as well, opening inner doors that expand and affirm everything we are and everything we hope to become.

PART II

ESSENTIAL NOURISHMENT

THE CHARACTERISTICS OF ESSENTIAL NOURISHMENT

All nourishment requires relationship grounded in love, and every relationship grounded in love constitutes nourishment. So what are some other characteristics of self-care in this context? What modes of being encourage a deepening and broadening of high quality exchange? If you are comfortable with a majority of the concepts outlined in the previous sections, and have practiced one or more forms of mystic activation to the point where you are experiencing some benefits, then I invite you to explore the following, more advanced elements of integral practice. Remember that, as you create a target zone of balanced effort in each maturity factor, you are inviting Love and Light into your being. You are creating a sense of safety, openness and skillfulness through which full spectrum nourishment can operate within and without. There is no point in rushing through any of this. To rush is simply to force ourselves into one mode of being – what I describe as mental spacetime – and that mode is limited in its facilitation of growth across other nourishment dimensions. In other words, the unfolding of our personal development builds on itself, and we can't skip any of the steps.

Harmony through Loving Relationship

It is rumored that when a Roman soldier burst in on Archimedes during the Siege of Syracuse, the famous mathematician was hard at work on one of his calculations. When the soldier demanded that the mathematician submit to Caesar, Archimedes angrily replied, "In a minute! I'm not finished..." And so the soldier ran him through with his sword. If this story is true, the course of human history may have been profoundly altered in that moment, for we now know that Archimedes had already laid the mathematical foundations for calculus – about a thousand years before those concepts resurfaced in Western Europe. As the invention of calculus was instrumental in the industrial and technological revolutions of the ensuing centuries, who knows where humanity would be now if those ancient events had unfolded differently? Such are the consequences of dissonance and conflict.

Let's turn this story into an allegory about nourishment. The Roman soldier can play the role of Healthy Body and Pleasurable Legacy nourishment, while Archimedes can represent Expanding Mind and Empowered Self-Concept. Both players can also represent Fulfilling Purpose to some degree. What if Archimedes had been more accommodating and humble? What if the solder had been more curious and less authoritarian? What if they had a mutually respectful, caring relationship? Instead of dissonance and conflict, there could have been harmony and support. Note that the only difference between these scenarios is simply the absence of fear and anger and the presence of love. In the same way, we must pay careful attention to how our nourishment centers interact with each other. Is my body urgently insisting I stop reading and go for a walk? Does my heart long to be somewhere deep in Nature, while my mind thirsts for a city's cultural happenings? Is my sense of purpose interfering with my emotional connection with people close to me? Have I sated my desires in one dimension so thoroughly that I have lost sensitivity to pleasure in others? All of these conditions indicate disharmony among nourishment centers. If I want to be whole, I cannot allow Archimedes to be impatient with the Roman soldier, and I cannot allow the soldier to use his sword.

Harmony is concordant balance – a symphony of nourishment where all dimensions interact with and support each other to create music that is pleasing to the essence of who and what we are. But that balance cannot be achieved through rigid adherence to time schedules for different modes of being or compulsory regimens of self-care. Forcing ourselves to go to the gym, pushing ourselves to learn a new skill, exposing ourselves to uncomfortable social situations to make new friends, experiencing pleasure without emotional content, creating situations where our spirit competes with our mind for attention…all of these things will not satisfy our underlying fulfillment impulses. We cannot force Archimedes and the soldier get along or work in harmony with each other. There needs to be genuine relationship there, a naturally evolved affection between parties. In a few pages, we will explore specific techniques to encourage this unfolding of affection. For now, suffice it to say that harmony will occur as we encourage dimensions to interact through integral practice. Just as it takes time to get to know someone, it may be a while before our mind accepts and appreciates our body, our heart accepts and appreciates our purpose, or our spirit accepts and appreciates our legacy. Over time, the soldier and the mathematician will be sharing meals, joking merrily with each other and basking in the warmth of true companionship.

But wait a moment. What is the difference between a necessary level of self-discipline and a grueling enforcement of unpleasant tasks? Or what is the difference between a healthy competitive tension and destructive and combative internal conflict? On the surface, subjective conditions can appear very similar. The difference is in the trust and caring infusing each relationship; the level of investment and compassion will create drastically divergent outcomes over the course of similar events. If I am truly in love with someone, my governing intention will be to lift them up, sustain them and give them space to grow. Likewise my Legacy impulses will support my Healthy Body impulses, my Playful Heart impulses will support my Expanding Mind impulses and so on. Nothing is competing for my energy, will or attention if I have fully embraced their interdependence. Society needs both mathematicians and soldiers, and any tendencies toward unproductive enmity will naturally be resolved through the rigors and nourishment of an integral practice that includes and engages them both.

When we employ harmonious frequencies of communication within all dimensions of nourishment, entrusting ourselves to the guiding discernment and energy of love-consciousness, the result is full-spectrum nourishment that grounds us in wholeness and perpetual transformation. In essence, the quality of our relationships determines the quality of our nourishment. As we nurture our being, we are infused with new energy, energy with which we can create and sustain loving relationships in every nourishment center. And as we grace each facet of our lives with love, we amplify the quality of our nourishment exponentially. So the cycle is complete: to nourish is to love, and to love is to be fully nourished. And that, in a nutshell, defines most of the supportive structures, objectives and strategies of *Integral Lifework*. Falling in love with life itself, we explode all barriers and limitations to being fully alive. Even as a generic sentiment or vague intention, this will greatly enlarge our existence. But when we apply a specific process – a conscious technique for deepening affection across all energy exchanges – we translate that intention into a concrete, indefatigable force for growth and positive change.

So what is that process? How do we create or enhance loving relationship? There are many steps, and it is important that we take them one at a time. First, we must evaluate where we currently are. Using that information, we can target the nourishment areas requiring the most attention. The *relationship matrix* was designed to begin this assessment. Take a moment to read through the definitions in each of the four quadrants in the matrix, and then try the exercise that follows.

RELATIONSHIP MATRIX

Level of Commitment

A. **Profound** – There has never been a question about this being a lifelong and mutually committed relationship, with the highest level of personal engagement

B. **Pronounced** – One of our closest and most important relationships, with a high level of personal engagement

C. **Moderate** – Bonds that facilitate personal health, status or success, like work relationships, doctor-patient relationships, or family members who aren't emotionally close to us; generally low to moderate engagement

D. **Mild** – Vague, lukewarm commitment to social expectations, such as conforming to laws or traditions; nearly as likely to be circumvented as engaged

E. **Dysfunctional** – Obsessive, addictive, codependent or compulsive engagement that is more destructive than constructive

Type of Affinity or Attraction

1. **Spirit** – An inexpressible but deep attraction that shares common ground in spiritual experience and a sense of spiritual connection

2. **Heart** – Sharing mutually important values, goals and attitudes, including spiritual ones, that indicate a felt emotional connection or attraction

3. **Mind** – Intellectual affinity; thinking alike, sharing similar tastes, or understanding each other's thought process with surprising ease, indicating a stimulating intellectual connection or attraction

4. **Body** – Enjoying how someone looks or moves, the sound of their voice, their smell, etc., indicating a physical attraction

5. **Sex** – Sexual attraction

Circle of Intimacy	Scope of Acknowledgement
I. **Devotional** – Worshipful connection that has no boundaries, is not attached to outcomes, naturally and perpetually shares all experience, and nurtures inexhaustibly II. **Soul Friend** – Deep trust, openness and honesty, with frequent synchronistic and supportive shared experiences, and porous boundaries that are few in number and frequently need not be communicated because they are intuitively understood III. **Companionship** – A comfortable closeness, frankness, mutual trust and support, and a desire for shared experience with few, often porous boundaries for interaction that sometimes must be clearly communicated IV. **Compassionate** – An unconditional acceptance of others with a desire to relieve suffering and promote growth, while maintaining less porous boundaries that often must be clearly communicated V. **Convenience** – Sharing common, cooperative goals for a limited duration, with the most, generally role-based and non-porous boundaries for interaction that are socially defined and tacitly understood	a. **Public** – Everyone knows b. **Immediate Community** – Only our closest friends know c. **Private** – I.e. "just us;" we only acknowledge it between ourselves d. **Self** – We know, but we haven't shared with anyone else, even the other person with whom we feel a connection e. **Unknown** – A relationship is beginning to take shape, but we haven't yet consciously acknowledged it to ourselves

---

Exercise: Relationship Assessment   For each of your nourishment dimensions, rate yourself in all four quadrants in your journal. For instance, in Healthy Body, what is your Level of Commitment to self-nourishment? Which description in the Circle of Intimacy quadrant best describes your attitude toward self-nourishment in this area? What Type of Affinity or Attraction do you have toward your body? In what Scope of Acknowledgement are you comfortable sharing your Circle of Intimacy, Level of Commitment, and Type of Affinity or Attraction towards your body's nourishment? Once you've captured this information, spend a few minutes reflecting on what it means. Then move on to the next dimension of nourishment. How would you rate yourself in the Playful Heart dimension, and so on? Look over the three-day nourishment assessment you did earlier to frame this exercise. And keep in mind that nourishment of any one dimension can involve many different levels, circles, types and scopes. This is not cut-and-dried or one-dimensional, so take your time. When you are finished, reflect on how you might have arrived at the current relationship you have with each nourishment center, and what choices you can make to move those relationships in more loving and caring directions.

Once you complete this exercise, you may come to your own conclusions about what constitutes an optimal orientation toward nourishment, and what status in each of the four quadrants tends to interfere. What is fascinating to me is how everything in life involves relationship and interaction on some level. Aiming for an "ideal" orientation is, I think, a worthwhile goal, but it isn't something that happens quickly, easily or consistently. If it did, we would have nothing more to learn. With that in mind, here are some suggested goals:

- **Level of Commitment:** Either Pronounced or Profound

- **Circle of Intimacy:** The more intimate, the more effective, beginning with Compassionate, then Companionship, then Soul Friend and finally Devotional

- **Type of Affinity or Attraction:** The more Types the better

- **Scope of Acknowledgement:** Public

What do you think? Let's take a look at each one. For Level of Commitment, we need the highest levels of engagement we can achieve, because engagement means attention, energy and focused interaction, without which nourishment will be incomplete. For Circle of Intimacy, if it is merely a matter of Convenience, our exchanges will be superficial and not very nourishing, but any of the other circles will provide ever-deepening infusions of nourishment. An unbound devotional intimacy in all dimensions is the ultimate goal of integral practice, but for most of us that usually takes some time to mature and relax into. As for the Type of Affinity or Attraction, clearly the more points of connection and exchange, the richer that exchange will be. Regardless, though, the more developed holistic nourishment becomes, the more it tends to engage all types of affinity and attraction at once. And finally, only a public Scope of Acknowledgement affords us a truly authentic life. In other words, if we feel the need to contain who we are and what nourishes us to a smaller scope of acknowledgement than what is fully public, something is likely amiss. We may be living in a hostile or oppressive environment, or perhaps we are still protecting ourselves with old survival personas. In either case, the flow of nourishment will be attenuated.

What do we do when we fall short of an ideal? That is inevitable, and in fact reliably enables our growth. But knowing where we stand in each quadrant for each nourishment dimension will spur our progress in *Integral Lifework*. It isn't the only metric to gauge our effort, of course, but it is extremely useful. Still, even with a strong, intimate and openly acknowledged relationship with every part of our being, there is still the question of how to love skillfully. How does a loving relationship manifest in each dimension? How does it translate into sustainable, transformative disciplines? We will be addressing these questions soon.

Dialectic Tension

All high-quality nourishment inherently contains dialectic tension. For instance, each dimension of nourishment benefits when the following two conditions occur concurrently or in close proximity:

1. The comfort of the familiar.

2. The excitement of the unanticipated.

Consider the ritual of going to your mail box. The ritual is ordinary and familiar, it is part of our daily rhythms, it represents a reliable service that reassures us; seeing our postal delivery person evokes a sense of stability and dependability – as Herodotus said: "Neither snow, nor rain, nor heat, nor gloom of night stays these courageous couriers from the swift completion of their appointed rounds." It's a fine, heart-warming comfort. At the same time, we are delighted when we discover unexpected mail. A postcard from a friend, the rebate check we thought would never arrive, the shirt we purchased long ago that was back-ordered, and so on. In the same action, we can experience both the comfort of the familiar and the excitement of the unanticipated. Another example in my own life is taking photographs – finding the right light and composing images through my camera's viewfinder is a comforting ritual, but it is usually occurring within new and exciting events or environments. The same dynamic exists when we read a new book in our favorite reading spot, or try a new dish at a familiar restaurant, and so on. When both of these elements are present in our integral practice, the energy exchange is powerfully amplified.

Why is this? I think it is because we enjoy both, and we need both. It also ties neatly back into our primary drives. The comfort of the familiar is essentially serving our drives to *exist* and *affect*, while the excitement of the unanticipated serves our drives to *experience* and *adapt*. We saw that this same tension was evident in the Motivating Change section. Looking over the sixteen fulfillment impulses, you'll also notice there are some natural dialectic pairs there as well. Discovery has a strong flavor of excitement and unpredictability, while Understanding allows us to translate what we discover into something tenable, reliable and settled. Autonomy is required to exercise our exploratory impulse and have encounters with the unknown, whereas Belonging becomes our anchor, the hearth and home to which we can return from our adventures. And so on with all of the fulfillment impulses. Although the specific pairings in the chart are just examples, the inherent contrast between those impulses that serve comfort and familiarity and those that serve unpredictable excitement is fairly consistent. By their nature, each impulse tends to supplicate one pair of primary drives above the other.

Thus, when our relationship with anything or anyone contains dialectic tension, the potential for enhanced nourishment is increased. Interestingly, however, the potential for dissonance and conflict is also increased. And this leads us to an important observation: that dissonance and conflict are sometimes natural and healthy components of the nourishment process – as long as they do not entirely overwhelm that process. In this context the phrase "a healthy argument" has new meaning. Sometimes the only way to express or experience an appropriate level of dialectic tension is through spirited debate or emotional turbulence. This ads necessary flavor and spice to energy exchanges. To feel fully alert and alive, our comfortable daily routines must be interrupted by the unexpected at least some of the time; we must welcome disruption to our homeostasis. Like so many other principles of nourishment, this is a finely balanced dynamic that varies subjectively. Each of us has a narrow band of tolerance for both boredom and excitement, harmony and discord, conformance and rebellion; somewhere between too much of one and too much of the other is just the right amount of each – or, more accurately, the balanced coexistence of each – which can then synthesize yet another level of nourishment. So within and between all nourishment dimensions, we entertain paradox in order to grow.

Dialectic tension also provides an explanation for certain other common behaviors. When our lives become too chaotic, we will tend to seek out comforting routines, activities and relationships to reestablish our sense of safety and equilibrium. When we become too comfortable or secure in our life course, we can either become irritable and dissatisfied (for no readily apparent reason), or impulsively create random challenges or crises for ourselves to reinvigorate an existence that has become too predictable. Returning to the idea of nourishment as relationship, consider the impact of dialectic tension on your closest friendships. Are there particular relationships you rely upon for excitement and challenge, and others that represent a haven of comfort and continuity? Have you experienced patterns relationship with one individual that provided you with both? The same sort of dynamic exists within every dimension of nourishment and necessitates careful evaluation of all our desires and appetites.

> Exercise: Dialectic Pairs   In the following fulfillment impulses chart, spend a few minutes musing over how each of the impulse pairings reflects dialectic tension in some way. For instance, Effectiveness vs. Perpetuation, Reproduction vs. Maturation and so on. Then consider how this applies to each of the twelve nourishment centers. These arbitrary pairings were created for this exercise; can you find other combinations of dialectic pairing that help make sense of your own experiences?

FULFILLMENT IMPULSE	ACTIVE EXPRESSION	FELT SENSE
Discovery	Observe/Explore/Expand/Experiment	Sense of adventure, risk, opportunity
Understanding	Contextualize/Evaluate/Identify/Interpret	Sense of purpose, meaning, context, structure
Effectiveness	Impact/Shape/Actuate/Realize	Sense of activity, success, achievement, accomplishment
Perpetuation	Stabilize/Maintain/Secure/Contain	Sense of safety, family, security, "home"
Reproduction	Sexualize/Gratify/Stimulate/Attract	Sense of attraction, arousal, satisfaction, release, pleasure
Maturation	Nurture/Support/Grow/Thrive	Sense of caring, supporting, growing, maturing
Fulfillment	Complete/Transform/Transcend/Become	Sense of wonder, awe, fulfillment, transcendence, self-transformation
Sustenance	Taste/Consume/Quench/Savor	Sense of fullness, enjoyment, contentment, satiation
Avoidance	Escape/Evade/Deny/Reject	Sense of fearfulness, self-protectiveness, wariness, stubbornness
Union	Accept/Embrace/Incorporate/Combine	Sense of "being," union, interdependence, continuity
Autonomy	Differentiate/Individuate/Rebel/Isolate	Sense of distinct self, uniqueness, freedom, personal potential
Belonging	Cooperate/Conform/Commit/Submit	Sense of belonging, trust, community, acceptance
Affirmation	Appreciate/Enjoy/Celebrate/Create	Sense of "I am," play, gratitude, aesthetics, inspiration
Mastery	Empower/Compete/Dominate/Destroy	Sense of strength, power, control, skill, competence
Imagination	Hypothesize/Consider/Extrapolate/Project	Sense of limitlessness, possibility, inventiveness, "aha"
Exchange	Communicate/Engage/Share/Interact	Sense of connection, intimacy, sharing, expression

Healing through Adventurous Being

Repetitive strain injuries probably predate the modern age, but with the advent of industrial production methods, work environments and technologies have created endless opportunities for the repetitive overuse of our bodies. Whether working an assembly line or typing on a computer keyboard, confining our movements to the same patterns over and over inevitably leads to traumatized muscles, tendons and nerves. From an *Integral Lifework* perspective, such trauma is not limited to physical repetition and strain. Confining ourselves to the same patterns of thought or behavior in any dimension of nourishment can lead to debilitating injury. We can become emotionally drained or calloused, or spiritually inept, or intellectually lazy; our relationships and exchanges can falter and fail. And yet we humans gain much comfort from the cozy routines we create for ourselves – those rutted paths that make our lives seem reliable, safe and secure. So what can we do to keep this from happening?

In short, we must learn to be fearlessly adventurous in every aspect of our existence. Every nourishment routine must include a provision for exploration, for discovering new modes of self-care that stretch us in uncomfortable ways. To avoid pain or discomfort and resist the shock and disorientation of novel and unusual situations is part of our natural, self-protective survival mechanisms. But when we allow those mechanisms to dominate any or all of our nourishment centers, it results in profound stagnation. Our energy exchanges become septic, clouding each facet of our being. And the only way to counter this is with conscious and focused effort. We must turn the fetid pool of comfort's darkening muck into a flowing waterfall of adventure that glitters in the sun. Despite all fear, resistance and avoidance, we must have courage to mix things up, try something new, change our environments and routines, immerse ourselves in an untested approach. We must take a few risks and let go of what is familiar and known. And we must do this regularly.

Where will we find the courage? In love, of course. In the compassionate affection we hold for ourselves and the widening horizons of interaction around us. In our resolve and commitment to the good of All. In the mastery of our most authentic and devoted intentions. In our grounding in clear purpose and a strong sense of self. And as we take those first steps that divert us from the rutted path, we will experience the exhilaration of discovery, the awe of new vistas and the satisfaction of tasty new flavors of experience, which in turn will fortify our efforts. Each fresh blast of fulfillment will remind us why we must renew ourselves through deliberate variation.

Of course, this exciting newness can become an addiction, luring us out of balance to the opposite extreme so that we are never grounded, never committed, never still or calm enough to fully absorb what we experience. Once again there is a narrow band of optimal function, a fulcrum's plane of constructive effort, which exhorts a careful balance. However, I have yet to encounter anyone who has not required an occasional reboot in at least one of their nourishment centers. We may hunger for newness in our strongest areas of self-care, while allowing our weaker areas to languish behind comfortable routines. So remembering the value of adventurous being as we create our *Integral Lifework Plan* or monitor our wellness over time will keep us flexible and strong in the face of new experiences.

Efficiency, Priority & Deprivation

One evening in my early twenties I sat down to schedule my daily priorities. I was having a challenging time accomplishing all the things I wanted to, and I figured allocating a minimum amount of time each day to my most important activities would help me be more productive in every area. The problem was, when I added up all those minimums, I ended up with twenty-six hours total...and that didn't include sleep! I think this is a challenge many of us face at some point. We simply have too much we desire to do in a day, and so something has to give. Particularly when we discover that some dimension of self is entirely undernourished, it can be distressing to consider how little time we have available to develop new self-care habits.

In *Integral Lifework*, the solution to this dilemma is a particular kind of efficiency that integral practice offers. As you will see when you develop a *Lifework Plan* for yourself, certain nourishment activities are able to nurture more than one dimension at a time. Also, as we combine different routines, natural synergies occur that increase the quality and intensity of each energy exchange. This kind of efficiency allows us to fit twenty-six hours of nourishment into a twenty-four hour day…without sacrificing sleep. Over time, as we fully integrate each new routine into a way of being rather than a focused doing, the whole process is simplified. When we are confident that all twelve dimensions are covered by the daily or weekly activities of X, Y and Z, any additional tasks or goals become extracurricular. That is, our time begins to prioritize itself with increasing clarity; we may selectively add icing to the cake, but the cake is always taken care of first.

Is there a priority for nourishment? The humanist psychologist Abraham Maslow suggested that certain needs must be met first before others can be addressed – his famous hierarchy of needs – and it seems as though this incomplete view still percolates through popular culture in the West. In reality, all twelve essential nourishment dimensions must be concurrently satisfied to some degree for health, growth and transformation to occur. Consider the ideas of fasting and giving away material wealth or possessions, which are common practices among many spiritual traditions. At first these appear to be deliberate acts of self-sacrifice, or even self-degradation in order to prove spiritual worthiness or discipline. But in reality they are just experiential proofs of a critical principle: that no single dimension of nourishment will ever fully nurture us. To realize this, we must free ourselves from our reliance, addictions and attachments to any one type of energy exchange; we must find a way to let go of whatever we routinely crave, even if it initially seems essential to our well-being. What we will discover in the midst of this freedom is that our overdependence on any one flavor of nurturing is often the result of fear-based reasoning or mistaken beliefs. We don't really need the emphasis or prioritizations we are accustomed to, we are just nervous about the consequences if they are taken away. So the answer to the question of priority is that, aside from temporary, targeted priorities for depleted areas – and the practical necessity of ordering our efforts – there really isn't any hierarchy at all.

At the other extreme, asceticism, suppression of natural desires or reckless abandonment of resources will of course have deleterious impacts on our ability to survive and thrive. Returning to the maturity model, this is yet one more factor that invites a delicate balance. When our *attachment style* drifts off-center, we can either become destructively detached or compulsively attached. If we decide to fast in some area, our intention should be to liberate ourselves from a harmful attachment, not replace it with another injurious imbalance. The reason this topic is important is that sometimes deliberate fasting or self-induced poverty can seem like the only way to let go. As many belief systems hold, such practices can be quite effective in this regard – at least in the short run. For until we taste the ambrosia of freedoms that result from sacrifice, we may remain skeptical at best – and willfully rebellious at worst – about even the possibility of abandoning any of our established habits and privileges. It really depends on the individual. The more we have – the more safety nets we or others maintain around us – the more difficult it can be to find something meaningful to give up. So sometimes extreme, short-term measures are useful to shake us out of our complacency and gain a conscious handle on our nourishment patterns.

As for one recent, cautionary tale, consider Jon Krakauer's *Into the Wild*. The main character, Christopher McCandless, is a young man who feels compelled to shed everything tying him to his past identity and affluence as he searches for self-purification. He burns or gives away all of his money, isolates himself from family and friends, abandons his car, and eventually hikes far out into the Alaskan wilderness. Whatever initially compelled him, McCandless eventually comes to realize that what is most important to him is not his fierce independence, his rejection of cultural programming or the self-empowerment of his journey. In his loneliness and isolation he recognizes the importance of human relationship, and his decision to return to society coincides with one brief journal entry: "Family happiness." Unfortunately, he did not make it back. This is self-sacrifice taken to an extreme that produced much pain and suffering for those who knew this young man. I am sure that McCandless did gain insight into his own inner workings and a clearer valuation of life's blessings, but the cost was exceedingly high. Somewhere between this sort of deprivation and the routine overindulgence in creature comforts in our modern world lies a realm of balanced sacrifice that will, if engaged thoughtfully and diligently, provide a helpful process of liberation and self-purification.

As another cul-de-sac in the spectrum of efficiency and priority, we can also become enraptured by new infusions of nourishment to dimensions that have long been neglected. Outsiders sometimes wonder why new converts to a particular belief system seem so destructive of their previous lives, casting off old habits in favor of newfound religious or philosophical fervor. The answer is simple: they were starving, and have finally found some food. And depending on their situation and the window dressing of the belief system they encounter, that food isn't always spiritual or philosophical. It might be the supportive community they have always craved, or the sense of purpose, or the values affinity they find in new friendships there. In other words, a channel of nourishment that had been depleted is now flooded with the water of life. And of course the same thing can happen with a new job, or a new hobby, or a new relationship. An explosion of water in a parched desert will seem like a life-sustaining oasis.

Often, because we have not yet learned balance or self-reliance, we will over-invest in these new discoveries so much that other nourishment centers are neglected. This, in turn, leads to depletion and a casting about for new nourishment – a pattern of frustration, indulgence and abandonment that repeats over and over again. With each new pattern of wobbly energy exchange we create inadequate substitutions for what we most lack. In our perpetual disillusionment we become a pendulum that can never find its center – or, perhaps more accurately, a roller coaster that never stops. If we do not consciously design efficient, full-spectrum nourishment, we will either cast about for new experiences that supplicate our thirst and longing...or resign ourselves to a slow, painful process of starving in the wilderness.

Restfulness

Last but not least, in order for our nourishment to be complete, it must embrace the quality of restfulness. Sometimes this can be accomplished by shifting focus from one nourishment center to another, providing a needed break from one frequency of concentration. At other times we simply have to cease all other forms of self-nurturing and enter into restful quiet. Restfulness should become a frequently revisited condition throughout all integral practice. We exercise and rest, laugh and rest, meditate and rest, make love and rest, socialize and rest and so on. For some people, restfulness can be challenging, because it implies stasis, a lack of productivity, an inability to dissipate internal energies, or a vague echo of purposelessness. However, achieving an authentically restful state is nevertheless part of all essential nourishment. As a counterpoint to restlessness, restfulness not only demands that we let go of busyness but also that we let go of the anxieties, assumptions and compulsions that drive our need to remain busy. This does not mean we collapse into an amorphous glob before a TV we aren't really watching, or consume alcohol until we become numb, our immerse ourselves in self-destructive recreation, or sleep through the day. Instead, we pointedly, consciously relax. We sit in a park and take in the sunset. We read a relaxing book, enjoy a humorous play, listen to our favorite music. We take a short nap in the sun. However we are able, we try as best we can to remain actively passive and uninvolved for a set period of time – just the right length to refresh and restore us, but not so much that it becomes a substitution for or escape from regular nourishment. This is yet another fulcrum's plane to navigate, but this time it's a narrow band of optimal *non-doing*.

Restfulness has some surprising implications. For one, it indicates that rest is required to absorb and process nourishment. Our being needs time to digest what it encounters, and this process can't be rushed. Restfulness also emphasizes the principle of impermanence for all energy exchanges. For example, the same routine or approach will not continue to provide the same level or diversity of nourishment over time. We need to change things up, rotate our crops, add some new spice, interrupt our routines, stay out of a rut – in other words, rest one form of nourishing activity for a while, even if it has been reliable for us, and begin another mode of self-care. We shift through different patterns of intake and output in order to keep our being receptive and pliable. In a way, this continual *letting go* trains us to grow. As we explore new avenues of nourishment, we strengthen our confidence, awareness and self-sufficiency, even as we humbly acknowledge that what has worked well for us before no longer offers the same intensity. And as in any relationship or exchange, this dynamic reinvention creates new horizons to explore and new accomplishments to celebrate.

The Twelve Dimensions in Depth

What does essential self-care look like? It is unique for everyone and even for the same person what constitutes appropriate nurturing will change over the course of time. But with a few descriptions and examples, I think you will get a clear picture of what each of the twelve dimensions are about, as well as how to create and integrate customized full-spectrum energy exchanges into your life. Consider for a moment the following levels of nourishment, which revisit the earlier concept of a narrow band of optimal function:

DEPLETION ←	OPTIMAL RANGE	→ EXCESS
1. Damaging 2. Empty Reserves 3. Partially Depleted 4. Dissonant	5. BASELINE 6. Harmonious 7. Healing 8. Transformative	9. Competing (Impeding) 10. Cross-Canceling (Retrograding) 11. Addictive 12. Damaging

One of the first tasks in *Integral Lifework* is to identify any dimensions that are outside of that optimal range, and work quickly to reset them to baseline with targeted integral practice. Throughout this chapter and again Part VI, we will explore ways of addressing different dimensions with targeted nourishment and thereby create harmonious – and ultimately transformative – interactions. Here is another metaphor for what baseline nourishment really represents: Consider that your life in all its complexity is a very rich, multilayered and demanding software program. In order for that program to perform well and provide your being with lots of cool and useful features, you need to maintain some minimum system requirements. That's what baseline nourishment is. Each of the twelve nourishment dimensions represents all of your system components – memory, storage space, processing speed, video chip and so on. Those components need to be both maintained and routinely upgraded to sustain each new horizon of growth you experience, and of course each depends on the others for full functionality. As a more organic comparison, imagine that you are both a complete, self-contained garden as well as the gardener who tends it; do you have adequate water, sunlight, soil and nutrients? Are you regularly planting new varieties of plant? Are you tending to those weeds? Are you harvesting the fruits of your labor or letting them fall to the ground? Again, all of these things interrelate.

As you read through this chapter, continue to spend time reflecting on how you currently receive nourishment in each nourishment center, how it is currently combined, and how it could be improved. You will undoubtedly discover some dimensions to be fully developed in your life, and others to be absent or greatly muted for no obvious reason. And that's just fine, because it's a starting point. Understanding where you are in this spectrum is the first critical step. After that, the adventure of a lifetime awaits you, for the results of a fully balanced, multidimensional regimen are truly miraculous and more than worth whatever effort is required to overcome barriers to self-sufficiency.

With all this in mind, let's take a peek at what generic baseline suggestions look like for each nourishment center. These represent the result of my own research, observations and hunches in each dimension, and are intended as a starting point for your own exploration of the kinds of energy exchange that work best for you. With so many conflicting strategies and principles flying around the ideosphere, it will be important to discover some solid ground for yourself as you move forward with integral practice. And that solid ground can only be reached through our own effort, introspection and attention to each nourishment center. Continuing to rely on what anyone else proposes – no matter how proven, scientific, innovative or initially satisfying they may be – will keep us in holistic infancy. At the same time, unless we are willing to venture forth into our first experiences of multidimensional nourishment, we will have challenges trusting that growth and self-transformation are even possible. So the steps outlined on the following pages are some possible first steps, a toe-in-the-water before we have learned to trust ourselves to swim out into open ocean.

1 - Healthy Body

I recall one of my *Integral Lifework* clients who always seemed to be in crisis. Deborah was in her sixties and struggling with a number of health issues. She was also trying to manage a very stressful conflict with one of her adult children, and grieving over the perceived loss of that relationship. Every time we met, she had a new story to tell about how one of her friends or relatives had betrayed her trust, sought to harm her, or otherwise caused her pain. When we got around to discussing her own health, she would quickly veer off onto the health issues of her friends, which she felt were much more serious than her own. In fact, whenever I probed a little around her self-care, there always seemed to be someone in her life that she needed to rescue, and that became the focus of our conversation, just as it had become the focus of most of her efforts. At one point, when the timing seemed right and Deborah expressed feelings of frustration and being at the end of her rope, I asked her a question: "What do you think would happen if you directed perhaps ten percent of the energy you expend helping others on your own well-being?" Deborah was silent for a moment; then she began to cry. "You know," she said, "that's exactly what I've always avoided. I guess even at my age, I still have something to learn." Nearly all of her life, she had tried hard to help others get through sickness and difficulties, and always at the sacrifice of her own happiness and wellness. Now, she decided, she would start caring for herself.

How we care for our physical body is really a metaphor for how we care for our entire being; it indicates the quality of the relationship we have with Self and the level of affection we hold for our own existence. If we cannot love the temple of spirit, the house of consciousness that is our flesh, how can we claim to love our own soul, the essence of who we are? Neglecting the nourishment of any part of us will always result in unhappiness, illness and pain, and nowhere is that more immediately evident than the physical self. So let's take a look at the main components of physical self-care. As with all other nourishment recommendations, these are just my opinions and are open to interpretations that work best for you.

Sleep. Sleep is the bedrock upon which our physical health is built; it is the anchor for all subsequent disciplines. Without appropriate sleep, all other facets of physical self-nourishment will fail. Although the optimal amount of sleep varies for everyone, the following guidelines are an excellent starting point:

- **Continuity.** Our largest chunk of sleep should be as contiguous as possible. That is, without internal or external interruptions. Although opinions in the scientific community have varied over the years, the optimum range seems to be about 6.5 to 7.5 hours. Less than that can be tolerated for short periods of time. Consistently more than that will negatively impact metabolism, health and possibly even lifespan. The recommendations that follow are all ways to encourage continuous sleep.

- **Consistent wake time.** Waking at the same time every day programs our body to cycle its internal rhythms around that wake time. If you need more sleep, go to be earlier rather than sleeping in. You will notice very quickly that waking at the same time every day helps regulate most other physical rhythms, as well as results in more overall energy throughout the day.

- **Avoiding caffeine and alcohol, especially near bedtime.** It is well documented that caffeine changes how we sleep, even to the point of serious sleep deprivation over time – even when the hours we lie unconscious in bed seem to be sufficient. Caffeine users always need caffeine to become alert not only because they have become dependent on the drug, but because they aren't sleeping well. Alcohol likewise impacts sleep in negative ways; although it may initially help us relax and even feel drowsy, it will ultimately reduce the quality of our sleep.

- **Cool down period.** About an hour before bedtime, we should let go of mentally or physically energizing activities in favor of relaxing ones. Going for a run, solving a cross-word puzzle or having an intense conversation are examples of energizing activities. Even watching a suspenseful movie or reading a stimulating book can interfere with preparing for sleep. Instead, spend some time reflecting on your day, or giving or receiving some light bodywork (a back rub, Reiki, etc.), or listening to relaxing music.

- **Consciously ending how we wish to begin.** How we end our day – what thoughts and feelings are with us when we fall asleep – influences what we think and how we feel during sleep and as we begin the day. So be conscious about this. I encourage practices like gratitude meditation, Reiki, or simply imagining what good things will happen tomorrow as helpful ways to fall asleep.

- **Reducing stress and increasing exercise.** There is no better way to relieve stress than to exercise, and no better aid to deep, satisfying sleep than relieving stress. We will discuss these in more detail later on.

- **Cat naps.** Ten to twenty minute naps when we feel tired during the day can have a delightfully rejuvenating effect on our energy and help us avoid sleep-sabotaging activities (like imbibing caffeine!). More naptime than that, and we may muddy the cycles that sustain us. Often it may seem easier to push through a tired moment, but this can lead to increased physiological stress, errors in judgment and so forth. So why not just...take a nap?

- **Avoiding sleep aids.** There is increasing evidence that sleeping pills not only interfere with the quality of our sleep but may have deleterious health impacts as well.[1] Really, almost any drug at all that we rely upon to help us sleep will have a negative impact on our well-being over the long run. And I would include in this category many OTC supplements.

Many people are blessed with a good, sound sleep each night, and for them these recommendations may seem like simple common sense. But it is very interesting to note that hardly any of the folks I have worked with over the years had been experiencing satisfying sleep when they first consulted me. Perhaps only one or two slept well. I think this is significant, because our quality of sleep can really be a measurement of how balanced other areas of nourishment are in our lives at any given time. When we are out of balance, our quality of sleep will suffer. When we approach self-nourishment holistically, our quality of sleep will substantially increase. Consider this in your own self-assessment. How rested do you feel on waking in the morning? How tired are you when you go to bed at night? Does your body feel relaxed and satisfied, or tense and achy? These are not only indicators of sleep quality, but our quality of life overall.

Exercise. In a society where many people are either sitting (at work, in a car, on a couch in front of the TV) or sleeping, adequate exercise can be a challenge. Part of this challenge is the psychological barrier of just doing exercise for exercise's sake. While this may be an inspiring adventure for some people, and even a professional goal for serious athletes, exercising for strength and health can be a major obstacle in an otherwise sedentary society. I myself tried a gym membership years ago, and found after a week or two that I would either require a personal trainer or some other motivational mechanism to keep me going. I just couldn't summon the energy to breathe stale, sweaty air and stare at silly sitcoms and infomercials while my muscles screamed for me to stop; that environment just seemed to be crushing my spirit. So I reverted back to activities where I could enjoy the exercise in a broader context: playing tennis, frisbee and basketball with friends, hiking in the mountains, swimming in the ocean, riding my bike for small errands, and so on. Doing these things outside in sunlight and fresh air excited me and helped my spirit soar. But as time becomes compressed by the demands of modern life, having enough freedom to casually achieve exercise in fun ways is difficult. That is, unless it becomes a higher priority, and that may not happen until we have experienced some serious interruptions to our well-being.

So what can we do? Exercise is a critical part of our overall health. Without it, our cardiovascular system becomes less efficient, we lose bone and muscle mass, we gain too much weight and, perhaps most importantly, any stress in our life has no healthy way to relieve itself; as a result, our overall well-being degrades. When clients come to me with frustration, anger or depression issues, some of the first questions I ask are about their exercise routine. Almost inevitably, they don't have one. And just as inevitably, when they are able to begin even a moderate amount of regular exercise, they begin to feel better emotionally as well as physically. So that brings us back to the question of motivation. When I lived in Frankfurt, Germany during my teen years, I observed something interesting about the people who lived there. They were surprisingly fit, by and large. Yet a majority seemed to regularly eat a lot of rich, fatty foods and drink generous amounts of high calorie beer. In addition, there were at least as many overweight people as there had been in cities where I had lived back in the States. And yet...so many of these Germans were lively, healthy, smiling, firm-bodied folk, whereas stateside obesity had generally been synonymous with irritability, flabbiness and immobility. What was the difference? Well, one readily observable difference was that the residents of Frankfurt walked just about everywhere. Need a fresh loaf of bread? Walk down to the local bakery first thing in the morning. Need some toothpaste? Walk to the local convenience store. Need a new frying pan? Walk to the local streetcar station, ride downtown to the pedestrian-only zone, and walk from shop to shop searching for the right one. And so on. In the evenings, city streets would be thronged with folks walking to a restaurant for dinner or walking back home. Because walking was the preferred mode of locomotion in these situations, motivation never came into question. Going out to dinner, shopping, and even commuting to work included exercise as part of a cultural expectation.

Probably as a result of these observations – and the fact that I joined my German step-grandfather on long walks every day – I am a big proponent of walking. I walk for about twenty minutes at least twice a day. The ancillary benefits are surprising. Walking near my home, I have gotten to know and even befriend many of my neighbors and local shop owners. Often my walks are elongated because I stop to chat, or because one or more neighbors decide to join me for a few blocks, or because I am walking to breakfast or dinner. I also know all of the neighborhood pets and they know me, responding warmly when I stop to say hello. And I get the sunshine my body craves when I walk outside. Afterward, my muscles and joints are loose and warm, any congestion in my lungs or sinuses has cleared, my posture is improved, my thoughts are more concise, and my mood is elevated. After my morning walk, I have more energy for the rest of the day. After my evening walk, I am more relaxed and able to sleep soundly at night. However, I do live in a part of San Diego where walking is not the most common mode of locomotion. In Frankfurt, Germany there were sidewalks everywhere and pedestrian overpasses or underpasses at busy intersections, but the streets of San Diego often lack any sidewalks at all, and crossing busy streets can be a scary proposition. Thankfully, right now I live in an area with access to boardwalks along the beach, streets with sidewalks and shady trees, and several restaurants, services and shops within walking distance. I made a conscious choice to include walking in my daily routine, and chose to live somewhere that integration would be easier. Movements like new urbanism and planned communities, which combine living space with work space, shopping and service environments, suggest a different future for America than continued suburban sprawl, and new potential for walking from place to place.

As exciting as I am about walking, walking alone is not a complete exercise routine. To fully benefit us, our baseline exercise should include each of the following components:

- **Increasing flexibility.** Gently and gradually stretching muscles and tendons beyond their habitual range of motion.

- **Strengthening.** Building up and sustaining muscle and bone density to support both normal day-to-day function and the occasional unusual demands on our body without increasing our risk of injury.

- **Moderate aerobic rate.** Increased heart rate (about 50% of our maximum heart rate) and breathing (faster and deeper, but not so fast as to make conversation difficult) to oxygenate blood and increase fluid movement through all systems of the body.

Walking at a faster-than-normal pace will easily fulfill the moderate aerobic component. But what about strengthening and flexibility? Here again we have many choices. For strengthening we could try free weights or isometrics. For flexibility we could try traditional stretching, Hatha Yoga, or George Leonard's ITP Kata outlined in *The Life We Are Given*. And of course we can combine things for efficiency's sake. We can introduce all components of exercise into our lifestyle. For instance, carrying groceries home from our walk to the store introduces a strengthening component. Choosing a hobby or vocation that regularly demands increased effort from our muscles is another route to strength. In my own practice, I use my flexibility routine as a time to connect with Nature in a worshipful way. Really, there are endless options for weaving baseline fitness into the fabric of our lives. A friend of mine rides her bicycle everywhere and doesn't even own a car. One man I know switched professions so he could spend more time outside and really use his muscles. One of my clients decided to ride his bike to work each day. Another started swimming again before work each day. Another client walks her dog at a favorite park as an excuse to get outside. There are so many mundane tasks that can become healthy exercise if we let them. Shoveling snow from a driveway, sweeping a sidewalk with a broom, or raking a yard by hand instead of using powered equipment or hired help. Taking stairs up to the fourth floor of a building instead of using the elevator. Washing a car with a bucket and sponge and waxing it with a cloth instead of running it through a car wash. Biking or walking to a nearby restaurant after work, instead of ordering in. Using those fifteen minute breaks at work to do some Hatha Yoga, or to walk to and from our favorite coffee shop instead of driving. The opportunities for moderate exercise are endless if we just shift our mindset from lethargic convenience to healthy effort.

For baseline physical fitness, only medium intensity exercise is suggested here. Of course, what constitutes medium intensity exercise of course varies from person to person, based on age, overall health and ability. But our available time, our level of stress, how tired we are from working a full day...none of these should influence our routine. It is, after all, quite easy to combine exercise with other nourishment habits, creating an increasingly integral practice.

Here's one last plug for walking: We can combine walking with interacting with others. I have frequently met clients at public parks to walk and talk. When I was a manager, I would walk with my employees outside when conducting one-on-one meetings. When counseling couples, I often recommend they begin resolving conflicts by discussing sensitive issues during a walk. There are all sorts of advantages to walking communication that ease us through difficult ideas, temper our inability to formulate words around our feelings, allow silent reflection upon what is being said without evoking an awkward silence, and so on. And walking can easily be wed to nearly any type of energy exchange.

We can meditate while sauntering, or sing, or compose a poem. It can connect us with a natural environment, with our community, with our sense of space and place. In this sense, walking is an ideal component of our overall integral practice.

Diet. Is there one optimized diet that benefits everyone? We are all different. Whether that difference is rooted in physiology, culture or family tradition is less important than the reality of the difference. Add to this that our nutritional needs change as we go through different phases of life, and the picture quickly becomes exceedingly complex. However, within this broad spectrum of variability, there are some simple guidelines for a healthy diet. A recently concluded four-diet study at the Harvard School of Public health offers an unsurprising guideline for controlling weight: eat less and exercise more. But beyond weight control is the question of overall health and well-being, and that is what I would like to address here. Some of the ideas in the following list are widely accepted principles, and some are more my own observations and opinion; see what you think and, if you are willing to give them a try, see how you feel after a month or two of following them.

Consider the type of relationship we had with food for several millennia as hunter-gatherers. We were close to the source, eating many things within hours or days of harvesting or hunting them. We had direct interaction with the plants and animals we ate, and were immersed in a transparently interdependent connection with the natural world. Even later on as farmers and herders we remained close to our food, in some ways increasing our level of intimacy with what we ate. In terms of preparation we were also intimately involved, grinding our own flower, baking our own bread, or maintaining close relationships with those who did. But in modern times, we have become disconnected from our food sources and many aspects of preparation. Any remaining relationship has been abstracted by an artificial distance from Nature – plants, soil and wildlife are "out there somewhere," barely acknowledged or appreciated as the fundament of our existence. The act of preparation is, for most people in the Western world, increasingly reduced to whatever is most expedient and convenient. Therefore, much of what informs baseline diet in an integral context is an attempt to reinitiate a closer, more personal connection with what we eat and drink.

- **Fresh, raw and whole.** Whatever you consume, if it came out of a garden yesterday or a local farm within the past week, it will offer you nutritional benefits beyond anything found in a can. Highly processed "food stuff" is not only laden with processing chemicals and preservatives, but a whole host of valuable nutrients have long since departed. Along the same lines, the more raw the food, the more nutrients are retained. Why cook, grind up, chemically treat or otherwise alter something that can be enjoyed in its natural form? The less processed and more whole the food is, the more nutritional value it can offer. Unfortunately, commercial food production in the U.S. has resulted in a broad availability and acceptance of non-nutritious food stuff; awareness is slowly growing about the resultant nutritional deficits and inflammatory impact of such quasifoods, and hopefully a reversal of the food stuff trend is gaining ground. The main enemy of fresh, raw and whole is of course convenience. To buy ingredients for making a salad at home isn't as convenient as buying a prepackaged one at a fast food restaurant. If you can create the opportunity – whether by growing fruits and vegetables, bartering with a neighbor who has a garden, or maintaining a relationship with a local farmer – try to cultivate at least some of your food close to home. As with many of the principles in this list, we can make a little extra time in our lives for our own well-being, and many of these steps can be combined with other nourishment dimensions as well.

- **Avoiding substitutes.** This is really a corollary to #1, but it is easy to overlook in the modern world. Instead of margarine, we can stick to fresh butter. Instead of aspartame, we can rely on organic honey. Instead of artificial creamer, we can use raw cream. Instead of engineered sugary or caffeinated drinks, we can quench our thirst with water. And so on. Just keep an eye out for chemically treated, manufactured substitutions for naturally available foods and try to avoid them. Thanks to government regulations, these food substitutes are easy to identify – they're right on the label. If there are several ingredients or processes with scientific names instead of a simple recognizable list of food items, you should probably avoid it. Why? Because this is not food, it's artificial, and it will alter your body chemistry, metabolism and overall health in ways that you cannot reliably anticipate. And that risk is unnecessary, because we can easily manage our diet with simple, unprocessed foods that have been ingested by humans for millennia. At this point in time, it is not clear to me that genetically engineered plants and animals are advantageous to human health, and they introduce potential risks to wild ecosystems, so for now I would place these in the "substitute" category as well.

- **Small, slow, frequent and well-masticated.** This is one of the more difficult principles, but it makes a huge difference in overall nutrition and diet management. If we eat smaller portions, consume them slowly and chew them well, spacing these smaller meals at regular intervals throughout the day with more frequency than just three major meals, we will tend accomplish many different things. For one, we will eat less, because we won't be ravenously hungry when we finally sit down to eat. We will also give our stomach time to recognize it is full, whereas rushed meals often lead to overeating. And by chewing our food thoroughly, we not only slow ourselves down, but also allow our teeth and saliva their rightful place in the digestive process, thereby reaping maximum nutritional benefit from our food...while enjoying it even more at the same time.

- **Making food time quality time.** It is essential to make meals meaningful times during which we focus on the taste, texture and enjoyment of our food. Have you ever eaten a quick snack in front of the TV, only to discover the snack has disappeared before you realized you had eaten it all? That is not a healthy way to eat. Why deprive yourself the pleasure of your meal by allowing such distractions? Focus on your food. In the same way, we can prepare as many meals as possible from raw ingredients. Why not become involved in the energy exchange with our food, reconnecting with the process of how our meals are made? If it just isn't practical to take this on yourself, then engage others in your immediate community who are involved in food production and preparation. In whatever way possible, become more intimate with your food.

- **Ingesting happy food.** I seem to be eating less and less meat, but when I do, I avoid anything that wasn't caught in the wild or is at least free range. Why? Because I believe millions of years of evolution do a better job providing nutritious food than all but the most enlightened farming practices – and captive animals are often not very happy anyway. If an animal is perpetually stressed, force-fed things it wouldn't normally eat, or is ill its entire life, I don't want to support that, but also consider what energies, hormones, microbes and chemicals these suffering creatures pass on to anyone who eats them. And the same goes for cheese, milk, eggs and so on. Do these come from animals that are emotionally and physically healthy and free, or from tightly caged, distressed critters in crowded, filthy factories? As just one example, one of the healthiest foods available to us is wild salmon, while most farm-raised salmon can contain excessive heavy metals, and their omega fat ratios can be closer to factory-raised beef than their much healthier wild salmon cousins. In the same way, some types of farming force plants to behave in unnatural ways or prevent natural interaction with their surrounding ecosystems. Why risk eating those "unhappy" plants either? In both cases, the organic and free range movements are a helpful start – but they are really only a start.

- **Fasting vices regularly**. Sugar, caffeine, simple carbs, alcohol, salty foods, carbonated drinks, chocolate, ice cream, butter, red meat....What do these have in common? Many people love them. In fact, kids of all ages prefer them to a more balanced array of nutrition. If we are given a choice between raw broccoli and a fresh, warm chocolate chip cookie, what do we choose? It's silly to think we will always be able to manage our intake of a favorite vice, so why struggle? Instead, we can continually fast a couple of these categories at a time, giving ourselves clear start and stop dates, and rotate through our list. This month no coffee, next month no soft drinks. This month no wine, next month no chocolate. This month no morning pastries, next month no desserts after dinner. This month no fatty meats or butter, next month no salty foods. By maintaining a continual, rotating fast of foods that aren't so good for us in excess, we will not only reduce our caloric intake to healthier levels, but also, in combination with other baseline diet principles, increase the overall quality of our diet. And then, when we begin to indulge ourselves after the fast is ended, in many cases we will find we won't crave the same quantities of the fasted item as we did before. In some ways selective fasting artificially duplicates cyclical patterns that exist in Nature, which our bodies not only tolerate but seem designed to expect. In other ways, selective fasting helps us take conscious control of our eating habits.

- **The rule of thirds.** This is not a scientifically validated approach, but I believe it can be a useful guideline. For all caloric intake for the day, consider obtaining one third from fruits and vegetables, one third from whole grains and protein, and one third from healthy fats. That alone is a helpful place to start. Once you get the hang of such a balancing act, you can refine it further. Within the first group, you could aim for a majority of intake from vegetables, with an emphasis on dark leafy greens. In the second group, try to obtain protein mainly from plants (nuts, beans, grains, etc.) and use whole grains (rolled oats, whole wheat flour, sprouted grains, brown or wild rice, etc.) that are as raw and unprocessed as possible. And in the third group, you might glean healthy fat from raw foods and wild animals as opposed to refined oils. Of course, many of these elements can be found in one type of food or other, so it doesn't take much effort to calculate the rule of thirds, especially with current food labeling standards and the plentiful resources available on the Internet. And once you get the hang of it, not only will your new habit sustain itself, but your body will likely start reminding you of its preference for balance.

- **Eating ethnically.** Having a diverse diet of course makes life more interesting, but what I am really talking about here is aligning your food intake either with your genetic heritage or with a particular type of ethnic food that seems to increase your overall health. For those like me who are genetic mutts, this may take some effort and experimentation – both in finding and preparing authentic ethnic cuisine, and zooming in on what works best for your body. American culture has a habit of morphing diverse and interesting dishes into mild-mannered, homogenized and commoditized qausifood. A delightful array of tasty German sausages become bland, chemically enhanced hot dogs. An equally varied selection of hearty, flavorful European breads become drab, tasteless white loafs. Spicy, fresh and interesting Italian, Chinese or Thai dishes become syrupy-sweet imitations of the originals. Where I live in San Diego, "Mexican" food, instead of representing the diversity of excellent and healthy dishes from the different regions of Mexico, has been reduced mainly to the vaquero (cowboy) fare of the wild West – with a few other traditional foods thrown in. In other words, finding authentic ethnic recipes or restaurants is not as easy at it first appears. But they're out there.

- **Activity breeds healthy appetite.** Over the years I have observed that intense physical activity tends to create appetites for healthier foods, and that, conversely, sedentary habits tend to inspire unhealthy appetites. Food can, of course, become a substitution for any other form of nourishment, but there seems to be something hardwired into our bodies to crave more salt, fat and sugar when we are consistently inactive. Perhaps this has something to do with the natural cycles of food during different seasons of the year. In any case, the more active you become, the more I believe you will – if you are tuned into your body – begin to desire healthy foods as well as attenuate excess appetite over time. I readily admit that I have no research at hand to back up this claim; however, I encourage you to give intense exercise a try and see if it helps you manage your food quality and intake.

- **Supplements are medicine, not food.** Regular, long-term use of supplements can have just as powerful an impact on our bodies as prescription pharmaceuticals. Rather than supplementing for a deficiency, I recommend gaining whatever is lacking from whole foods that are eaten raw. There will always be exceptions – such a sublingual B12 for folks lacking B12 cofactor, etc. – but even in those cases, I would encourage using the lowest dose that is effective. Even water-soluble vitamins can have a negative impact on well-being if taken in excess. If something has a positive short-term impact, consider slowly ramping off of that supplement to its minimum effective dose, just as you might do with a powerful medication.

With all of this said, the real key to the success and health benefits of any diet lies in our capacity to listen to what our body is trying to tell us and to avoid using food as a substitution for other nourishment. For me, after years of struggling with food allergies, digestive problems and interrupted sleep, I finally began listening to what my body was trying to tell me and stopped medicating away physical and emotional discomfort with caffeine, alcohol, simple carbs and fat. After cutting most of the major offenders out of my diet – red meat, hard alcohol, caffeinated soft drinks, unfermented soy, gluten, sugary sweets and a host of other inflammation-producing foods – I consistently have more energy, better sleep and fewer symptoms. How did I know to remove these from my diet? By paying close attention to my bodily sensations, smells, energy, complaints, cravings and so forth; by tuning in to my physical being. And whenever I am disciplined enough to shift my biology into a more alkaline state for a few weeks, all of the physical maladies I have accumulated evaporate and I feel incredibly healthy. But again, my particular diet isn't a prescription for anyone else – it's just what my body responds to. The key is listening to what my body is trying to tell me. If I had not begun paying careful attention to my body, I would have become more and more ill; that is, my body's complaints would have become louder and louder. And lastly, as with all of these principles, keep in mind this can be a slow process of transition from old habits to new.

Resources: Try a web search on the core concepts in each of the dietary principles listed and see what you can uncover. I also recommend reading the book *In Defense of Food* by Michael Pollan.

Rhythm & Resonance. The natural rhythms of Nature are everywhere, intersecting with everything we do and mirrored in everything we are. Lunar cycles and menstruation, the Earth's rotation and the circadian rhythms of the body, the seasonal tilt of the earth and changes in human mood and activity – these correlations are an immutable part of our existence. Alexander Tchijevsky even observed that solar cycles correlate with societal trends, noting that some of the more tumultuous times in human history coincide with the highest cyclical levels of sunspot activity. And of course age-old astrology asserts that the astronomical cycles of planets and stars have distinct influences on individual propensities and cultural patterns. Whether we believe these correspondences to have meaning or significance is a matter of personal choice, but to acknowledge and reconnect with them on a conscious level – regardless of what we believe – is to reconnect with something primal, vital and energetic. When we tune in to natural rhythms and alter our patterns to resonate sympathetically with them, we experienced a fluidity of being that improves the quality and accuracy of our navigation through each moment. As we attune ourselves to Nature, all the energies of Nature flow through us both more tranquilly when there would otherwise be conflict and cacophony, more freely and more fiercely when there might otherwise be resistance.

As with much of the rest of the world, the highest concentrations of human population in the U.S. are within cities. Cities where dirt is paved over, plants and animals are carefully confined and groomed, where sun and moon and sky are obscured by human industry and artifice, and where the most basic awareness of Nature has been drowned out by noise or muted by disconnection. So for most of us, achieving reconnection and resonance with natural rhythms requires deliberate effort. What follow are some sample activities that acknowledge those rhythms and begin a process of reconnection. As such, they can provide a healthy baseline within this channel of nourishment:

- Using a lunar wall calendar or a daytimer that notes lunar phases, actively track the phases and orbit of the moon over the course of the month. When the sky is clear, search out the moon to witness her arc, features and changes. Become familiar enough with her cycle that if someone were to randomly inquire about it, you would be able to answer out of current awareness.

- Several times each week, spend five or ten minutes watching the sun rise, set or both.

- Acknowledge the solstices and equinoxes each year in some way. By celebration, ritual, prayer, socializing or some combination of these, honor those times for the real changes they bring to our quality of life on Earth.

- At least once a month, spend an extended period of time far away from human habitation in some natural environment. Go slowly, observing the details of your surroundings, noting the quality of light, the smells and sounds, the taste of the air and its feel on your skin. At some point, just sit down, close your eyes, and welcome Nature into you as the part of your being it really is.

Why do I think these cycles are so important? As just one example, consider that without our orbiting Moon, life on Earth would be very different – if it existed at all. The gravitational interaction between the Moon and Earth created and continues to maintain the Earth's magnetosphere, which protects our planet from the potentially mutagenic radiation in solar winds. And although its impact is not completely understood, the tidal action the Moon produces in our seas has likely had a crucial role in distributing nutrients and both concentrating and sorting the building blocks of life. Without tide pool zones, would life have evolved so robustly or been able to transition to live on land at all? In addition, moonlight seems to have significant impact on everything from plant seed germination to animal behavior. It appears that our scientific understanding of the Moon's influence on Earth life is slowly catching up with the worshipful appreciation ancient cultures held for this Deity in the sky.

As you reconnect with the cycles and subtleties of Nature, an awareness of the natural world will slowly begin to grow inside you. What the moods of the sky or smell of the air portend for weather. What animals are trying to communicate to each other and to you. When it might be prudent to stay indoors or away from others, and when it might be fortuitous to venture forth and engage. The least productive time to make major decisions and the most productive time to act on them. And so on. This channel is included in the Healthy Body dimension because it is more physiologically based than anything else. What we are doing here is aligning our will, thought and actions with what our body already knows...and has known all along: that our interior energies follow the same complex, cyclical patterns that the exterior energies of Nature do. So, instead of resisting that natural resonance, we can consciously facilitate and reinforce it. And like so many other components of well-being, the proof of what may at first seem hypothetical benefits will come about through practice.

Touch. Being able to touch and be touched by another person is a critical nourishment factor, supporting and enriching our existence from soon after we are born until our final hours in this world. I place touch right up there with breathing and hydration as a fundamental energy exchange. Of course, what constitutes appropriate and acceptable touching is something we must always navigate carefully in each relationship, environment and culture. Because each person's conditioning and sensitivities, we all experience touch differently, but the need for human contact is always there. As a baseline, I like to take predictable daily touch in social contexts and amplify them just a bit. A handshake becomes a real connection by looking into someone's eyes and really seeing them, really feeling them, as we hold their hand. A hug, a shoulder-pat, a fist bump, a ruffling of hair or any other socially appropriate gesture becomes an opportunity for real connection several times a day. The depth of that connection is set by two things: each person's intention and each person's receptivity. If we feel deep compassion and caring for someone, that will translate from our being to theirs through touch. If I am open to such loving kindness, then I will feel it through the connection someone offers to me.

In Western culture, physical intimacy that is non-sexual is an anomaly among some age groups, communities and sub-cultures. As a result, when affectionate touch backed with compassionate caring is first experienced, it can be misinterpreted as sexual, invasive or awkward. Likewise, when we offer such intimacy it may trigger wariness or sexual feelings in us. I have a group of male friends I have been meeting with every few weeks over the past four years or so. I have always given these men full frontal hugs whenever we have met individually. As a group, however, these men didn't feel so comfortable giving or receiving hugs in public. At first, they were a bit tense and self-conscious, sometimes making jokes to cover discomfort. Eventually, they began to relax and, within the last year, I find that if I forget to offer a hug I am engulfed in one initiated by them. So in this instance, I chose to push back at status quo restrictions with my physical affection – within certain limits. There are, of course, all sorts of complex rules about appropriate contact between the sexes, between adults and children, between ex-lovers, gays and straights, bosses and employees, teachers and students, health practitioners and clients....Yet however we can do so, it is imperative we find ways to have meaningful touch between us.

In addition to daily social contact, I would also include as part of our basic nourishment more extensive connection in relationships where that is expected and promoted. For instance, therapeutic touch with a licensed practitioner, a backrub or foot massage from a close friend, kisses and cuddling from family members and so forth. In my own practice, I have found self-administered Reiki to provide energy exchanges in this channel as well. For a few hours every week, we need to experience touch that is pointedly intended to provide deeper nourishment, healing and support, and experience it in both giving and receiving ways. If we can approach sexual affection in this way, lovemaking can become a natural extension of nourishing touch; however, for many different reasons beyond the scope of this book, sex has additional layers of mental, emotional and psychosocial complexity that can sometimes interfere with authentic intimacy or confuse our most compassionate impulses. So I would recommend not pushing the envelope there as part of baseline self-care. Yet however we connect physically with our loved ones, we must discover what our comfort level is in the spectrum of mutually caring touch, and find the most productive ways to explore more open, honest and compassionate intimacy.

2 - Playful Heart

Our ability to feel is a huge part of being human, and to regularly experience a broad array of emotions can itself be nourishment. To express those emotions – whatever they are – in creative ways deepens the breadth and subtleties of our emotional vocabulary. All emotions are important in this way. In addition, there is one facet of our emotional life that deserves special attention, because it heralds the profound success of being alive: Joy. To feel joy on a daily basis is to announce to the Universe we are alive and well, at the same time reminding us and everyone around us of the wonder and delight of this amazing feat.

Emotional Awareness. Emotions are intended to get our attention, to help us navigate our personal circumstances and make decisions about that great big world out there. So being able to tune into our current emotional state is a very useful skill. Having clear emotional awareness also prevents strong emotions from completely taking over our consciousness and overwhelming our ability to manage our behavior. One method of enhancing emotional awareness is to close our eyes and find the physical locus of a given emotion. Where does anger occur within you? Where is happiness felt? What about sadness or excitement? Another is to enter a meditative state where we observe our emotions arising within, spend some time letting them wash over us without judgment or any impulse to change them. Another is to develop to expand our emotional vocabulary, exploring the difference between similar emotions like grief, sadness and loss. During mystic activation, emotional awareness can become very acute, detailed and subtle. Listening to the feedback of others about our perceived emotional state can also be illuminating; when people ask us why we appear agitated or sad, it can remind us of a state to which we have unconsciously become acclimated. So there are many ways to increase emotional awareness. The important thing to remember is that we must eventually be able to check in with our emotional state at any given moment, and understand what it is we are feeling and, ideally, why we are feeling that way.

Emotional Experience. Have you ever listened to music that brought you to tears? Attended some event that got you excited and inspired? Seen a movie that made you laugh out loud? Been filled with wonder at some site in Nature? Felt an emotional connection to the characters of a book? These are the result of choices to experience emotion. The emotional content of anything is not outside us, but within us, and we seek it out because we want to feel. Of course there are always natural emotions that occur from day-to-day, from moment-to-moment, but we often let those pass through us without really noticing them or giving them space to grow. But when we consciously choose to evoke feelings through absorbing some experience, we are seeking to exercise the emotional breadth of our being. We stretch, we exert, we run and fall down. And our emotional being parallels our physical being in every respect. To become conscious of this desire for exercise and regularly indulge it is the baseline of emotional experience. In fact, if we don't exercise our emotions we will tend to create opportunities for expression in unconscious ways. We might create conflict in our relationships, or start seeking the excitement of new friendships because we believe something is missing, or become depressed because we no longer seem to feel as deeply about things. In a way, anger, anxiety and depression are natural consequences of an atrophied emotional life – they can evidence our heart trying to struggle free from immobility.

How can we plan our emotional life more consciously? One question I often ask my clients is this: What activity or hobby did you really enjoy when you were younger that you no longer do? For one person it's sailing, for another it's flying a kite or building model airplanes, for another it's playing with play-dough or using finger paints, for another it's spending time camping out in Nature or traveling to foreign places. Somewhere along the way, an activity that brought us much joy and contentment faded from our life. Often, it was a childhood interest that we eventually dismissed because we wanted to be more accepted or appear more adult. Or it may have been something we felt we no longer had time for once we found ourselves working full time or starting a family. Perhaps as we entered a new committed relationship, we let some activity fall to the wayside to make more room for our partner. This unintended sacrifice of joy is more common than you might think, and it almost always results in unresolved grief and loss buried deep within.

Here are some other forgotten joys my clients have shared over the years:

> "I used to sew a lot. I don't know why I stopped…I used to love sewing."

> "Juggling. I'd forgotten all about that. And doing magic tricks. I was obsessed with it till about high school. Then I gave it up. I guess it wasn't as cool anymore."

> "I had season opera tickets for years, but my husband hated opera. So I stopped going. I'm sure he wouldn't mind me going now. I just haven't thought of it."

> "Just reading for pleasure. I don't read anything nowadays except for work stuff. Some of my happiest memories are being curled up with a good book."

"I would draw pictures every day but I was never very good. I wouldn't show them to anyone. Maybe that's why I stopped. What was the point? But drawing did make me happy."

"Probably running. I used to run everywhere when I was a kid and loved it. I guess in Junior High or so my friends said I should try out for track. I did...but I didn't enjoy the competition. After a year I quit the team and stopped running altogether. I never thought about just running for fun again."

"It's a little embarrassing now. I used to take my sister's dolls out into the back yard and act out these elaborate stories. For hours."

"I learned piano when I was pretty young and played for a long time. Then in college I focused on other things – my career, dating. I moved into my own place and didn't have a piano. I always played for myself anyway. I miss it."

And with each of these recollections, similar emotions rush to the surface for each person. Their faces light up with joy, become concerned with puzzlement, or darken with the sadness of loss. And, without exception, once they eventually began reengaging their forgotten joys in some fashion, they found a wellspring of emotional nourishment awaiting them.

> **Exercise: Recovering Joy**   What have you given up that once brought you joy and contentment? Why did you give it up? Could you start again without disrupting your life or anyone else's? Is there a similar activity that could fit into your daily life that would bring you joy now? Begin imagining how you might reengage in such an activity, and then gradually schedule it back into your life. Start with perhaps thirty minutes just one day a week, at the same time and place, and see how that goes. Then, after a month or so, try thirty minutes twice a week. Could you combine this with other nourishment activities? After a couple of months, give that a try.

Creativity. What is creativity? An expression of self, to be sure, but even more so an intimate connection with self on many levels. To express our heart we must know our heart, and the creative process inspires us to deepen our awareness of – and conscious relationship with – our emotional interior. Creativity can also connect us with our intellect, our physical need for self-expression, and our spiritual sensibilities. As such, creative endeavors are a naturally integral practice. However, in modern American culture, creativity is often relegated to a chosen few who are encouraged, in their position of grand celebrity, to indulge every creative whim to the delight of a rapt audience, and then receive huge monetary rewards for doing so. But this mass consumption of creativity is not the same as being personally creative, and to a great degree this cultural tendency has undermined the importance of individual creative efforts by substituting a shared experience of consumerism. In order to nourish our creative needs, we should spend at least twenty minutes each day engaged in some sort of creative endeavor. This could be anything, really, as long as it has three fundamental characteristics: 1) complete, unrestrained emotional freedom; 2) genuine expression of our most intimate substance; and 3) a belief that our creative offering has inherent value. Freedom, genuineness and belief.

The creative impulse can be expressed in any medium by anyone. And a medium can be anything. I recall the movie *Edward Scissorhands*, where Edward seems to always choose artistic media that are inherently impermanent. Ice sculpture, hair styling, topiary...whatever he creates will quickly change or pass away. And that really captures the essence of the effort: to be enthralled and satisfied with the process of creation. For an example of unrestrained creativity, just observe young children going at it with play-dough or finger paints. They throw their whole being into their creative expression, intent and enthralled in the activity – regardless of their qualifications or experience. And the result? A smear of blue and yellow paint at the corner of a piece of paper. A misshapen lump of clay that plays a very important part in some elaborate and meandering imaginary story. An ever-expanding mess across the living room floor. An unabashed eagerness to share their efforts with the world. This is the quality of effort we need recapture as adults when we pursue baseline creative nourishment.

Skill is not a prerequisite for creative effort. In fact, it is the mistaken belief that skill is necessary that often snuffs out the creative spark in people. "Oh, you wouldn't want to hear me sing. My singing voice is terrible. I can't even stay in tune!" "I tried writing a computer program once, but it didn't work like I expected." "Oh, I don't know how to draw. Never could do it well. My pictures don't look anything like the real thing." "I'm just not a creative person. I've tried a lot of different things – pottery, painting, acting, writing – and I haven't mastered any of them." And so on. The expectation that our efforts should resemble some famous artist's work – or anyone else's work, for that matter – can rein us in to a complete stop. In reality, writing in a personal journal every day can be a bravely creative act. As can making up a silly song while we are taking our morning walk, or adding some random spices to the dinner we are preparing, or rearranging the furniture in our home or the plants in our garden into to a more pleasing flow, or inventing a new type of bottle opener that is only useful in our own kitchen. It doesn't matter if those efforts are ever appreciated or approved of by anyone else…what matters is our remembering to unleash that part of us that longs to create.

That said, skill can be a useful compliment to our creative endeavors. As we delve deeper into our creative self, the challenge of applying more advanced or complex skills to the process can be rewarding. A new glass-blowing technique, for instance, or a new way to strum a guitar, or advanced technical knowledge that informs a new invention, or a writing class that helps us craft our prose. There is a delicate balance to be forged between enslaving our creativity with too many technicalities or rules, and not advancing our creativity because we neglect the technical craft of our endeavor. Somewhere between these two extremes is another narrow band of optimal function that will nourish and inspire our creativity. This balance will, of course, be different for different avenues of self-expression, depending on our natural aptitudes and abilities. The more things we try, the clearer our path will become – well, unless we are blessed with the curse of being good at everything. Regardless, however, we should spend as large a portion of time each day possible engaged in creative activities.

> **Resources:**   If you find exploring your own creativity challenging or completely foreign, I recommend two books. The first is *Drawing on the Right Side of the Brain* by Betty Edwards. The second is *The Artist's Way* by Julia Cameron, which takes a distinctly spiritual approach to the creative process.

Playfulness. Much like creativity, playfulness invites us to return to a childlike state. The key to playful experiences is that they are unstructured, free of deadlines, goals and rules that crowd out joyful inspiration. Playfulness almost always involves laughter. Not only the knowing chuckle at a good joke, but the carefree giggling of being tickled. There always seems to be a physical aspect to playfulness as well. To roll around on the ground with a puppy, or throw water balloons at each other, or play hide-and-seek, to jump up and down with excitement. Playfulness means engaging the world around us without any agenda other than to let go, remain open, and enjoy it. Social conventions are cast away, responsibilities are set aside, and our whole being devolves into silliness. There is nothing respectable or restrained about playfulness. As for specific activities, there is joking around, goofing around and otherwise having fun. About the only restriction we might place on playfulness is that our fun not cause harm to anyone or anything. We could be a bit out-of-control, bouncing all over the place at random, but our impulsiveness is not intentionally destructive. Regular playfulness is essential to physical health, and so we should find any and every opportunity to be playful – at least five or ten minutes each day at a minimum...but, really, we will benefit even more the more we can keep it up.

Emotional Intimacy. As with physical intimacy, emotional intimacy must be navigated according to social expectations and boundaries. In *Integral Lifework*, I advocate the idea of falling in love with pretty much everyone and everything as an extension of the love we feel for our own essence. And that, of course, is an important distinction. We cannot authentically fall in love with anyone or anything until we have learned how to love our own being. As we open ourselves to trust, emotional closeness and intimate connection with others, we can then be safely grounded in the self-nourishment of compassionate affection we hold for our innermost Self. We are not expecting reciprocation, and we are not even dependent on acknowledgement of our love – we love because it is a natural function of who we are. Falling in love with All that Is becomes an extension of our gratitude for being, our wonder and delight in life itself. So intimacy is really just emotional honesty about a joyful feeling that encompasses all existence, offering itself confidently to each unfolding moment. If I am intimate with this breath of air, this piece of stone, the leaf of this plant, the skin on the back of my hand, the muscles around my knee cap, a child's carefree smile, the mischievous glint in a friend's eye…then I am intimate with my whole being and the wholeness of life all around me. And as I unfold with openness and honesty about my own state of being, this will evoke a desire for openness and honesty in others. Intimacy resonating with intimacy, grounded in love. What is the baseline for this channel of nourishment? As often and as deep as we can comfortably go, within the confines of our cultural and situational constraints, we should do just that. Then, when we are ready, we can open up and expand our emotional being just a little bit more each and every day.

Intimacy issues have frequently been the focus of the couples counseling I have done. When two people have committed to celebrating a high level of intimacy (at or above Companionship in the *Relationship Matrix*), but find that intimacy has been undermined in some way, it often has to do with trust. When we don't feel completely safe in trusting someone, we will have challenges with intimacy, so in order to improve emotional intimacy we need to rebuild mutual trust. This is equally true with the emotional intimacy in any relationship – if we trust someone completely, we will open our hearts, minds and lives to them. And yet this cannot depend entirely on the worthiness of others; it cannot rely solely on them earning our trust. Instead, we must also address our fears surrounding our own vulnerability. We must ask ourselves: "What is the worst thing that could happen to me if I trust this person?" Often, the only clear answers are that we might be disappointed, that our time or resources may be wasted, or that we could be socially embarrassed in some way. Are these sufficient reasons not to trust other people? It's an interesting question to consider, especially if we rarely offer intimacy to others or find the intimacy we do experience unsatisfying.

At the other end of the spectrum, what if we are very trusting and open, but find ourselves in relationships where intimacy is not reciprocated?

In my experience this usually is caused by one of two circumstances. On the one hand, we may be drawn to people who are inaccessible, withdrawn or aloof in their relating to us, which is really a way of protecting ourselves from authentic intimacy and playing out old patterns from our childhood. On the other hand, we may be subtly broadcasting an unhealthy dependency on the intimacy we desire. We see here once again the principle of the narrow range of optimal function. At one extreme, we can be rigid, self-protective and fearful in our inability to experience or attract true intimacy, or, at the other, we can be needy, dependent or codependent in our unhealthy craving of intimacy. Only when we find the fearless, self-sufficient middle ground of wholeness, wellness and loving kindness for self will we be able to offer and receive intimacy in supportive and enriching ways.

> **Resources:**   One technique often employed to increase emotional intimacy of two people or a group is a battery of trust exercises. By searching the web for "trust building activities" you should find a number of useful sites. Give some of these activities a try with someone with whom you already share a mutually agreed upon Circle of Intimacy, and see what happens.

3 - Supportive Community

Developing a supportive community begins with finding people whose values resonate with our own. This of course requires a clear understanding of those values, and doing values-related explorations like the previous Values Alignment Exercise and regular meditation will assist with that process. That is not to say we shouldn't also cultivate relationships with people whose values differ from our own – in fact, its good to have both types of relationships as party of our community. Once again, though, this is about establishing reciprocal trust.

Friendship. What is a friend? I believe this term has been widely misunderstood in modern American society. A friend is someone who not only reciprocates our affection and trust, but also shares the same level of involvement in each of the four quadrants of the *Relationship Matrix* described in the previous section. For a friendship to exist, it should:

- Experience a mutual **Level of Commitment** at or above Pronounced.

- Experience a mutual **Circle of Intimacy** at or above Companionship.
- Experience a **Type of Affinity or Attraction** in at least two of the first four areas (the affinities or attractions need not overlap, but each party should hold at lease two towards the other party).

- Experience a **Scope of Acknowledgement** that is at least Private or above.

This level of involvement is fairly easy to assess, especially if both parties are willing to evaluate the relationship using the Relationship Matrix. What is both unfortunate and common is a lopsided involvement, where one person perceives more mutuality in each quadrant than the other, or a confusion of what is really less than friendship for the real thing. For instance, a Moderate Level of Commitment does not constitute friendship, nor does a Compassionate Circle of Intimacy. Sharing a purely sexual Type of Affinity or Attraction can be satisfying, but that alone is not friendship. These are all functional acquaintances – important to our nourishment in other areas, perhaps, but not as friendship. And, of course, the higher the level of mutuality in each quadrant, the closer and more important the friendship becomes.

Is there an ideal number of friendships that provides ideal baseline nourishment? I think this varies from person to person, but in my experience very few people can sustain more than three or four close, active friendships outside of their immediate family at any one time. By active I mean friends that we interact with regularly and who are part of our weekly or biweekly routine. Past friends with whom we seldom interact do not meet the "active" requirement for friendship nourishment, no matter how close they have been at one time. So for many people, five active friends are just too many to handle. There are exceptions, but remember that these friends are part of our most intimate circle of connection and will require a fair amount of time and energy. These are the folks we can count on being present and involved with us in both inclement weather and fair, amid both crisis and mundanity, and whom we would not hesitate to support or help in any we can. At the other extreme, it is common for some folks to believe they can only maintain close friendship with one person. This usually restricts nourishment, however, simply because no two people can share deep connection and mutual nourishment on every level.

People have interesting ideas about this channel of nourishment. For instance, one client visited with a grandmother in her dreams, and felt closer to her than anyone living. Another befriended a spirit guide through meditation. One person considered their hair dresser among their closest friends. Another presumed they had an especially strong bond of friendship with their coworkers and relied heavily on those relationships. Some people consider their animal companions to be their best friends. And so on. What is happening here? Understandably, we will tend manufacture friendship substitutions where there is really be a different kind of connection (a lesser Level of Commitment or Circle of Intimacy, fewer Types of Affinity or Attraction, etc.), because our heart knows we require such intimacy to thrive. Not that these other relationships aren't important – they are very important and part of our overall support system. But they do not fulfill the role that at a truly profound friendship does.

As to how we can cultivate true friendships, that becomes relatively easy as we explore relationships through our Interests Affinity and Values Affinity interactions. So let's cover those next.

Interests Affinity. This is perhaps the easiest group for us to engage. Whatever our interests are, wherever our passions wander, we can always find affinity groups with whom we can interact. Whether hiking, books, movies, travel, language, exercise, food, architecture, history or crossword puzzles…there is a group of people somewhere who share our interest. This is such a common way to connect with others that whole organizations have formed around interest groups. The Internet is of course a great way to find such connections. The next step is simply to show up. Not that this is an easy first step, but when we find our courage in the necessity of our own nourishment and the care we have for our well-being, showing up becomes easy. And of course we don't have to rely on existing groups or connections, we can create some from scratch. For instance, I once started an art salon in my home with a free ad in the local alternative newspaper. But perhaps the broadest and strongest shared interest available to all of us is our own personal history; once we open up to others and listen to their own stories, thoughts and feelings, we create bridges of empathy and affinity. As Barack Obama wrote in *Dreams from My Father:* "There was always a community there if you dug deep enough...There was poetry as well – a luminous world present beneath the surface, a world that people might offer up as a gift to me, if I only remembered to ask."

Values Affinity. It can be more challenging to find groups that share our values. The first step is clearly identifying our own values and perhaps which stratum of moral valuation we gravitate towards in each area of interest. That is, we must define the scope of our values as well – the arena of affection within which we are most comfortable expressing our values. What is most important to us, and what arena of action are we able to promote those convictions? In Part IV we will explore this idea further. For now, consider the intersect of your own values with affinity groups you have identified for baseline interests affinity. For example, if I enjoy outdoors activities and value the preservation of Nature, there are plenty of organizations that intersect the two. The same would be true if I enjoy working with my hands while helping the homeless or impoverished, or expressing myself artistically while educating underprivileged kids, or public speaking while lobbying for political reform, or cooking food while strengthening my community. There are so many opportunities out there, and if there isn't an ideal intersect already available...well, create one. When I first started teaching classes on mysticism, I had no idea that many of the people who attended my classes would eventually become some of my most cherished friends.

Celebration. A close relative of playfulness, celebration is really about ritual. Whether it is a regular pizza night with friends, a Sunday worship service at the same place each week, a gathering in our home to watch our favorite TV show, or a skyclad dance deep in the forest under each full moon, we need to anchor our lives in regular rituals that connect us with each other and our inner life. We should create whatever excuse possible to celebrate. And by celebration I mean joyfully cutting loose with laughter and gratitude in the presence of those we consider our community. There is a natural nexus between social expectations and celebration – attending a party at work, or watching a local sports game, or joining our relatives for a birthday or holiday – but often our participation in these rituals is constrained by social expectation. We must behave a certain way or risk being ostracized from the group. So creating our own celebratory rituals on our own terms becomes an important part of communal nourishment routines.

Neighborliness. There are still communities in America where new arrivals to the neighborhood are welcomed with fresh baked goods, where the next door neighbor shows up with a shovel to help when they witness you out digging in your front yard, where people watch out for each other and parents watch over each others' children without thinking twice about it. Often these communities are small, tight-knit and rural, but there are plenty of folks who have consciously recreated such characteristics in densely populated urban areas. Sometimes this in a structured or formalized way, such as in the cohousing movement, but just as often individuals and families make a deliberate choice to act a certain way – a neighborly way – towards others, and the kindness becomes infectious. The following are some small but significant ways we can introduce neighborliness into our immediate environment:

- Greet people in your neighborhood when you walk by them.

- Offer to assist neighbors in small but meaningful ways when the opportunity presents itself.

- Accept offers of small but meaningful help from your neighbors.

- Get to know your neighbors – their names, interests, concerns, histories, etc.

- Create time for impromptu conversations with your neighbors.

- On random occasions, give small gifts to your neighbors that resonate with their interests.

- Acknowledge and thank others for their courtesy.

- Avoid negative judgments of others in your heart and negative gossip about others in your words.

Some of these may seem like common courtesy to readers who were raised with certain communal expectations. To others they may seem like empty and meaningless gestures that only impede efficiency or personal security in a fast-paced, transient lifestyle. But really this is about the fundamental social cohesion that facilitates connection and exchange between all people. The shorthand for this is practice is *cooperative effort*. Do we wish to live in a competitive society or a cooperative one? Do we wish to be true citizens who advocate for and contribute to the well-being of the Whole, or entitled consumers who abdicate their communal responsibilities? Most of us long for cooperative support and are eager to offer it, but because of the coddling and dependency engineered by consumerist, commercialized Western culture, there is a lot of interference to deal with. As a result of dependency-producing capitalism paired with certain perceived expectations and entitlements, many people in the West project responsibility for their own well-being and the well-being of society as a whole on political leaders, big business, healthcare and anyone but themselves. They desire instant community in a can. But regardless of that interference, if our aim is to create a supportive community, and we acknowledge our responsibility to work toward that end, neighborliness is a great starting point for our efforts.

Face Time. In a world of cell phones, texting and on-line chats, technology has perpetuated an illusion of interpersonal connection that too often supplants physical proximity. In-person interaction offers us a level of exchange that is not yet possible by any other method. The nuances of expression, the subtleties of scent and chemistry, the unconscious honesty of body language – all of this reinforces the importance of spending face time with our friends, neighbors and community. A convenient baseline is at least two hours of face-time per week with individuals and groups that represents our primary community of support. To whatever degree we are able, if we replace other forms of communication with face time, we will strengthen the bonds that create healthy and nurturing community.

Avoiding Substitution. In the modern world it is relatively easy to avoid communal relationships with other people, and instead prioritize other types of interaction in an attempt to generate the same sense of connection or belonging. We may come to see books or music as part of our community, or the fictional characters in a computer game or TV show, or the commentators on our favorite news program, or even inanimate objects. Our need for a supportive community is so great that in cases where our repeated efforts to connect or integrate are thwarted, or we lack the skills or immediate opportunity to interface with others, we will simply fabricate a community from whatever is conveniently at hand. By doing this, however, we short-circuit the opportunity for the high-quality exchanges that truly sustain us, and over time deplete our nourishment in this dimension. If there is never a time in our lives where we graduate from our beloved doll, toy car, stuffed animal or favorite pet to real human playmates, we will remain emotional children. We need not discard or deny those beloved relationships, but we must augment them in order to grow.

Avoiding Exclusivity. In the same way, we can inadvertently overemphasize one type of relationship to the exclusion of others. For instance, we might expect our immediate family, a romantic relationship or our work relationships to provide us with all of our essential nourishment in this dimension. And such a distorted expectation has unfortunately been amplified by decades of entertainment media that tend to model this behavior. But such habits a tremendous strain on too few points of connection, so that eventually either those connections disintegrate under the undue burden, or we become dissatisfied and frustrated that our reliance on them has provided us inadequate nourishment. The answer, simply put, is to have a broad and diverse community of support, with widely distributed interdependencies built in. No one person or group of people should ever become our exclusive means of emotional connection or communal nourishment.

Diversity and Inclusiveness. As important as it is to include people in our community of support that agree with our values and share our interests, it is also important to include some folks whose views, values and interests are different from our own – or even conflict with our own. If we surround ourselves with like-mindedness, the strength of our convictions will never be tested. So at least once or twice a week, consider initiating interaction with people you fundamentally disagree with. Once a month, attend a lecture or group discussion that presents alternate viewpoints to your own. Befriend people whose values are different from yours – invite them out for a walk or a meal. Spend a small but meaningful amount of time exposing your being to communities that impede or oppose the societal goals you value. Then see if you can not only tolerate but learn to enjoy and grow from these interactions. Find the common humanity in your opponents and celebrate it; find the good that resides in every human heart. Try to fall in love with the diversity that might otherwise antagonize your well-being.

Shifting from Modern Tribalism to Interdependence. When we begin to identify strongly with any one group, we risk the pitfalls of converting our community of support into a tribe of conformance. In the simplest terms, tribalism synthesizes an "us versus them" mentality, lauding the benefits of the self-selecting group and diminishing and excluding everyone else beyond its confining circle. In fact, the only difference between a tribe and a cult is the rigidity with which those boundaries are drawn and enforced, and the vehemence with which we control the "us" and demonize the "them."

Some writers have suggested that modern tribalism is a stage of societal or interpersonal evolution, and I believe this is sometimes the case. However, modern tribalism can also become just one more substitution for authentic nourishment. When the fulfillment impulse of *belonging* combines with other fulfillment impulses like *effectiveness, perpetuation, mastery* and *exchange*, the urge to create a stable mechanism to satisfy all of these at once can be overwhelmingly strong. Tribalism appears to satisfy all five impulses, albeit in superficial and self-limiting ways. In one way it approaches integral practice – attempting to combine many forms of energy exchange into one discipline – but it is ultimately inefficient and counterproductive because it naturally excludes diversity and calcifies interaction into fixed patterns of conformance. Perhaps most importantly, tribalism tends to place perpetuation and protection of the tribe as the highest priority, far above more compassionate human characteristics. In this way it eliminates or antagonizes nourishment in many other dimensions.

What is the alternative to tribalism? One is to become more individualistic and reject conformance to any group, striving toward the illusion of complete independence. But this is a really step backwards into a cocoon of imaginary control and delusional self-determination. Whether we can fully appreciate it or not, we are members of our community and our daily lives are shaped by interaction with that community. The required shift is, I believe, in the opposite direction. We must discover a larger field of identification instead of a smaller one. We will explore this in more detail in the *arenas of affection* section, but consider the earlier discussion about governing intention, where the good of All becomes our primary focus. Once we begin to identify with larger and larger circles of self, we begin to act in harmony with those more inclusive exchanges of energy. If I identify as a member of the human race, why would I differentiate between different skin colors, nationalities or belief systems? If I identify as being an integral component of the Earth's ecosystem, why would I differentiate between human activity and any other force of Nature? If I identify as a mote of awareness afloat in a vast consciousness that spans the Universe, why would I differentiate between human consciousness, animal consciousness and the consciousness that manifests in other regions of space or in other dimensions entirely? As you can see, the larger and more inclusive our realm of identification, the more an "us verses them" orientation is diminished. But in terms of building community, how does this work in a practical sense?

If I believe in the inherent value and sovereignty of every person, knowing with certainty that they play an equal part in the concert of life, then I enter into an interdependent exchange with them as an equal. Remember that our ideal fulfillment orientation is neither protective nor dependent, but self-reliant. So each exchange is a choice to engage in mutually beneficial interaction. As we construct a wider and wider network of mutually beneficial interactions, we build a community based on those interactions. We synthesize a values affinity there, an interest affinity here, some celebration over here, then leaven the mix with neighborly kindness…and what is the result? An ever-changing community of interdependent, mutual support. And because this community is perpetually dynamic, there is no cultish self-identification with that community and there are no static boundaries to enforce or defend. Everyone and everything has a part to play, wherever they are. At the same time, each of the connections we generate demands our integrity, commitment and authentic love. This is not about moral relativism or relationships of convenience, it is about being fully present and engaged in each and every interaction from a place of belonging and centeredness, in relationship with something much vaster than those interactions. Instead of allowing our self-concept to be defined by our relationships with others, we relate to others from a clear centered self-concept grounded in a connection with our conception of the All – the essence of things, the ground of being, etc.

It seems prudent to raise one important caveat regarding interdependence, and that is to recall the principle of *quality input* for all nourishment. The more interactions we have, the more we must discern the appropriateness of our investment; it would be difficult to make it home from the grocery store if every interaction required equal prioritization. So we can prioritize according to those aforementioned choices. Is this interaction part of my chosen community or not? If not, do I have the space, time and energy in my life to explore this interaction? Does the potential of this relationship tie into my other nourishment dimensions? Am I able to effectively and authentically love this person in this moment? And so forth. I have found interaction with strangers to be a delight more often than not, so when I do have the time, energy, etc. I am happy to engage others. But if I am having dinner in a public place with a loved one and my intention is to demonstrate my devotion to them, is engaging a stranger in that context appropriate? Probably not. What if I have students or clients awaiting my arrival as I pass through a crowded parking lot? I am sure you see my point.

Social Boundaries. What are social boundaries? In the context of supportive community, these boundaries are personal safety zones that we broadcast around us so that others can know where they may tread with confidence, where they should approach only after humbly asking our permission, and where they shouldn't tread at all…ever. There are many different types of boundaries, and it is important we are clear about where each line is drawn in each of our relationships. There are time boundaries, communication style boundaries, information boundaries, emotional intensity boundaries, expectation boundaries, involvement boundaries, intimacy boundaries, physical boundaries...there are boundaries for every facet of our being, each one defining how energy should be exchanged. And depending on where a relationship plots within each quadrant of the Relationship Matrix, those boundaries will be different. The knack for this is to be clear about them for ourselves, and then direct and honest with others with as much diplomacy as possible.

I remember one incident many years ago with a neighbor in Seattle that illustrates several points about boundaries. Whenever I was outside working in the yard, my elderly neighbor (let's call him Henry) would suddenly appear and, after watching me for a few minutes, ask me what I was up to. I noticed that he always stayed on his side of the property line, so I was also careful to stay on my side as I worked. These were usually brief but pleasant communications that seemed, for the most part, to be relieving Henry's concerns about my activities. Over time, it became clear that Henry wasn't interested in idle chit-chat or creating a neighborly relationship, he just wanted information. Despite my attempts to ask him about his day, the neighborhood, his life, whatever...the information only flowed one way: from me to him. As a result I became less invested in our conversations, excusing myself politely on several occasions, saying I was short on time and just couldn't explain everything I would be working on that day.

Then, one day, I awoke to pain radiating through my abdomen. It was so intense by body was going into shock, and I knew it. After a half-hour of trying to figure out what was wrong and failing, I called for an ambulance and sat waiting for them on my front steps. When they arrived, Henry came bounding out his front door and yelled over to me: "What's wrong with you?" And without much thought about the sting in my words, I croaked through my pain, "It's none of your damn business."

For the remaining time I lived in that house, Henry never approached me again...about anything. At first, I was a little relieved. Then I found out something that changed my view of everything that had happened. I overheard Henry speaking with his adult son in their driveway. The conversation was about Henry's wife, Lily, and how she was very worried about the new retaining wall I had recently installed. According to Henry, she was worried about a lot of things, and very insistent that he find the answers right away. Henry's son was encouraging him to relax and not get so worked up about Lily's concerns, but Henry angrily defended her and rejected his son's counsel. She was disabled and in poor health, he reminded his son, and was stuck in that house all day long; she relied on Henry for everything. So Henry's son dropped that topic and began offering opinions on the retaining wall instead. I was surprised to hear any of this. I had never seen Lily and hadn't known she lived there.

Let's look at all the boundaries defined in this little story. First, there is the information boundary Henry set with me: he declined to share anything about himself or his wife in any of our conversations, which resulted in me remaining unaware of his overall situation. He also demonstrated a physical boundary by never crossing our property line, which resulted in me being careful to respect his space as well. I set a time and information boundary with Henry when I disengaged from his questions as quickly as possible. Then there was the information boundary I set with him about the details of my medical condition, which, probably because I was so forceful, resulted in Henry disengaging from any more interaction with me. Henry then demonstrated an emotional boundary with his son by defending Lily's concerns, making it clear that their marital relationship would remain outside his son's realm of influence. This resulted in his son shifting focus to a discussion about the retaining wall.

This is how boundaries are constantly communicated – sometimes consciously, sometimes not. Developing our own boundaries and respecting those of others is part of social and emotional maturity; they are they acknowledge acceptance of our own adulthood. In the maturity model discussed in Part I, the fulcrum's plane in this area is a permeability of self that is neither a hardened bomb shelter nor openness without gates or walls. We must carefully engineer a balance between extremes and be vigilant to maintain them. And yet, if we aren't clear and careful about how we receive or communicate our boundaries, they can have unintended consequences.   For instance, my gruff retort seemed to discourage Henry from seeking me out again on any topic, which was not really my intension.   Henry's inability or lack of willingness to make our conversations more of a two-way exchange of information made me less sympathetic to his inquiries.   Henry's stern emotional boundary with his son may have closed the door to what sounded like wise counsel.   In each case, the boundary may have been appropriate, but how it was conveyed undermined the possibility of mutually supportive relationship.

Because of the vast cultural and generational differences inherent to large, transient, heterogeneous communities in the U.S., it is imperative that such boundaries be clearly communicated and – to whatever degree is plausible and reasonable – mutually respected. As with so many other areas, here too there is a narrow band of optimal function.   When interpersonal boundaries are too numerous or too extreme this leads to alienation, isolation and depletion; when they are too few or too porous the result is overwhelming and debilitating intrusion on our self-governance. Somewhere in the middle is a happy medium that allows cooperative community without annihilating individual well-being. The baseline for this component, then, is simply an awareness of this ongoing process.

> **Resources:**   One book you might consider on the topic of generating community is *Creating Community Anywhere* by Carolyn Schaefer & Kristin Anundsen. There have been and will continue to be plentiful technology-based community building resources and tools, from Facebook to Yahoo or Google discussion groups to Meetup.com or Craigslist and Twitter – though we must be careful not to supplant real community with such technology. And of course there are many of non-profit organizations that specialize in engaging people of similar values or interests in communal activities.

4 - Expanding Mind

Mind is consciousness, so the Expanding Mind nourishment dimension is really about expanding the shape, size and complexity of our consciousness. Why is this important? Because consciousness is the single most significant contributor to our well-being and the well-being of everything with which we interact. For whatever reason, the Universe has conspired in favor of our consciousness. It is therefore our privilege – and perhaps even our duty – to train our consciousness to return the blessing; our consciousness should conspire in favor of the Universe. This is something at which our mind is naturally gifted, but often we constrain or confine that gift, either rigidifying its processes until our thoughts are limited to the same repetitive patterns, or interrupting self-examination with perpetual, rapid cycles of distraction. When this happens, nourishment is not occurring in the dimension of mind. So what can we do to encourage its expansion and flexibility? The following are some ways to approach this.

Mindful Openness. Mindful openness has three prerequisites: flexibility, curiosity and confidence. If we are incurious or insecure, we will tend to be close-minded and reactive in our thinking. Likewise if our thinking has calcified into fixed patterns or we have limited our understanding to information we have already learned, we will naturally resist open-mindedness. We can easily assess our level of openness by observing our reactions to new information or environments. Do we reflexively reject whatever new things we encounter, or do we allow ourselves opportunities for learning and interaction? To achieve baseline openness we must practice the relaxation of reflexive rejection and regularly allow new information to pass through the doors of our mind – that is, to enter our consciousness through our senses. The mindful aspect comes into play when we evaluate the new information; can we continue to question our past conclusions in the face of contradictory evidence, or do we reject anything that doesn't readily integrate into our current understanding? The following charts compare and contrast a mind that is actively and thoughtfully open to a mind that struggles to remain passive, avoidant and closed-off.

PASSIVE, AVOIDANT, REFLEXIVE & CLOSED

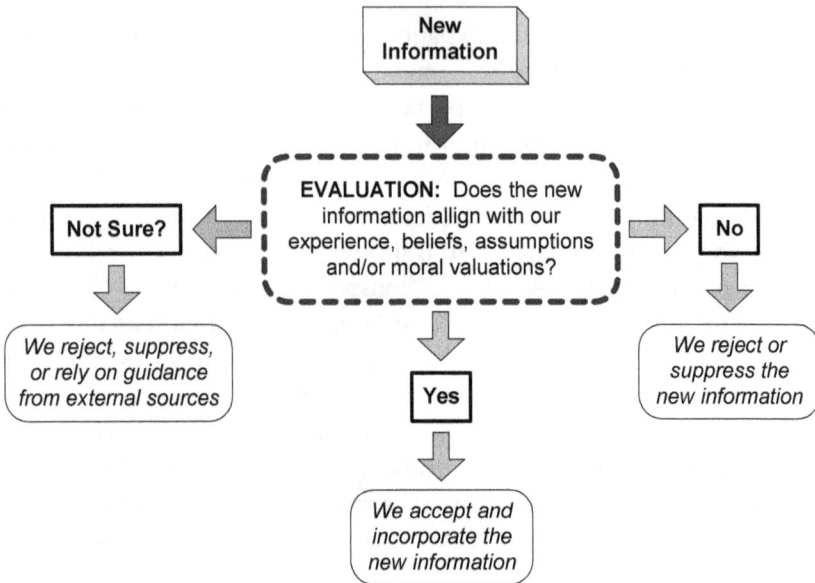

New
Information

EVALUATION: Does the new
information allign with our
experience, beliefs, assumptions
and/or moral valuations?

Not Sure?

No

We reject, suppress,
or rely on guidance
from external sources

Yes

We reject or
suppress the
new information

We accept and
incorporate the
new information

Why is mindful openness important? On the one hand, if we allowed all
new input to flood our consciousness without thoughtful consideration,
we would either be overwhelmed or carried hither and thither on each
new wave of data. On the other hand, if we deny ourselves the
opportunity to consciously evaluate new information, and instead try to
block it out, there is no telling what will trickle into our unconsciousness
and reshape our thinking without our knowing it. In other words, if we
can't find the optimal range of function within which we can appraise
new data without being overwhelmed by it, we will be influenced by
that information without realizing what has happened. No mind is truly
closed, and organic growth will occur whether we are actively engaged
or passively resistant. The difference here is that we can influence the
shape, texture and expansiveness of our own mind when we maintain
mindful openness.

ACTIVE, QUESTIONING, MINDFUL & OPEN

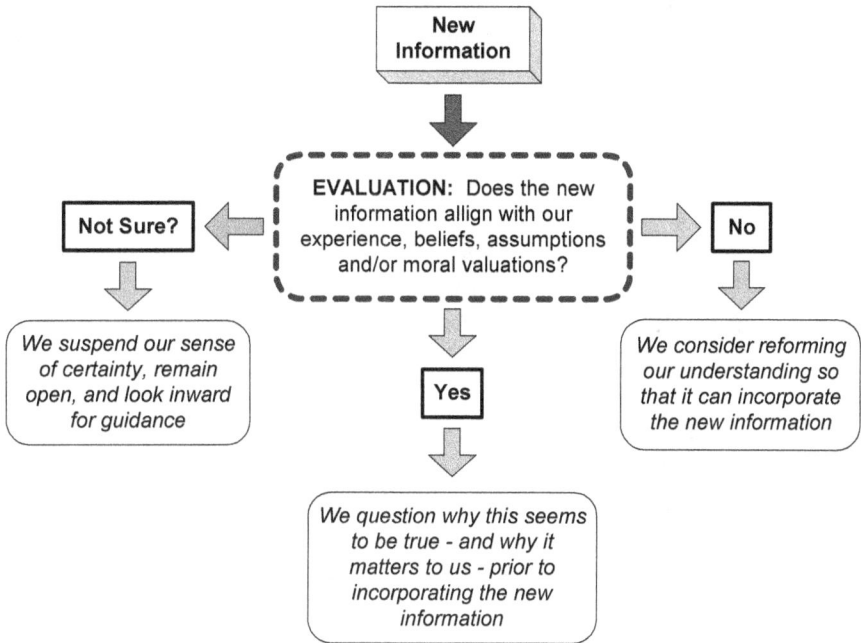

New
Information

EVALUATION: Does the new
information allign with our
experience, beliefs, assumptions
and/or moral valuations?

Not Sure?

No

We suspend our sense
of certainty, remain
open, and look inward
for guidance

Yes

We consider reforming
our understanding so
that it can incorporate
the new information

We question why this seems
to be true - and why it
matters to us - prior to
incorporating the new
information

Stimulation. Mental stimulation is anything that excites a response, that engages our mind and invites our curiosity and imagination. How will this book end? How can I solve this puzzle? How do I learn to perform this new task? What is around the next bend in the road? Mental stimulation usually occurs along with one or more of the following mental processes:

- **Concentrating.** Paying rapt attention to any one thing – such as reading a book, playing a game, constructing or creating something, meditating or praying in a focused way, and so on.

- **Problem-solving.** Solving a conundrum or puzzle, in whatever mode, method or medium we can, stimulates and strengthens our cognitive function and helps us create helpful structure for our thought process.

- **Applied learning.** Whether it be a new craft, language, skill or area of expertise, learning something new is a thrilling way to stimulate the mind. What differentiates applied learning is that we put whatever we have learned into regular practice, so that the learning loop is reinforced. For instance, when we learn how to prepare a certain meal, we will prepare that meal at regular intervals over time.

- **Teaching.** Teaching others is a powerful mind stimulator. Whenever we teach, we are challenged to think about our subject matter in new ways. And by sharing our knowledge and skills, we enrich the world around us. For the teaching to be meaningful, the learning can likewise be expressed and applied in some way that is meaningful to the student.

- **Imagining.** To daydream or fantasize about interesting possibilities may come naturally to some, but to others it can seem a distraction or waste of time. In *Integral Lifework*, it is essential to cultivate our imagination as regular component of our baseline mental stimulation. It is of course most helpful to imagine positive and constructive things – things that perhaps contribute to nourishment in other dimensions.

As with mindful openness, here too there is an optimal range and a balanced level of input. Too much stimulation and our mind becomes bruised, overwhelmed or perpetually distracted; too little and our faculties languish. The optimal range for each person varies, but, as one example, think about how long you can engage in any one mental activity. To achieve baseline stimulation, we should be able to sustain mental effort that involves one or more of the processes above for at least two hours each day, and touch on all of these processes over the course of each week. It is also important to consider which habits and activities interrupt or interfere with these processes. For example: TV, alcohol, poor nutrition, depression and stress are all well-known antagonists of healthy brain function.

Resources: There is some promising research being done on neuroplasticity that has already resulted in several scientifically validated enhancement techniques, including software programs that improve overall brain function. The key to these techniques seems to be making such exercise fun and game-like. For more information on this topic, research neuroplasticity and "brain fitness" on the web, and be sure to verify any claims of outcomes by checking for independent research. It may also be worthwhile to explore the influence TV has on brain development and function, in particular its contribution to ADHD in America's young people.

Structure. Structure in this case refers to regularity of energy exchange in all dimensions. Without becoming inflexible about them, we need routines and rhythms that help us ensure that regular essential nourishment is occurring. Our mind is the initial purveyor of such routines, recognizing and facilitating their critical place in our lives. Certainly we must attune our senses to the promptings of each dimension if and when they become undernourished, but our mental discipline is what governs the overall flow and balance of self-nurturing. What this means is that we create a system of reminders that keep us on track. Different systems work well for different people. I use a daytimer to plan out many of my nourishment routines, augmented with post-it notes, and reminder items left in conspicuous places (sneakers placed in front of the front door, a book I intend to read placed on top of my computer keyboard, a healthy snack on an end table, and so on). Knowing that my mind has perhaps the largest impact of all on every aspect of my well-being, I train my mind to support holistic nourishment. This is of course no less true for the expansion of mind itself, and learning to pattern my day around healthy, self-sustaining activities also helps pattern my mental processes around this same goal.

| **Resources:** | I'm a fan of Stephen Covey's work when it comes to structure. Many of his principles have helped me organize nourishment in my life. Things like the Covey's urgency vs. importance quadrants, scheduling priorities rather than prioritizing my schedule, and many other tools and principles found in his literature have been immeasurably beneficial to my integral practice. As one starting point, you might consider his book, *The Seven Habits of Highly Effective People.*

Crosspollination. All of us have areas of intellectual interest that we find particularly rewarding, but if our tendency is to focus on those areas of passion or affinity exclusively, we may end up depriving ourselves of a much richer tapestry of interrelated and mutually invigorating information.   Although Western educational institutions often pride themselves on diverse curricula, touting the benefits of broad liberal arts education, the reality is that U.S. culture encourages and rewards specialized and narrowly confined expertise above more generalized knowledge or diversified skills. There are exceptions, but for the most part success in any given field is predicated on our level of specialization in that field. Increasingly, I believe this tendency is being recognized as a weakening rather that strengthening influence for both individual competency and societal welfare. The more isolated ideas, practices and specialized fields are from each other, the less potential for complimentary or revolutionary synergy exists.   To enable more synthesis and less fragmentation and isolation, we must regularly expose ourselves to new ideas in areas where we might have little to no initial interest – we must cultivate new connections and relationships between what first appear to be disparate or unrelated bodies of information. This applies to our own cognitive processes as well as our vocation and society as a whole.

How can this be achieved in a practical sense? By picking up a magazine on a topic we know nothing about and flipping through its pages. By clicking links on a news website that explore areas with which we are unfamiliar – or to which we might even harbor mild aversion.   To dialogue regularly with people who hold views that differ from our own, or whose experiences and interests offer perspectives we have never encountered. To attend lectures, read books or watch media that we know may challenge our views or expose us to new ways of being and doing. To allow our curiosity to lead us into places we have never been. And how often should we do this? At a minimum, at least once a day; the amount of time we spend expanding our mind in this way is less important that the initial impulse to do so and the moderate amount of effort required to follow through.

Stability.   There are many forms of instability that can affect nourishment of mind. Certainly imbalances in other dimensions of nourishment can lead to breakdown in healthy cognitive function. For example, emotional stress can disrupt our ability to concentrate or remember. Excessive physiological stressors can likewise impede our ability to think clearly – a paucity or excess in nutrition, physical activity and so on. In fact I believe that many psychological disorders are the result of imbalanced nourishment in other areas of our being. Of course, there may also be fundamental structural barriers to mental well-being over which we have less conscious control. But what we are aiming for here is the strength, reliability and trustworthiness of our mental processes. Once we achieve stability, we have the confidence to move forward in healthy and supportive ways. If those processes become destabilized for any reason, our ability to successfully self-nourish in this and other dimensions will be greatly curtailed.

Another way to describe stability is consistency. Am I able to consistently stimulate, expand and strengthen my mind? If so, this indicates an appropriate level of stability. If not, what is impeding that nourishment? Am I too anxious? Impulsive? Obsessive? Lazy? All such impedances point to deeper imbalances or barriers to nourishment, and we will address those in upcoming chapters. But in many cases, all that is occurring is that we are undervaluing the importance of self-care, and our own indifference undermines the stability we require to thrive. And the remedy for such indifference, as you might anticipate, is love.

Psychic Boundaries. Our psychic self is the realm of contiguous mental energy within which we operate most comfortably. That comfort level determines the efficiency and strength of our mental energy, and is in largest part defined by our level of moral development. As we will explore in the Arenas of Affection, Arenas of Action section, successive moral development defines an ever-expanding self-concept, so that distinctions between "self" and "other" become fewer and fewer. However, until those boundaries are redefined through a natural maturation process, we must be careful not to extend our mental energies or the stirrings of our will beyond our current capacities. And that is what psychic boundaries are: the recognized limitations of a distinct sense of self. Once we relax into a level of self-awareness that clearly identifies such boundaries, it is our responsibility to operate within them.

This may seem abstract, but it has very concrete applications. Consider Reinhold Niebuhr's prayer: "God grant me the serenity to accept the things I cannot change; courage to change the things I can; and wisdom to know the difference." Or Epictetus's warning: "Whatever you prize which is beyond your will, you have inasmuch destroyed your will." Our objective in creating and maintaining psychic boundaries is simply to recognize our own limitations and where our efforts are best applied. At the end of each day, I can look back over my thoughts and actions and quickly identify where I have overstepped my bounds. That is, where I worried about something beyond my control, where I became disheartened by consequences that could not be anticipated, or where I became frustrated because I strove to obstruct or alter a current much larger than myself.

And of course psychic boundaries work both ways. They are not just boundaries for my thought-energy or will, but also deliberate walls that corral and filter the forces all around me. If I am conscientious and directed within my realm of influence and identity, focused and secure within my chosen purpose, then the chaotic energies assaulting the walls of my domain will find no foothold or refuge there. No matter how permeable or vulnerable I may feel, the push and pull of someone else's desires or the random disruptions of my environment will not alter my course, diffuse my intentions or change my core practices. Why? Because in fully understanding and embracing who I am, what my life is about, where I am going and how I intend to get there, I have created a safe and secure bubble of identity that extends just as far as my moral development allows, and no one and nothing may enter that does not conform the principles and nature of that inner landscape. And if that purpose and its facilitation are grounded in true love, then all must pass through the door of love to enter or exit the influences of my being.

So to cultivate baseline psychic boundaries is really to recognize our own limitations, and then to live within those limitations. If we do this, our energy will concentrate itself and our efforts will become more effective. If we don't do this, our energy will dissipate and our efforts will become ineffective.

5 - Fulfilling Purpose

It is so easy to have our purpose dictated to us. By parents who want the best for us and project their hopes and dreams onto our lives. By lovers or partners who feel we should support their personal purpose and vision. By friends who depend on us to join them on their own adventurous journey. By employers who feel we should invest our time and energy in their mission statement. By educators who see our potential in their field and want to encourage it. By believers of various faiths who gladly enjoin us to adopt their worldview. By salespeople who have a vision to share that involves just a small investment of our time, energy and finances. By societal institutions with decades of momentum to pull us in into their wake. This bombardment from external sources is unending. And if we hitch a ride with any one of these influences, we may at first feel inspired and on fire with a sense of direction in life. But given enough time, we will begin to question that commitment. And eventually we will discover that, in our heart of hearts, we don't feel very fulfilled or purposeful at all.

When I was in my late teens, I opened myself to the Universe and cried out with my spirit "What am I doing here? What is my purpose? Please show me the way!" For the next few months I was overwhelmed with opportunities I had never encountered before. I was invited to an Amway rally by a friend, learning that one choice was to get rich through multi-level marketing. The next day I met a Scientologist who invited me to take an "e-meter" test to clear myself of negative energy; so I did that and discovered L.Ron Hubbard had an intricate methodology to address my every concern about purposefulness in this life. Then a young woman invited me to a presentation by her mentor, an evangelist of Reverend Sun Myung Moon, who had another set of answers for me – and a very persuasive pitch that involved being locked in a small room for several hours. And the opportunities just kept materializing. Once-in-a-lifetime investment schemes. Immersion in a presidential election campaign and the broader political process. A few choicely subversive political demonstrations. Volunteering with various organizations to help the poor, to save the environment, or to fight discrimination. By the time the holidays arrived to distract me from my quest, I was exhausted and more confused than I had been before I started searching. So I took a break from it all, and in the simple quietude of a still, thoughtful moment, I suddenly realized I was looking in the wrong place. The answer was not outside myself, but within myself. I just had to listen carefully to the subtle promptings within me, and filter out all the imperatives and sales pitches I had invited to worm their way into my being from the outside.

Listening to our innermost intuition is not, however, a path we are often encouraged to take. There are societal and cultural expectations, the expectations of our family and friends, and the expectations that spring from core beliefs about ourselves and the world in which we live. In my case these were to go to college, get married, buy a house, have one or two kids and raise them up to repeat this process. To facilitate this lifestyle I was to acquire the reliable income of any career that had a higher-than-average social respectability and pay, and which I could perform moderately well. And I did attempt this path...but it just didn't mesh with the essence of who I am. From years of managing dozens of employees in different business environments, counseling innumerable clients, and researching some relevant statistics, I would also propose that trying to meet such externally imposed expectations usually results in pervasive feelings of failure, disappointment, entrapment and mind-numbing futility for all but a very lucky few.

So if the answer to question "What am I doing here?" can only be found within ourselves, how do we access that? How can we escape from the enculturation that distracts us from those interior resources? How can we evade the seemingly random conditions and events that lead us into a life our heart doesn't want and our soul doesn't need?

Vision. Our first step is to introduce some vision into our lives. I will suggest a means of accomplishing this here, but in many ways this is an ideal exercise for a solitary physical and spiritual retreat, away from our normal environment and relationships. Also, this is an iterative process; we may attempt to actualize one vision only to encounter new life experiences and interior resources that reshape our life direction many times over. But there must always be a conscious beginning, so the following are some steps that will encourage those creative juices to percolate. These could be part of a therapeutic dialogue, a natural extension of the mystic activation exercise, the focus of a personal weekend retreat, or part of any number of other methods. For now, however, don't be concerned about how you will accomplish each step, just digest these ideas as the instigation of a larger process that you can embrace when you are ready to do so.

Exercise: Dowsing for Light

1. **Create an inviting space.** Sit somewhere quiet where you won't be disturbed, close your eyes, take ten deep, slow breaths, and relax. Wipe your inner slate clean of "must haves" and "have tos" and "can't dos." Let go of self-limiting assumptions and any negative self-talk, and create an empty stage of imagination that can entertain ridiculous and delightful possibilities. As a matter of setting your intention, just say "no" to "no."

2. **Crank open your intuitive spigot, then let it flow.** With eyes closed and attention directed inward, ask "What is my purpose?" Hold out the bowl of your consciousness to catch the stream of insights, sensations, images and ideas that arise. Let that flow accumulate in your mind without diverting it or turning off the source. Keep asking the question. Try not to edit or grasp onto what comes up, and don't worry about writing it down or remembering what you encounter. Just keep going, keep asking and searching and letting the flow continue.

3. **Watch for your reflection.** Somewhere in that upwelling of ideas is a true reflection of who you are and what your life is about in this moment. You will recognize this event when you experience it. You will feel its certainty and rightness. You will sense its brightness and intensity. You will want to linger there to absorb its warmth. And you will feel both content and inspired because it happened by. Breathe deeply and evenly.

4. **Repeat this exercise once or twice a month for at least twenty minutes.** As you develop greater concentration, you might want to cast the net inward for an hour or more. As you go deeper, you can begin to refine your vision with additional questions. "How will I express or accomplish this?" "What resources will augment my efforts?" "What specific outcomes should I plan for

in the upcoming weeks?" Really, you can ask anything you want about how to fulfill your purpose. They key is to keep asking, remaining open, and letting whatever arises from within stream lightly across your mind and heart.

This visioning process will flow naturally from our inward attentiveness and any practices that tap into our innermost intuitive compass. If we aren't accustomed to sustained interior awareness, it may at first be difficult to let go and let things flow. To strengthen those intuitive muscles, you might consider practicing a mystic activator for a few weeks prior to attempting this exercise. The type of perception-cognition induced by mystic activation is close kin to intuition, and is excellent preparation.

Over time, it will eventually become important for you to discover any shared ground of common purpose with the rest of humanity. Can you imagine what might be a universal vision for all people everywhere? What do you suppose binds us together in a communal effort and unified objective? What profound accomplishment is available to all people, and might even justify and empower our existence all by itself? What governs the outcome of all vision and purpose, weaving itself into every meaningful action? This can be answered intellectually, but as you pay close attention to your heart of hearts, the answer will blaze forth as a clear conviction and imperative, an umbrella of shared purpose under which we subordinate and align our own individual vision.

Will. A life vision without an investment of will behind it is like a pleasant dream – we may be enthralled and enticed by it for a little while after waking from sleep, but we quickly forget its substance and return to the habits of our day. What is will, exactly? In *Integral Lifework*, will is the combined power of the body, mind, heart and spirit to translate *volitional impulses* from those quarters of our being into meaningful and supportive action. In this context, will is not desire, nor is it action or the final fulfillment of our wants, but the mechanism that instigates action and fulfillment whereby all whims and wishes can be manifested in our lives. The volitional impulses within us may be conscious or unconscious, formless or fully formed, always seeking the energy and substance of actuation. But for our will to effectively channel these impulses into existence, they must issue from the core of our identity, beliefs and values. They can never be externally or superficially generated. This is why the vision we generate for our lives must also issue from an authentic center. And once the power of our will is engaged, other forces converge to amplify and harmonize with the objects of our will. So we should take great care with this process, for when begun it is difficult to quickly change course.

Imagine that every time you burst into song, the melody and meaning of that song is absorbed by countless agents all around you who then rushed off together to turn your impulsive creation into a beautiful symphony – with chords, harmonies, variations and so on. Our will is like that song, broadcasting our intentions and desires to the Universe. So you can see that having a baseline will to actuate our purpose and vision is very important; if the voice of our will is weak, diluted or off-key, it will either not be heard or its melody and meaning will be misinterpreted. How do we achieve a useful baseline? By learning to develop a neutral and quiescent state of being that allows our will to remain neutral and fully energized until it is consciously applied. We will call this baseline *willingness*, or a *neutrality of will*. And we can achieve this state by perfecting the following four disciplines:

1) **Quiescent vitality of body.** Releasing all tension and stress, relaxing and strengthening all physiological systems through moderate exercise, increasing overall flexibility and energy, and healing illness and injury.

2) **Quiescent vitality of mind.** Reducing the seemingly arbitrary cacophony of thoughts rattling around inside our head to a state of readiness, openness and stillness; while at the same time healing any self-defeating or antagonistic ideations.

3) **Quiescent vitality of heart.** Relaxing our acquisitiveness, anxiety, anger, desire to control outcomes, and any other compulsive or insistent emotional activity; while at the same time healing guilt, shame, grief or other emotional burdens.

4) **Quiescent vitality of spirit.** Achieving a state of intuitive readiness and spiritual receptivity, activating spiritual perception-cognition

without judging or interpreting the phenomena we encounter; while concurrently working through any residual negative karma.

When we achieve a modicum of aquiessence and vigor in all these areas simultaneously, our will can concurrently approach a point of energized stillness, gathering strength as it readies itself for a more directed and conscious application. With proper intention, attention and diligence, we can achieve all of this over time through daily integral practice – most notably through various forms of mystic activation.

Metrics. At one extreme, we could find ourselves sailing through life, confident we are fulfilling our purpose without any means of measuring if we are doing so. At the other extreme, we might have grave doubts about our effectiveness and be equally in the dark. So how can we be certain? How can we measure the fulfillment of our own purpose? One approach is to create intermediary goals and reasonable timelines to fulfill them, with clear checklists for dependencies and the order of our efforts. Another is to surround ourselves with honest, straight-shooting folk and allow them to hold us accountable to our aspirations. Yet another is to enter into formal relationships with professionals who role is to help us complete our objectives. We can do all of these things, but none is as important as checking in with our own internal compass. Is this decision I am making right now in alignment with my life's purpose? Only in my heart of hearts will I find the answer. So regularly checking in with the authentic, innermost center of my being is the most reliable way to measure my overall progress. As long as that interior connectivity remains open and strong, I will know if I am remaining on-track and have the clarity to make supportive decisions. The following are some methods for doing this.

| Exercise: Checking In On Purpose |

- Before you go to bed at night, right down a couple of questions about how you are gong about your day, framing them within your sense of purpose. For instance: "Is this career path I am taking really helping me fulfill my purpose, or is it interfering with it?" or "Is the romantic relationship I am in supporting the purpose of my life, or distracting me from it?" or "Does the recreation I am engaging in today align with the vision I have for my life, or not?" or "Are today's activities an expression of who I authentically am?" And so on...whatever is relevant for you in the moment. Then, when you wake in the morning, ask yourself those questions first thing, before you have started your day or even fully awoken, and note the feelings and convictions that surface in response.

• When you are about to engage in some activity or other, take a moment beforehand to look in a mirror and ask yourself about the purposefulness of that activity. Then answer these same question aloud with a simple "Yes" or "No." Be sure to look yourself in the eye when you ask and answer, and note any physical responses that might contradict what you say (eyes shifting to one side, hands clenching, shoulders tensing, etc.) and the emotions you feel within.

• Enter into the stillness of non-judgmental introspection techniques found in the many exercises among these pages, then offer the same sorts of questions to that space, waiting patiently and openly for responsive emotions, sensations, images or intuitions to arise.

On particularly challenging days, we may need to do this type of internal check-in several times. At other times, perhaps only once or twice a week. Sometimes the momentum of our decisions will seem to carry us far, far down the road toward our goals without us feeling the need to measure our progress. Yet we must still regularly confirm that our compass is true and our footing is sound, lest we lose ourselves in the fervor of our aspirations.

Inspiration & Renewal. Finding inspiration to energize our vision is also our responsibility and privilege, as is remembering to regularly remind ourselves of the core beliefs and values that propel us toward our goals. We can think of inspiration and renewal as food for our will, the sustenance that angles us forward and lifts our feet; it is closely bound to other dimensions of nourishment. For instance, inspiration and opportunity for renewal are dependent on:

- The values-affinity relationships we make in our community.

- The acuity of our emotional awareness.

- The breadth of our mental stimulation and crosspollination.

- The regularity of our spiritual grounding and connection.

As with every other dimension of nourishment, Fulfilling Purpose is intimately interconnected with all other dimensions. The greater our commitment to fortifying each nourishment center, the more these efforts combine to interdependently replenish all dimensions at once. If I neglect any areas of self-care, I will inadvertently undermine my capacities and abilities in other areas. This is why our integral practice must become an all-inclusive way of being; a gem with many facets that is formed by a single, unifying substance; a flying carpet that we experience as a unified whole rather than an assemblage of distinct strands of thought, feeling or action. So inspiration and renewal are really inseparable from all other aspects of nourishment – what renews and inspires us is what sustains us in every respect, and by consciously surveying our nourishment routines we can selectively mine them for the food our will requires. Today this will mean reading a book or taking a class, tomorrow meeting with a close friend or affinity group, and next week a few hours of deep meditation to reconnect with the essence of our being. In these regular events, as guided by our compassion and a commitment to our governing intentions, we generate all the energy we need to fulfill our purpose.

What happens when we don't have a life purpose? Does it really influence our nourishment? This is a fascinating area of focus for me. What I have observed is that when people lack purpose, they create crises and other exciting distractions for themselves that ultimately sabotage energy exchanges in many other areas as well. They also tend to allow other, external influences to take over their motivation and well-being. What is going on here? I think it is a simple case of substitution. We want to be energized by purpose, we want the excitement of the challenging, unpredictable journey a life of purpose provides, while at the same time being comforted by the continuity of that purpose. In other words, if we don't actively generate a vision for our efforts, we will create substitute dialectic tensions that a life of purpose would otherwise provide.

6 - Authentic Spirit

In *Integral Lifework*, our connection to the ground of being is considered a constant spiritual reality – we can never be separated from it because our essence is part of Universal Essence, our individuated soul is part of Collective Soul, the joyous spark of our being is but a fragment of the Divine Whole. Any presumption of separateness is therefore a useful but artificial construct. We maintain our separateness to accomplish growth – to explore consciousness, to create interpersonal edification and synergies, and to develop the societal structures necessary to support complex systems of cooperative effort, to further encourage the evolution of our soul and the Universe itself. But because the connection with the ground of being is often only peripherally perceived, fleetingly experienced, uncomfortable to accept and difficult to assimilate, the recognition of that connection often remains latent and disempowered in the depths of our awareness. By bubbling this intimate sense of interdependence and belonging up to the surface of our perceptions in a conscious way, we can begin to harmonize our thoughts, feelings and actions with an underlying reality. In other words, we can conform our consciousness to the felt experience of spiritually being, and infuse all our choices with the content of that experience and consciousness. In this way, over time, we begin to live authentically in concordance with our spiritual center – we begin to live in harmony with our soul.

However, belief in this presupposition is not necessary to nourish ourselves spiritually, it just creates a convenient backdrop against which we can rationalize certain practices that, in truth, may initially seem confusing, disorienting and perhaps even pointless otherwise. Spiritual practice in some form has persisted around the globe these past millennia for a reason. Some might argue that spirituality has been perpetuated as an opiate to dull natural curiosity, advance sociopolitical agendas and perpetuate religious authority. Clearly there have been

historic abuses along these lines, though in response I tend to
differentiate spirituality from religiosity – the former being defined by
our relationship with the ground of being, and the latter being defined
by adherence to religious dogma or conformance to the culture of a
particular faith-based tribe.   But whatever our prejudices and
experiences, there remains within us a spiritual dimension that longs to
be fed. In order to receive such nourishment, we must at least try to
open our hearts and minds to its enduring and ineffable Light. And with
appropriate intention, attention and follow-through, we do not require a
specific flavor of religion to receive spiritual food.   Again, having a
religious framework may provide a helpful context for the unfamiliar
experiences that spiritual disciplines generate, and this should not be
discounted. But, as a foundation for holistic growth, what we do require
is a more general sense of faith that spiritual nourishment processes are
important for our well-being, and cannot be substituted with
nourishment from other dimensions.

Connection. How can we consciously connect with the ground of being?
How can we bubble this innate spiritual condition up to the surface of
our awareness? There are many avenues, but nearly all of them involve
either spontaneous spiritual intuition or deliberate mystic activation.
Most of us have experienced seemingly random events during our lives
when we have been struck with a sense of oneness. In childhood we
may have felt intense moments of oneness with a parent or a sibling.
Perhaps we were struck with a peak experience of oneness out in Nature,
during periods of intense concentration, or in the midst lovemaking.
Maybe there have been times in our life when one event after another
has woven together with every other in surprising synchronicity. All of
these are echoes of the connection with all-being. They are hints at an
underlying sameness of our essence and the essence of everything else.
However, in order to achieve baseline nourishment here, we cannot rely
on such arbitrary occurrences. Instead, we can treat this dimension as
we would any other nourishment center and design a structured means
of self-care. And that is what mystic activation provides; for most,
beginning with even five or ten minutes of mystic activation practice
each day will produce significant benefits.

Grounding. In *Integral Lifework*, grounding means translating the ineffable into the practical as quickly and effectively as possible. Each spiritual epiphany is therefore manifested as an immediate personal choice of supportive action, and each new level of awareness is applied to the mundane daily tasks that comprise our existence. There is no better example of this than the quality of our interpersonal relationships. If I have plumbed the depths of mystical union but cannot demonstrate compassionate affection for my loved ones, then my spirituality is not adequately grounded; there is a disconnection between my spiritual practice and my daily life. Likewise, if I cannot be patient, attentive, understanding and engaged with others, really caring about their condition and experiences, then whatever heights of spiritual awareness I have achieved are quite literally inconsequential. The energy of spiritual nourishment naturally supports and expands love, so unless my spiritual practice results in loving intentions and actions, that energy is effectively wasted – dissipating into unfocused background radiation. In the most practical sense, every spiritually-centered activity must have consequences in how we live our lives from moment to moment, from person to person, from self to other.

Of course, if we fixate on translating our spiritual experiences into meaningful action, we will probably overextend or deplete ourselves rather quickly. Once again we must find the narrow band of optimal function between inactivity and overcommitment. Midway between these extremes is a calm overflowing of recognition and appreciation of spiritual connection into an effortless, unselfconscious expression in action. We're no longer trying, we're just being. So part of baseline grounding is letting go of urgency and compulsiveness while still engaging the world around us with new spiritual information. I encourage people to manage this balancing act by linking spiritual nourishment practices with specific decisions or preparation for action. For example, that practitioners of the healing arts sanctify themselves and their practice space through mystic activation prior to each session. For artists to do the same before the act of creation; for teachers before they lecture; for managers before a work meeting; for lovers before making love; for builders before construction; for mechanics before they repair a vehicle. To include spiritual practice in and around our daily activities integrates our spiritual self with the rest of our life. In other words, we consecrate all action with spirit.

Once this process becomes comfortable and habitual, there is one more obstacle to overcome. Such well-intentioned habits can sometimes lose their potency and meaning through empty ritualization over time. We can begin to take for granted the repetitive inclusion of spiritualized intentionality, and the same disconnection we experienced without any spiritual practice at all can reassert itself. So we learn to integrate without minimizing meaning, we celebrate inclusion of our spiritual being with gratitude and love, honoring connection with the ground of being without becoming preoccupied with – or desensitized to – the form and pattern of that honoring. And as with all other processes of maturation, love will help us find ways to walk the tightrope of authentically being and continually becoming whatever spiritual truths we encounter deep within.

Generosity. Generosity accomplishes many things. For one, it loosens the manacles of avarice and acquisitiveness around our heart. For another, it exercises compassion for our fellow beings. Generosity also allows us to enter the flow of positive, supportive work that is greater than ourselves; it expands our arenas of affection and enhances the progression of our moral development. Yet giving skillfully is not as straightforward as it may initially seem – it requires discernment, patience and attentiveness. Simply dropping some money in a hat on the street may balm our conscience a bit, but what if they money we give is being used to support a drug or alcohol habit? What if we are destroying someone's ability to heal, grow or thrive through our giving?

Years ago I spent many hours each week reaching out to the homeless in Seattle. Because so many were alcoholics, I decided not to give money but instead offer to buy them food. I had no idea what I was in for. The disappointment, dismissal, condescension and even rage when I offered to buy them a sandwich was shocking. They needed some booze, they would say, and not giving them what they asked for was, in their view, disrespectful and controlling. On two occasions I was even physically threatened because I wouldn't provide alcohol instead of a meal. There were some takers for my informed generosity, of course, and there was even gratitude, but here too my expectations were foiled. One example in particular comes to mind. A man was seated on the sidewalk, looking old and tired. He asked for money and I told him I would rather buy him a sandwich. At first seemed indifferent to my offer and looked away, but when he saw that I wasn't rushing off, that I might even be genuinely concerned, he engaged me. He told me a little about himself and how he had ended up on the street, how he had struggled with alcohol and drugs and just couldn't beat them. I sat by his side and listened. After a while, I offered to get him his sandwich. "No," he began, and I braced myself for a negative onslaught, but he continued, "You listened to what I had to say. That's enough." In that moment I think I learned what true giving was.

How can we be truly generous, then? It begins and ends in authentic compassion, and our skillfulness depends on thoughtful effort. Letting someone else decide what beneficial giving is can be a counterproductive and sometimes dangerous road. So we must inform ourselves, experiment a little, and decide what is best, but ultimately we must engage those in need on a personal, empathic level. Our time, our openness, our mental energy, our compassion, our sincere effort – these are priceless contributions. To look someone in the eye and give of ourselves in the time of their need is to say "I love you." So volunteerism is an excellent route, especially when we can interact directly with those receiving services. Even then, however, we should first research the charitable organization to learn about its mission, its effectiveness and its administrative overhead. It is incumbent upon us to give wisely, however we choose to give.

For a baseline, consider giving ten percent of your free time to a cause which benefits something you value and for which you will gain no prestige, recognition or even thanks. In other words, give freely, give personally, and share yourself in a way that does not expect anything in return. As with all integral practice, where at first we may encounter resistance in ourselves, this avenue of nourishment will eventually become second nature.

7 - Restorative History

To live fully in the present we must acknowledge our past. Each of us has a story, an intricate map of successes and disappointments, adventures and crises, joys and sorrows that stretches back into our earliest childhood. And all of these events, perceptions and experiences have contributed to a complex amalgam of core material that influenced our development and continues to shape how we process information and relate to our environment from moment to moment. So self-nourishment has to include the formative flow of our Restorative History. Sometimes this will mean reprocessing past experiences with new tools, sometimes releasing imperfect perceptions or embracing new conclusions about what happened long ago, and sometimes acknowledging the influence certain relationships or moments in our history will inevitably have on our well-being. Like any other, this nourishment center can be either neglected or overemphasized, so our goal is to find the fulcrum's plane of processing the past with just the right attitude and investment to help us be healed and whole in the present.

Since all nourishment channels within Restorative History rely on memory, how can we access that memory? Often we can recall relevant core material without any assistance or special techniques. In other cases, we may need some help. In my *Integral Lifework* practice, the Restorative History dimension has been explored with any number of tools, including guided imagery, verbal probes, somatic memory accessing techniques, hypnotherapy, or other forms of therapeutic interaction. Sometimes a homework assignment of memoir style journaling can rekindle associations that were deeply buried, and it is in that spirit that the following baseline practices are offered for each channel of this dimension. Whatever the approach, the objective is not to force anything to the surface, but to create a safe environment for past perceptions and experiences to bubble up on their own when we are ready.

Accomplishment. Take a moment to think about accomplishments you were most proud of when they occurred, going back into your past as far as you can. That is, a focus not necessarily on the accomplishments you are proud of now, but on those that made a big impression at the time. For me, this might include things like riding a bike for the first time without training wheels when I was four, learning to read when I was seven, escaping the wrath of a neighborhood bully when I was eight, performing my first solo musical gig when I was thirteen...and so on.

No matter how insignificant those early accomplishments may seem to our adult mind, when we experienced them they were huge. They were critical in how we came to view ourselves and the possibilities for our future, and in many ways they still do, at least symbolically. One suggestion for this channel is to write down as many accomplishments as you can remember...no matter how silly or fleeting the accomplishment appears from your current vantage point. Later, after they have been captured on paper, we can then regularly revisit our accomplishments, remember them, laugh over them and in whatever way possible enjoy them anew.

Moving forward, we can begin recording our accomplishments on a weekly basis. Again, this doesn't mean capturing what would impress the general public or even what we would consider a significant milestone years down the line, but rather the lesser victories that reassure us of our ability to realize desires and goals. For example, the exercise routine we managed to complete each day this week; spending time with a friend we have been meaning to visit; getting all of our bills paid on time; and so on. Once we begin to track our accomplishments from our earliest memories into the present, we confirm our ability to accomplish what we set out to do as part of our identity – as proof of our integrity.

Grief. The amount of grief many of us carry around inside us is astounding. Grief over losses both great and small can accumulate over time until it becomes an enormous burden, a physically felt weight that crushes our spirit. Feelings of grief are of course a natural response to life events, but sometimes the grieving process is interrupted, suppressed or prolonged in ways prevent us from healing from our loss – ways that arrest the lessons and growth that losing something dear to us can offer. So this nourishment channel is about identifying what grief over past events still resides within, and encouraging that grief to resolve itself in organic, supportive and healing ways.

As with our accomplishments, a good starting point for this process is to capture the events in our past that evoked a sense of grief for us at the time each event occurred. Some common examples are listed here to help you identify those occurrences in your own past. These are among the grief-inducing events that stuck with my clients as potent and influential moments from a lifetime of memories:

- Loss of a favorite toy in childhood.

- Death of a beloved pet in childhood.

- Parental anger or disappointment.

- Absence of a parent in childhood (as a result of job travel, divorce, substance abuse issues, illness, etc.).

- Loss of a beloved home environment in childhood (as a result of moving, natural disaster, divorce, etc.).

- Absence of love in childhood home environment (as evidenced by conflict, tension, disinterest in a child's well-being, lack of affection, etc.)

- Lack of acceptance or tolerance (among our peers, our family or society at large).

- Loss of a close relative (as a result of moving away, a familial spat, a death, etc.).

- Loss of a close friend (as a result of moving away, parental restrictions, a falling out, a death, etc.).

- Betrayal of trust by a close friend or relative.

- Failure and alienation in an important relationship in adulthood (romance, partner, close friend, family member, key workplace relationship, etc.).

- Patterns of disappointment (feeling as though no one ever seems to care, that expectations are seldom met, that failure occurs more often than success, that goals are never reached, etc.).

- Personal illness, loss of function or dysfunction (this could be physical, mental, emotional, social, etc.).

- Change (the passage of time, changes to places we have lived, our own natural aging process, people moving away, etc.).

- Inability to self-nourish in some dimension (for instance, feeling a lack of purpose, being physically unhealthy, an inability to create a legacy, etc.).

All of us have experienced pain and loss in one or more of these areas. Some people have experienced pain and loss in all of them. And yet the resulting grief is expressed uniquely for every person – there isn't a set sequence for the grieving process. Nearly always, however, our grief has a felt component. In the early phases of grief, it might be anger, or resentment, or sadness, or anxiety, or fear, or an overwhelming emptiness – and the more intense the grief, the more intense the emotion. So take a moment to catalogue some of the events in your own life that have caused grief, and pay special attention to all the emotions that associate with that memory. Are there any memories of loss that bring up especially strong emotions for you? If so, write those emotions down along with the memory. Spend some extra time just allowing those feelings to surge through you, and be patient with yourself, providing uninterrupted time and space to practice these recollections and emotional associations.

This is the beginning of processing old grief, and if we revisit this exercise regularly (perhaps three or four times each year), it will provide a sufficient baseline for us to track our progress. At some point, the emotions associated with even the most painful loss will begin to shift towards a softer, less intense sadness, a more relaxed and accepting peace of mind, and ultimately an acquiescent sense of love and gratitude. Keep in mind that for certain traumas – especially the loss of a parent, sibling or child, or either repeated or extreme abuse when we were young – our grief may resist processing altogether and our emotions may shut down completely. So these may require some therapeutic assistance to work through, and, when we are ready to do so, we must make that attempt. All grief requires our loving attention, and the natural resolution of grief into peaceful acceptance and, ultimately, gratitude is a necessary outcome for our self-nourishment to be complete. We will explore this idea further in Part IV, Understanding & Managing Barriers to Wholeness.

Parental Relationships. How we were parented as a child has a special place in our personal history. Why? Because our parents modeled many things for us. Their own beliefs about the world. How to treat other people. Patterns of self-care. We first learned how to love ourselves from our parents – however they cared for us when we were young becomes our default pattern for self-care as adults. In fact, our own identity and self-worth is intimately wrapped up in how we perceive our parents, and the quality of our current relationship with them will reflect the quality of relationship we have with different parts of ourselves. If we are angry at a parent for things they did in the past, then we are angry at part of ourselves that we unconsciously identify with them. If we are ashamed of them, we are ashamed of a part of ourselves. If we resent them, we resent a part of ourselves. And so on. Our family of origin – the people who had the greatest influence on our childhood development – has an enormous impact on our self-concept and our mental and emotional cycles. In the distinct sense of self-nourishment, *they are us.*

It follows, then, that to become fully healed and whole, we must attempt to create a relationship with our parents that is healed and whole, and to honor the contributions they have made to our lives. For someone who has become completely alienated from their family of origin, this may be a daunting prospect. And for those whose interactions with their family of origin often generate pain and antagonism for them, this might seem unhealthy or entirely counterproductive. There is also the possibility that we believe the relationship we have with those who parented us is just fine, when in fact it may be codependent or dysfunctional in some way. So these can be particularly difficult waters to navigate, and garnering some therapeutic assistance with the process may be helpful. However, there is a way to begin, a way to achieve a useful baseline in establishing healthy rapport in our Parental Relationships.

First, take a moment to reflect on the feelings you have for your parents or other significant players in your family of origin. Are they mostly positive? Is there some lingering resentment, frustration or sadness there? Is there anything you'd like to say to them, but which you have so far been unsuccessful in sharing? Regardless of your initial response to these questions, take some time out of your day to write a letter to each person who played a significant role in your early childhood. It doesn't matter if they are still alive or are a part of your life right now, just compose a letter as if you are confident they will receive it. It is also helpful that this letter be hand-written. Make sure you have privacy, solitude and adequate time to write these letters, and spread them out over a week or two if necessary – there is no need to write them all at once. As you write each letter, try to include as many "I feel" statements as possible. For instance, "I feel angry about how you treated me at grandma's that summer..." or "I feel so grateful that you made sure we had dinner together as a family every night..." and so on. Try to avoid blaming or accrediting statements ("because you said *X* I did *Y*," "you made me *Z*," "your actions did *A, B* and *C* to me," etc.) and focus on your own emotional experience of each situation instead. Once you finish each letter, set it aside for three or four days, then read it again, adding any details you feel are missing.

When you are satisfied a letter is complete, try one more thing. Stand facing an empty chair, imagining the letter's recipient is sitting in that chair. When you are ready to do so, read the letter aloud to them. Make sure they pay attention as you read. Notice what feelings and physical sensations arise, and allow those feelings to flow freely out of you. Make sure you finish reading the letter, even if it takes several tries. Perhaps you will find you have more to say than what you wrote – if so, just go with that. Share everything inside you. Sometimes this exercise can feel artificial or awkward, and other times it will stir up all kinds of emotional intensity. Nearly always, it will be beneficial and healing.

This is a great baseline practice. Beyond this is exercise are attempts at real contact with your family of origin. We can reshape our ongoing relationships with them, offering their contributions to our history as we see them. Once again these would be couched in "I feel" statements rather than accrediting or blaming statements. Such real-world dialogues are the ultimate goal for this channel of nourishment, but it may not be practical or even achievable in the short run, and may require assistance and support to work through. In fact, it may even endanger our well-being to rush into such intense contact, no matter how healing the intentions. So start with the letters and, giving these missives ample time and space, see where that process leads. Many people find it helpful to revisit their letters later on as well, or to write new ones when some of their feelings about the past have changed. By doing this, we are not dwelling on the past in obsessive or stuck ways, but allowing the importance of our past to exist in the present, acknowledging the fact that all our past experiences add up into who we are today.

What await us at the heights of this particular process are feelings of forgiveness, gratitude and love, which in turn allow us to more fully integrate and appreciate the contributions of our family of origin to the person we have become. To have respect for ourselves, we must find a way to respect those who parented us, even if they're efforts were ineffective or hurtful. To have compassion for ourselves, we must have compassion for those who raised us, however that can be achieved. To honor our whole self, we must honor the family of origin from which we incorporated so many facets of who we have become.

Other Relationships. Although family of origin relationships have a major impact on our development, other relationships over the years may have also held much importance to us, and those relationships should be honored for their contributions as well. How we go about honoring them will depend upon the nature of their contribution – it might have been supportive, antagonistic, or both. We can begin simply by making a list of people whose relationship had a major influence. For example, here are excerpts from my own list:

- My dog Puma in Eugene and Florence, OR when I was four and five.

- The elderly woman who made candied orange peel next door in Eugene, OR when I was five.

- The staff at the children's hospital in CT when I was eight.

- Ann Z., Gary W. and other faculty and staff at my elementary school in Amherst, MA when I was ten and eleven.

- My friend Dean F. and his family in Belchertown, MA between ages ten and thirteen.

- The foster family I lived with in Belchertown, MA, when I was thirteen.

- Jerry M. and many of my other teachers at FAHS in Frankfurt, Germany throughout my high school years.

- My fellow thespians in Frankfurt, Germany throughout my high school years.

- Tim K. and his family in Frankfurt, Germany throughout my high school years.

- The friends I made at the Churches of Christ in Seattle, WA in my late teens and early twenties.

- My discipleship relationship with Milo H. in Bellevue, WA between ages eighteen and twenty-one.

- My ex-wife, Shannon, during the years that we were married in Seattle, WA.

- My cat, Taya, in my early twenties in Seattle, WA.

- My fellow folk band members during my twenties in Seattle, WA.

- My therapists and doctors in my twenties and thirties in Seattle, WA.

- The stranger who on impulse gifted me his copy of *Chop Wood, Carry Water* in a Seattle café when I was thirty-two.

- My mentors and supervisors at various jobs in my twenties and thirties in Seattle, WA.

- The close friends I made in my twenties and thirties in Seattle, WA.

- The participants of my classes in San Diego, CA in my early forties.

I could go on, but you get the idea. It may at first seem odd that cats, dogs, counselors, spouses, lovers, coworkers, bosses and friends all seem to share the same space, but the point of this exercise is to acknowledge the influence these forces of Nature have had on us over the years. In my own list, some of this influence was positive and supportive, and some of it painful or antagonistic, but all of it contributed to my learning and growth in some way. Merely recognizing this fact is nearly a sufficient baseline for this channel of Restorative History. To complete the process, we can journal a bit about why each influence was important to us, how we feel about their contribution, and so on. In my case, I have written poems or songs about some of them, or recounted these influences in my classes, or compiled slide shows about these times in my life, or maintained many of these relationships, or contacted certain folks just to thank them. In some way, we must keep these connections alive in our being, so that we continually remember how we arrived in the present. Ultimately, we can arrive at gratitude and love for all the multifaceted contributions to our journey, which in turn helps us integrate the most healing and supportive aspect of these relationships into our current modes of being.

Guilt, Shame or Pain. Shame, guilt and pain are natural self-regulators of thought and action. They exist to help us navigate the expectations of our relationships, our community and society at large as those intersect with our own values. Returning for a moment to the Fulfillment Orientation component of nourishment prerequisites, healthy guilt, shame and pain are part of balanced self-reliance in the fulcrum's plane. As we drift toward the protective side of the spectrum, we may suppress and deny any guilt, pain or shame, and exhibit callousness toward the needs of others or, if we become fixated on acting with disregard to all external expectations, we may even exhibit narcissistic or sociopathic tendencies. If we drift toward a dependent fulfillment orientation, we can develop a reflexive guilt, pain or shame response to any situation where we believe we have failed to maintain dependence or codependence. In other words, healthy levels of pain, shame and guilt resolve into healing and supportive action for ourselves and others, and unhealthy levels pain, guilt and shame undermine well-being by reinforcing disempowering dependence or denying we have any responsibility or accountability.

With that said, guilt, pain and shame are part of our past experience, and understanding how these emotions have played out in our lives will illuminate how we can fine-tune our fulfillment orientation. Take a moment to recall the times in your life when you were deeply ashamed. Being publicly chided or reprimanded for doing something socially unacceptable when we were young is always a good starting place for searching our recollections, as are incidents where someone we have loved or respected has expressed aversion, disgust or dismay over what we have done. If you can, catalogue these out in your journal, describing why you felt guilt or shame in those moments. Be sure to differentiate unknown judgments from known ones. For example, instances where you were learning for the first time that some relatively harmless or innocent thing you had done was supposed to be shameful indicates an unknown expectation. Whereas trying hard to conceal some activity from others because you knew it was considered shameful or wrong – and then having your activities exposed in some way – is more of a known expectation; even if we justified or rationalized our actions to ourselves and others at the time, if we knew we could be ostracized, ridiculed or punished for it, we still chose to take that risk. After you make your list, tally up your known versus unknown expectations, and think about any current patterns of behavior that might be a consequence of those experiences.

What we can assemble from parsing our past in this area is a list that differentiates the kinds of circumstances or experience that evoked pain, guilt or shame. These might include:

- **Victimized** – Guilt or shame about circumstances that were externally imposed and beyond our control.

- **Innocent** – Guilt or shame about outcomes we did not know at the time had a social expectation of guilt or shame.

- **Compulsive** – Guilt or shame about fulfilling strong nourishment imperatives or impulses that we did not know how to manage at the time, but which we knew or suspected were socially unacceptable.

- **Deliberate** – Guilt or shame about situations we initiated knowing they would result in outcomes that defy social expectations.

Considering all these differences, what quickly becomes clear is that only the last category, *deliberate,* presents a reasonable situation for guilt or shame to exist at all. After all, we can take responsibility for our choice to knowingly create circumstances that do not conform to social expectations. And in that case the pain, guilt or shame is a healthy response, intended to prod us toward changing our choices and behaviors. However, in the first two, *victimized* and *innocent,* we cannot be held culpable at all. The guilt, shame or pain may feel real to us, but those feelings are neither rational nor reasonable. The only category that might give us pause is *compulsive,* but even here, the measure I use for personal accountability is this: if we refuse to seek help with our compulsions and don't even try to manage them, then it is reasonable to feel pain, guilt or shame about them; but if we actively seek help to resolve such issues and try our best to manage them, the fact that such impulses arise within us is not an occasion for guilt, pain or shame. In certain circumstances, it may even be the case that social expectations at the time were unreasonable, and the conditioning to feel shame, guilt or pain over some innate proclivity remains equally unreasonable. We will discuss some examples of this in a moment.

What this means is that a majority of the time, the pain, guilt or shame associated with past experiences are irrational and unreasonable responses. They feel real, but they have no authentic basis for persisting in our history. For example, such feelings are common for people who suffered emotional, physical or sexual abuse as children. They may even have been told at the time to feel guilt or shame for what they were experiencing, even though they had no control over what was happening, which was of course just an added component of the abuse (or a projection of the abuser's own pain, guilt and shame). So how can we reprocess these experiences in light of this knowledge? There are many powerful therapeutic methods for doing this, and if the feelings and associations are potent enough, it may be useful to obtain the support of a skilled therapist. I will offer one of my favorite methods as a self-directed exercise – this is usually a guided visualization and has many variations, but if you take your time with it, it may lead you to interesting places of healing and strength.

Exercise: Supporting Our Younger Self

1) Find a place to sit where you things will be quiet and undisturbed for about twenty minutes.

2) Sit comfortably with your eyes closed, breathing deeply and regularly. Briefly focus your attention on the muscles all over your body and imagine each one relaxing and softening. Do this for five minutes or so, until you feel as relaxed as possible.

3) Imagine you are sitting in a circular room with a high ceiling, with doors regularly spaced along the circular wall; try to color the walls a soft peach or pale pink color, and the doors white with gold knobs on them. The floor could be wood or marble.

4) Behind each door is a scene from your past. Without opening the door, begin preparing a scene behind one of the doors that involved you directly when you were young, and evoked guilt or shame in some way. Just know that the scene is there without necessarily visualizing it completely. Perhaps you might hear what is going on through the door, or merely can anticipate what you will find there. Keep breathing regularly and try to relax. The door will not open until you are ready.

5) When you are ready, approach the door. Feel the gold handle in your hand. Listen for a moment and prepare yourself for what you are about to see. Keep breathing regularly and try to relax.

6) Open the door and look at what is happening. Perhaps you will see the scene you expected. Perhaps you will see something else. Just go with the flow whatever you discover and remain in the doorway. Know that you are safe and let yourself feel whatever emotions arise.

7) Now enter the scene beyond the door and locate your younger self. Get as close as possible to your younger self and try to get their attention. Sometimes they will be despondent, or turn away, or be preoccupied with what is happening...whatever

state your younger self is in, just be a presence next to them.
Offer them your calm, caring, wise, adult companionship.

8) Once you get your younger self's attention (by catching their eye
with a gesture, speaking to them, touching their shoulder, etc.),
hold out your arms to offer them a hug. Whatever happens,
keep breathing, remain as calm as possible, and be patient. If
your younger self runs into your arms, hug them tight. If they
just want to hold your hand, then let them do that. If they just
want to talk to you, then have a conversation with them.
Perhaps they'll have some questions for you, or the may be an
opportunity for you to explain why there is nothing here for
them to feel guilty or ashamed about. Whatever their actions or
emotions – sadness, anger, panic, fear, laughter, excitement – just
let their energy wash over you and be a comforting, stable, calm
and caring presence for them.

9) If others in the scene begin to interact with you, gently disengage
from them and focus on your younger self. You may have to ask
these others to leave if they won't disengage. You want to spend
time with your younger self right now.

10) At a point when your younger self is calm and comforted, and
when you have established positive and warm rapport with
them, tell them from your heart: "I will always be here for you.
I love you. You can always count on me." Give them some time
to absorb this. Repeat it if necessary.

11) Now tell them you have only a few minutes left before you have
to go, and let them decide what they want to do with the rest of
your time together. Assure them that you will be back soon.
Spend those last few minutes being encouraging and reassuring.
Then return to the circular room, closing the door behind you.

12) Open your eyes and reflect on your experience for a few
minutes. Perhaps capture some thoughts in your journal.

13) Being true to your word, try this exercise again another day,
perhaps with a different memory in mind. By doing this once or

twice a week, work through each of the past experiences that have evoked guilt or shame for your younger self.

Now, what about those environmental conditions that evoked guilt or shame? What about unreasonable societal expectations? What if everyone in our childhood environment thought that being an artist or musician was a silly waste of time, but that is what we always knew were called to be? What if that environment ridiculed or persecuted certain racial characteristics we have? What if we knew we were gay or bisexual and those orientations were considered unacceptable or deviant in our community? And so on. This could even be about something seemingly trivial, but the introduction of guilt or shame through social judgments can have a monumental impact on our being. We can reprocess these in much the same way we did our other guilt/shame triggers in the Supporting Our Younger Self exercise, with the addition of our adult self reassuringly explaining to our younger self why this condition, attribute or situation is really acceptable and okay. We provide nourishment to this channel by offering a caring and supportive relationship to all the younger selves languishing away behind those closed doors. Through falling in love with the vulnerable child of those long past events, we strengthen ourselves in the present.

An important caveat in such visitation with traumatic material from our childhood is that we shouldn't push ourselves too quickly or to hard to confront certain things in our past. If we cannot approach these interactions in a relaxed way, if we cannot feel safe or adequately self-managed when offering compassion to our inner child, then we may actually do more harm than good. We might compound our earlier injuries by acting them out in the present. We might decompensate, losing our ability to contain or manage chaotic emotions, depression or destructive impulses to the point where we undermine healthy function. So it behooves us to take this slowly, carefully, and caringly. There is no need to rush, push ourselves, or force ourselves to engage this process alone. Additionally, when we encounter childhood proclivities that we decide are intolerable or unattractive to us even in the present, and cannot resolve the guilt or shame we feel about them, this may require an entirely different approach; something we will discuss in the Empowered Self-Concept section.

Exhilaration. Those moments when we have felt most alive also tend to imprint themselves on our memory, and often can inform how best to nourish ourselves in the present. For instance, just as we discussed in the Emotional Experience channel earlier, there are often a series of distinct experiences in our past that brought us joy, elation and excitement, which we have either chosen to excise from our modern routines or which have slowly faded from our conscious recollection. As we return to those moments, we can learn a great deal about what would stimulate a similar response in us moving forward. Usually these fall into a few distinct categories:

- **Taking risks** – Knowing that we are putting ourselves at risk in some way, but pushing ourselves to take the chance anyway. These might be physical risks such as skiing, white water kayaking, mountain climbing, hang gliding, etc. Or social or emotional risks such as telling someone for the first time that we love them, confronting a friend about something they don't want to face, revealing our true personality or proclivities in a public situation, etc. Or even intellectual risks, such as letting go of some preconception or prejudice, admitting we have been deceiving ourselves or were mistaken about something, etc.

- **Exploring new things** – Seeing new places, trying new foods, learning new concepts, immersing ourselves in new and different experiences, and so on.

- **Breaking patterns** – Sometimes, simply interrupting a routine or deviating from a plan of action can be exciting. Skipping out on some commitment, staying up later than usual, getting up earlier than usual, taking a different route to a routine destination, responding in unpredictable ways to predictable situations and so on.

- **Being "naughty"** – This is really just taking risks, exploring new things or breaking patterns, but with the added backdrop of assuming (or knowing for certain) that our choice or action is socially taboo, doesn't conform to the image we project of ourselves, has to be concealed in some way...or is outright illegal.

The kinds of choices and activities that exhilarate us most will reveal themselves in the patterns of our past. So look over the categories above, and take a few minutes to write down some of the moments in your life when you were the most exhilarated, where you felt the most alive and engaged in what you were doing. For most of us, there were probably some marked periods of time in our past when exhilaration-seeking behavior reached a climax. For me, this includes a series of adventures I had when I was six, seven and eight; and then again in my late teens; and again for a few years after my divorce. During these stretches, I did some pretty crazy things. When you look back on your own exhilarating moments, consider how you could adapt some or all of their characteristics to the activities you do now – or even a few new activities. Of course, as adults we can be aware of the consequences to ourselves and others for our choices and actions, and unleash our exhilaration without contradicting our values or harming anyone involved. If we find that we have tended toward destructive or self-destructive consequences when we were the most exhilarated, we can seek out an appropriate therapeutic relationship to help us reshape those impulses without losing the excitement in our lives. However we arrive there, even a couple hours a week of renewed exhilaration can awaken our vitality through this nourishment channel.

Empowerment. Our empowerment began the first time we acted out some impulse, and the desired result was realized. First we tested this empowerment within the familiar confines of a world defined by our parents. Then, as we individuated from the influence of our parents, we began to test the limits of our will in the world at large. In friendships, work relationships, romantic involvements and our role in the community we experimented with the influence of our will. Along the way -- if we had a relatively healthy and constructive experience – we also learned the limitations of our power. Based on these experiences, we developed parameters for our personal empowerment, boundaries for our will and some idea of what is possible for us to achieve from day to day. To understand how this channel of nourishment functions in the present, we need only decide to advocate for our power in some situation, and notice our thoughts and emotions in reaction to that decision. Are we anxious? Fearful? Excited? Aggressive? Do our reflexive thoughts support our decision? Undermine it? All of this relates back to experiences of empowerment throughout our history.

Which is why it is so important to reflect on those moments and work through how we felt about them at the time.

As with the other channels in this dimension, making a list and notes about each experience of empowerment in our past can be helpful. Another exercise that can help us tune into this area is to take a moment at the end of each week to reflect back over moments of empowerment we experienced in the last few days. What did they feel like? What conditions contributed to our power? How attached are we to those experiences and why? Did those moments facilitate our nourishment or support the nourishment of others? Why or why not?

Tranquility. When have we felt most at peace? What conditions precipitated that experience? What associations from those experiences still evoke tranquil feelings in the present? A certain smell? A time of day? Being in a certain place? If we can access tranquil memories, it can help us create peace in the present and assure us that equanimity or contentment are something we have experienced before and can experience again. If we believe we have never been at peace, the lack of confirmation that this is available for us can undermine any attempts to create it. A good baseline for Tranquility is to cultivate at least three vivid memories of times in the past when we have been completely relaxed, content and unperturbed. Those memories are almost certainly there, somewhere in our psyche, no matter how challenging our life has been. As with so many other areas of nourishment, it is easy for us to look outside ourselves for a source of tranquility, but when we focus inward for that source, we will eventually discover a wellspring of peace just waiting to be tapped.

8 - Pleasurable Legacy

What will we leave behind for those we love? Whether we do so consciously or not, every action and interaction, every choice and accomplishment contributes to the legacy of our existence. We constantly create memories for others, influence their decisions, reinforce outcomes in their lives and help synergize formative experiences that will endure long after we are gone. So what will the themes of that legacy be? How can we assure that our investment of energy in a moment or over a lifetime will contribute positively to the well-being of others? These are the questions we answer within the Pleasurable Legacy channel of nourishment.

At first it might seem that this nourishment center is directed outward. However, as with all other dimensions, we must first perfect whatever gifts we wish to offer others within our own being. Our Legacy therefore becomes a natural overflowing of self into the world around us. As we discover joys and passions in our life, joy and passion promulgate through our actions and interactions into the lives of others. At the same time, as we stabilize and secure the transmission of joy and passion, we do so to ensure the successful perpetuation of that transmission for as long as possible – in this life and after we are gone. Thus we nourish ourselves and others at the same time, which is the hallmark of a Pleasurable Legacy.

The most prevalent example of this can be found in how our species reproduces. In the joy and passion of falling in love with someone, we create a bond that attempts to assure a stable, devoted and supportive environment for our children. And when we in fact begin to expand that family, we increase the security and stability of that environment so that our children can experience joy and passion of their own. We build a nest so they can be safe until they are ready to take flight. We want them to grow and flourish, taking great pride in their successes and fostering their abilities to eventually create a stable and thriving family of their own. All our relationships, intuitions, decisions and risks are vetted through the filter of hope that the pleasure of our experiences can be perpetuated through continuing generations. For me, paraphrasing the lines of the Weavers song "Kisses Sweeter than Wine" pretty much sums up the whole process:

> *"Well now that we're old and ready to go*
> *We get to thinkin' what happened a long time ago*
> *Had a lot of kids, a lot of trouble and pain,*
> *But then, whoops oh lordy, we'd do it all again*
> *Because we had kisses sweeter than wine*
> *We had, mmmm, kisses sweeter than wine...."*

And of course this pattern is not restricted to biological reproduction, but also the perpetuation of inspiring and satisfying ideas, feelings, perceptions, experiences and so on. A work of art, a shared adventure, a right of passage, a kernel of wisdom, a challenging but rewarding responsibility – any of these could be part of a Pleasurable Legacy. When we say we want "what's best" for someone we care about, we are really saying we want to secure whatever we believe will provide them with skills, opportunities and resources that afford them joy in life, and the supportive stability to sustain that joy over time. And to transmit those things fully and completely, we must begin by modeling them ourselves.

Enjoyment. If the chief theme in Pleasurable Legacy is enjoyment, how do we cultivate enjoyment in a way that contributes to our legacy? Mainly we do this by demonstrating, sharing and encouraging that enjoyment with those we love at every opportunity. If we do this lovingly and responsibly, we will always empower them to generate such experiences on their own and not create dependence on us or competition with us. For example, if I desire that a loved one inherit a pleasurable sense of accomplishment, I might include them in a project or process that leads to shared accomplishment, celebrate that accomplishment with them, then encourage them to pursue a project of their own. In my own life, I experienced this very pattern with my German step-grandfather, Joachim, who loved to work in his shop building and repairing things, occasionally helping me with my own projects and always encouraging me to use his tools and knowledge without necessarily inserting himself into my process. I remember the first time I broke down and rebuilt my 10-speed bicycle in his shop. I was thirteen and had no real clue what I was doing, and Joachim was careful to make himself available but not to intrude on my efforts. When I emerged at the end of the day with a bike that worked perfectly, I was ecstatic that I had actually finished the job by myself. Joachim, in his characteristic way, simply shrugged and said, "Well yes, of course you did," as if he had never doubted my abilities.

To build a baseline in this area, it is imperative we cultivate legacy-driven enjoyable experiences each and every day. It is not enough to set aside what brings us pleasure for weekends, holidays and vacations.

And, with respect to this channel of self-nourishment, it is also insufficient to experience pleasure for pleasure's sake without the guiding context of creating our legacy. So yesterday I spent time working on a joint project with a work acquaintance, a project we are both excited about and that we both hope will benefit others. Today I will take a book I enjoyed when I was young over to a friend's house, and we will take turns reading it aloud to her children. Tomorrow I will make dinner for some friends, preparing a meal that is one of my favorites, and which I know they will also relish. And so on. Each point of enjoyable contact adding to the legacy I leave for others and they leave for me.

Passion. What is passion? In this context, passion is the heightened, highly energized engagement of our whole being in a specific focus or activity. When we are passionate about something, we are intensely absorbed in it, channeling all our attention and effort into a single process that satisfies that absorption. To find areas that we can be passionate about is one of life's greatest blessings, and to share that passion with those we care about is one of life's greatest joys.

I remember being spellbound as a child observing my father have animated intellectual debates with his friends. In these moments he was more expressive, more engaged and more intense than at any other time. He was passionate about ideas. To his credit, he always allowed me to participate in these discussions, even though I had little to offer at that young age. Sometimes this irritated other adults who participated in his discussions, but my father made sure I was included and that my thoughts were heard. Over time, I of course caught the intellectual passion bug myself. As I grew up, I loved to find people with whom I could explore ideas, and began to hear in my own emphatic discourse the same intensity and flexibility of thinking my father modeled. Eventually, as an adult, I could even engage my father in such discussions. So this became one of his legacies to me. Because of his including me in his passion and enjoyment, I now have passion and enjoyment in my life.

As a baseline, here too we can devote time each day to things we are passionate about, and included others in our process whenever possible.

And we should realize that whenever our passion falters, this can endanger our legacy.

Security & Stability. With both enjoyment and passion, there is a range of sustainable function within which either may be facilitated. When we fall short of that range through lack of effort, or overextend ourselves in fixated or obsessive effort, joy and passion rapidly dissipate. What can help us manage this balance are the steps we take to create security and stability in our lives and the lives of our loved ones. The security and stability channel is supported by four factors:

- **Space** – Our ability to create clearly communicated boundaries around nurturing physical space so that we and those we love can feel safe in that space. For instance, having a designated place for regular meditation, creative work, physical self-care and so forth; sanctifying our bedroom or sleeping environment by making sure no argument or hostility occurs there; sharing family meals in the same place each day; having a designated area for games and playfulness; and so on. The more we can depend on such defined spaces, the more relaxed and expansive we – and everyone else – can be in those environments.

- **Time** – Our ability to manage our time so that it, too, has clear boundaries. Time boundaries are really about our integrity with intentions we have set for ourselves or communicated to others. For instance, that we will finish up work on some project at a specific time; meet with friends and a specific time; only spend so many hours each day in recreational activities; donate a certain number of hours to help a friend with their needs; share meals at a certain time; get up at a regular time; and so on. In each case, when we fulfill the intentions we set and communicate, we build security and stability into our environment – for ourselves and everyone who relies on us to follow through on those intentions.

- **Relationships** – Security and stability also manifests in the spectrum of trusting relationships we cultivate. Can we feel safe around everyone in our lives? Can those we care about feel safe around everyone in their lives? Do our relationships support and facilitate our legacy? Do they create synergies that amplify enjoyment and passion? If we can't confidently answer all of these questions in the affirmative, we must reevaluate our choice of friends, partners and community. Without a broad base of trusting relationships, it will be challenging for our legacy to thrive.

- **Resources** – Somehow, we must feed and clothe ourselves and have adequate resources to facilitate our legacy. This will depend on where we decide to live, what skills we learn to materially support ourselves, and our habits of spending, consumption and saving. These choices will determine what resources are available to us over time. In my own life, I decided at various junctures not to pursue a college degree, to put down roots in Seattle, to live alone, to invest all my savings into my own business, to take time off from full-time work to write books about mysticism, to change careers at least twice – all of which greatly affected resource availability over the following years. My choices allowed me to pursue one legacy, but curtailed my ability to pursue others. It is important that we become conscious of the consequences of such decisions as we make them.

Here again we must discover our optimal range of function. If our efforts at security and stability become too rigid, controlling or obsessive, they will defeat the intended purpose and create insecurity and stress for us and everyone around us. If they are too lax, ambiguous or poorly communicated, they will likewise undermine any sense of continuity, regularity, dependability and safety. Between these two extremes is a realm where our legacy can be perpetuated in a relaxed and safe environment.

9 - Flexible Processing Space

It has often been observed that each of us has a unique way of experiencing life – that is, a unique way of processing each event or tidbit of information we encounter. One person sees a lovely, glowing orange sunset while another sees an upsetting impact of pollution in the evening air. One person is inspired by a certain kind of music while another is depressed by it. One person enjoyed the dinner party while another feels it was a waste of time. One person experiences a conversation as an uncomfortable confrontation while another considers it a lively and stimulating debate. And so on. And it often seems as though many of these reactions are hard-wired, deeply seated in personal beliefs and either genetic or social programming. In other words, that they are the result of chained associations unique to each person. While this is true to some degree, I believe something else is happening here that is dependent on both the *processing space* being accessed at that moment, and the *frequency* of the information itself. By processing space I mean the part of our being through which a majority of the information is being funneled, absorbed and interpreted at that moment. And by frequency I mean the very literal wavelength, harmonic or type of energy that is being exchanged.

First let's explore what is meant by processing space. There are many more than the five outlined below, and each of them overlaps and interacts with all the others in whole or part, creating a complex matrix of nuanced processing capacity in every person. But for the sake of simplifying and understanding types of processing space in a usable way, they have been narrowed down here to what happens mainly within our head, heart, body, spirit and soul. Each of these engages a unique form of perception-cognition native to our being, each one necessary to interpret and process various aspects of the world around us. Over time, we naturally tend to gravitate towards the processing spaces with which we are most comfortable, or which we believe have helped us the most during the course of our life, and use them as our primary mode of interaction within each dimension of nourishment. Each processing space also operates at a specific, subjective rate of time. That is, time runs faster or slower for us when we are functioning in a particular processing space. So what we are really talking about here is unique spacetime of perception-cognition.

Mental Spacetime. This is future-oriented, fast-paced analytical processing. Here we are focused on effective action or reaction to immediate circumstances, using our analytical abilities to make what we interpret to be rational, sensible choices. Most of us don't need to consciously practice this or incorporate it into our daily experience, since we are constantly pressured by externals to operate in this mode. We plan our week out in a day-timer; we focus on the next task to accomplish; we engage in animated discussion about some topic of interest; we quickly rationalize our choices so that our actions are justifiable; we absorb the evening news and pass judgment on the world. In Western culture, much of our daily routine occurs in mental spacetime. And since mental spacetime is highly valued in Western society – that is, to make quick decisions, communicate clear goals, have decisive reactions, be competitive with others operating in this mode, and so forth – Westerners tend to dedicate much more of themselves to this processing space than is necessary or beneficial to their well-being. When we neglect to consciously shift into other modes of interior processing, we inevitably disconnect from a wellspring of alternative insight and nourishing function within ourselves, as well as from the healing, growth and transformation that is available through our other manifestations of being. In fact, we disconnect from some of the critical substance of our own humanity. In terms of exchange, this mode allows us to connect with others on mainly verbal, symbolic and intellectual levels.

Emotional Spacetime. This is past, present and future-oriented and generally slower-paced emotional processing. Here we feel our way through situations, knowing intuitively that we can't rush certain experiences or decisions. When we heal from grief and loss, for example, much of that healing occurs in emotional spacetime. When we fall deeply in love, our affection develops within this processing space. And where in mental spacetime it may be easy to dismiss a hunch or intuition as superstitious silliness, emotional spacetime accepts the importance of such input, feeling its way through the moment. This processing often happens unconsciously. But paying conscious attention to this spacetime both honors the intuitive component of self and integrates felt experiences into our being. If we ignore or suppress it, heart-based processing can become arrested or confused, and an important input stream to our wisdom and discernment will be crippled. Examples of consciously entering emotional spacetime include the gratitude meditation in the next section; praying from the heart; journaling about intensely personal or emotional issues; attentively feeling the music to which we are listening; free-flowing creative expression; replaying significant memories from childhood; daydreaming; certain guided meditations; falling in love; or dwelling the felt experience of the current moment. When people share love, laughter, tears, anger, joy or other strong emotion with each other, they are connecting in emotional spacetime.

Somatic Spacetime.   This can be either very slow-paced somatic processing, or fast-paced reflexive responses; in both cases, however, somatic spacetime is usually oriented to the past or present.   On the slower side, when stress or trauma occurs in our lives, somatic memories are created that we carry with us for years.   Processing those memories – bringing them into conscious awareness – is one reason why accessing somatic spacetime is important.   Another is that our body has intelligence, wisdom and guidance for us should we choose to listen to it. If we don't listen, our body's efforts to engage our attention may become more and more extreme, until serious illness or other chronic conditions develop.   On the faster side, our bodies can react very quickly to threats, attractions, the perceived body language of others and so forth – more quickly than we could ever consciously react.   So shifting into our body's processing space can rapidly accelerate our awareness, or slow it down to the speed of breaths and heartbeats.   Shifting into somatic spacetime can occur during therapeutic bodywork, certain types of yoga, in body-centered psychotherapy, during physical listening meditations, when trying to identify an emotive locus in our body, when we invite the palpable presentation of intuitive promptings, during physical intimacy, while practicing martial arts, or any time we are completely absorbed in physical activity.   We can connect in somatic spacetime with others through things like playing sports, having sex, giving or receiving body-centered therapy, or sharing other intensely physical experiences.

Spiritual Spacetime.   This is time-space suspended spiritual processing, meaning that it has no anchor in sequential time, moves independently of most concrete or tangible reference points, and is a sort of spiritual intuition.   I like to call it *gnostic* processing.   Sometimes entering spiritual spacetime seems like complete stillness without even the possibility of movement, and at other times processing in this spacetime seems faster than light, spanning incredible distances in an instantaneous leap.   Many schools of meditation and interior spiritual discipline encourage access to this space, but it can be experienced spontaneously during prayer, as a natural component of wonder and awe, as an ineffable *aha* when peak experiences occur in other processing modes, during the course of a dream, during intense moments of pleasure or pain and so on. Exchanges in this processing space can occur during group mediation and prayer; during shared experiences of intense intimacy or intense crisis; or in the sudden, unexpected recognition of a kindred spirit.

Soul Spacetime. This could be described as the eternal present, an arena of spacetime that is entirely free of processing – it just is. This is becomes an important concept in certain spiritual disciplines, in particular the advanced mystical practices that cultivate immersion in a kind of non-awareness or non-being that harmonizes with the Absolute. At the center of this processing space is a completely transparent connection, exchange and merging – with the essence of the Self and the essence of the Universe, with the All, the Transcendent Reality, the ground of being.

In one way, all spacetimes are simply modes of interior processing that are always present and available to us. We interpret our experiences unconsciously through an internal nexus where all of these modes coincide. We can, of course, suppress or interrupt this natural synthesis. Things like stress, obsessive thought or behavior, incomplete or indulgent nourishment in one or more dimensions, the consumption of mood or mind altering substances on a regular basis – all of this can interfere with the natural rhythms in each processing center and their combined synergistic power. Likewise, when we begin cultivating each mode of perception-cognition as a distinct, conscious experience, major shifts will occur that increase potential synthesis, stimulating processing on many levels at once. Through practice we can consciously integrate all of these modes into an input stream that informs our wisdom and discernment, especially in ways that nurture all essential dimensions of being at the same time, so that our efforts are not only healing and skillful, but transformative. So, at a minimum, it is extremely helpful to develop specific awareness in each spacetime mode so that we can live more effective and fulfilling lives. Once this is accomplished, we can shift between each spacetime with increasing ease, flexibly engaging any situation from multiple perspectives. This flexibility becomes a powerful ally in our efforts to nurture ourselves and express compassionate affection through every thought and action. To master each mode of perception-cognition and access them on-the-fly in any situation allows us to love more truly and effectively.

Returning to the idea of relationships and communication, each processing space also has its own unique language and mode of exchange. Clearly, one component of high quality relationships is that such unique modes of exchange – the particular language of one or more processing spaces – will be fluid and fluent. If you've ever held hands with someone you care about, you know that very important communication can occur in non-verbal ways, so we aren't just talking about talking. In fact, verbal communication that facilitates connection in mental spacetime quite well often becomes decreasingly efficient as we move through other modes of being. In emotional spacetime, we may be able to describe what is occurring with words, but heartfelt laughter or the sight of a grieving person's tears are far more potent communicators in that realm. The same is true of somatic spacetime, where sharing physical intimacy exchanges energies and sensations that the body understands perfectly, but the mind and heart must reinterpret at different frequencies. In fact, intense physical pleasure or pain tends to override processing on all other levels. And when we arrive at spirit or soul spacetime, words really lose relevance altogether. These are spiritual and existential exchanges that are understood intuitively and experientially by spirit and soul alone, to be reinterpreted later in other spacetimes. Emotions and sensations offer reminders of these experiences, evoking distant echoes of abstract concepts on the cognitive plane, but the actual communication – the actual energy exchange – is occurring mainly in a non-verbal, non-emotive and non-sensory way by the spirit and soul.

Take a moment to consider the relationships with others in your life that operate on different levels or modes of exchange. Has there ever been someone you were physically attracted to, but with whom you had very little else in common? Or someone you could have stimulating conversations with, but couldn't connect with on an emotional level? Years ago I had a close friend with whom I played Frisbee on a regular basis. It mattered little what either of us was doing when the other called to go play, because that connection was so important to us we would usually make room for it. We could talk about certain things, of course, and evoke a vague emotional companionship around some of our shared experiences, but really our friendship was all about Frisbee. This may seem trivial on the surface, but it really wasn't. We could depend on each other for that connection, and it was something we had not found in other relationships. And when, after nearly a decade of tossing a plastic disc back and forth, our relationship ended, I felt a real loss. Since then I have tried to reignite a similar connection through tennis, basketball, hiking and so forth, but nothing has come close to the intimacy of what my Frisbee friend and I shared. How could that be? I think it is because we could send and receive on the same frequency of communication within somatic spacetime. In sharing a frequency, a wavelength of exchange, we could synch up precisely with very little effort in that spacetime. This kind of connection can occur in any spacetime, and makes the flow of energy (and therefore nourishment) that much more free and uninhibited.

This seems like a good time to offer some asides about close relationships. Too often in our culture we are encouraged to find the be-all and end-all soul mate that will satisfy all of our needs. That is, discover someone who will connect with us fluidly on every level, who speaks all our favorite mode-of-being languages fluently, and who matches or resonates with our favored frequencies. Likewise we can be discouraged when our closest friends cannot offer us exchanges in more than one or two spacetimes. Such high expectations inevitably lead to frustration, disappointment and sadness. And when we try too hard to force a few close relationships to generate all the nourishment we desire, we also inevitably become depleted in one or more areas. When we mix frustration, disappointment, sadness and starvation into one huge avalanche of hurt, the strain disintegrates what few authentic and nourishing connections remain. More than any other single contributing factor, I believe this is why relationships fail; not because they cannot provide mutual and essential nourishment, but because we expect them to generate more nourishment, on more levels and at more desired frequencies, than is realistically possible. If we understand more clearly how those exchanges occur across all of our relationships, and how to address deficiencies, then we would neither abandon our connections nor force them to conform to an unhealthy ideal.

Clearly, changing our expectations is critical, and often this requires unlearning what we have been taught about relationships from some pervasive cultural fantasies. But even more important than this deprogramming of expectations is creating a diverse community of supportive relationships in a conscious way, and resisting any tendency to constrain our interactions to a smaller and smaller set of exclusive, all-consuming connections. There will be those where our primary exchange is in mental spacetime, and others where the sharing is from the heart, or body, or even spirit. It is even possible to encounter and expand our soul connections with others. In a way, it is our privilege to discover what levels of connection we can achieve with each and every person we meet. There may be boundaries to this effort – because of our personal commitments and what is socially acceptable for our times – but consider the revolutionary idea of falling deeply in love with everyone around you, and then attempting to express that love on every level imaginable without rigid expectations of how this should be accomplished or with whom. Why do I suggest this? Because when we fall in love, our ability to synchronize in different spacetimes is greatly enhanced – because our frequencies of exchange in each processing space either harmonize (interacting in a pleasurable and constructive way) or converge entirely. Without love, there will inevitably be disconnection and dissonance.

Of course, because of how we are wired and the society in which we live, certain types of exchange will likely be reserved for our most intimate relationships. Commitment and special relationship status also create a sense of safety for intimate exchanges, and this is very important for both interior and communal growth. So our closest friends and our romantic partnerships are not intended to be casualties of a diversified processing space approach, nor are socially appropriate boundaries of conduct intended to be breached. On the contrary, when we relieve the pressure on those closest to us to provide for all of our needs, it encourages freedom and joy where once there was oppressive confinement. There is an implied balance of openness and commitment here, based on whatever our own close relationships and those of others can honestly tolerate, but the idea is to recognize what connections we have and what connections we have yet to create. From that point, the world around us turns into a very interesting place as new horizons simultaneously arise.

When authentic, open exchange occurs on any level, this constitutes a high quality relationship. When the exchange endures and deepens over time, or expands into other modes of connection additional processing spaces, a relationship of an ever higher order is created. If I connect with someone on all levels for even a fleeting instant, that is meaningful to me. And when I realize that I am surrounded by a supportive community of such multi-faceted relationships, this is both a great honor and a purposeful accomplishment in terms of mutual, full-spectrum nourishment. There are of course many other significant components of relationship that must be present for full-spectrum nourishment to occur, and you can review these in the High Quality Relationship section in Part I.

Spacious Energy. Creating baseline nourishment practices in the Flexible Processing Space dimension is really much simpler than it may first appear. One straightforward approach to this nourishment center is the creation of *spacious energy* in our lives; that is, a relaxed easing of focus on our habitual processing space. Rather than concentrating our energy in any one spacetime, we encourage the total energy of our being to flow freely through multiple processing spaces. Each person will have a particular activity that promotes this freedom, and our main experience will be characterized by feelings of safety, relaxation, letting go, heightened enjoyment and a sense of personal expansion. Here are some sample techniques that help cultivate spacious energy:

- **Time alone in Nature.** Spending time wandering the open desert, wending our way along a trail in the woods, sitting in an alpine meadow or on a deserted beach or otherwise immersing ourselves in a wild, natural environment will begin to evoke spacious energy.

- **Combined meditation techniques.** Certain types of meditation that combine elements of physical movement, mental concentration and emotional or intuitive sensitivity will help us free the energy of our being.

- **Unstructured solitude.** Another approach to encouraging spacious energy in all processing spaces is to have a solid block of uninterrupted time where we have no agenda, no responsibilities, no structure and no contact with anyone else. This could be sitting in a chair at home, going for a walk, going for a casual swim, or engaging in some activity that relaxes us without forcing us to constrain our focus to one type of spacetime.

- **Body-centered therapy.** Although this relies on a therapeutic relationship to initially encourage or structure spacious energy in our lives, having some assistance to our own efforts can be a useful gateway to new modes of being. There is such a wide range of therapies available I hesitate to include any of them here, but any approach that tunes us into our body in a relaxed way will help us expand energy into multiple processing spaces at once. Mirka Knaster's book, *Discovering the Body's Wisdom*, is an excellent introduction to the wide range of techniques available. For me personally, some of my own gateway experiences occurred through Reiki, Hatha Yoga, craniosacral therapy and Hakomi.

It takes time and effort to shift from focusing all of our energy in one or two processing spaces into a more tranquil, all-inclusive mode. If we can spend half an hour each day or more in activities that encourage spacious energy, we will begin the necessary relaxation of our habitual processing patterns.

10 - Empowered Self-Concept

How we perceive and define ourselves from moment to moment has a pronounced influence on all other dimensions of nourishment. In *Integral Lifework*, self-concept is a complex cloud of factors shaped by answers to certain types of questions – questions which, as exercises in self-awareness, can be quite illuminating. Once we understand how we define ourselves to ourselves, we can also see how we naturally gravitate toward certain areas of nourishment while tending to ignore or neglect others. We can also begin to enrich our self-concept with greater confidence and deeper awareness in new areas. This is what nourishing our Empowered Self-Concept will achieve.

Although each person's construction of self-concept is unique, there are some common themes all of us can explore. For example:

1) Do I believe my choices have an impact on the course of my own destiny?

2) Am I content with my physical wellness, appearance, vitality and strength?

3) Do I have a sense of humor about myself – especially about my own weaknesses?

4) Do I think of myself as smart, well-educated and/or experienced?

5) Do I have a strong sense of purpose from day to day?

6) Do I believe I am lovable? Do I believe I am well-loved?

7) Has my past contributed in positive ways to my well-being?

8) Can I be silly, goofy and carefree when I choose to?

9) How connected do I feel to other people, the All, the ground of being, the Divine, the Absolute, the Universe?

10) Is there something I know will remain from my efforts after I am gone? Something that the world – or at least those I love – will remember me by?

11) Is my physical and emotional intimacy deeply satisfying to me?

You may notice that these questions in fact directly relate to other nourishment centers. That is because much of our self-concept is constructed from how we are able to nourish ourselves in other dimensions. If I believe my body is unattractive or lacking in vitality and strength, I might tend to either overcompensate for that body image with extra effort, or neglect my physical well-being altogether. If I don't feel connected to other people or the ground of being, I might tend to either undervalue those connections or strive to remedy my lack of connectedness through extraordinary effort. If I feel I lack a strong sense of purpose, the same two choices are available: to expend much effort in establishing a purpose, or to ignore my purposelessness by making it unimportant. For every question that relates to a specific dimension of nourishment, these two extremes can establish themselves as lasting patterns and inform an enduring image of self. And so we circle back once again to the narrow band of optimal function; somewhere between these two extremes is the most constructive, healthy and relaxed self-concept, where we both embrace who we are, and are inspired for healthy, self-supportive reasons to grow and change.

| Exercise: Self-Concept | Take a moment to look over the
questions above and try to answer them. How do the answers to
these questions compare to the answers in the earlier exercise
where you estimated your self-nourishment in each of the
twelve dimensions? Are there differences? Why do you think
that is?

Self-Awareness

Are we self-aware? This is one of those situations when, if we have a
well-developed awareness of self, we may tend to doubt the clarity or
completeness of that awareness – and if we are absolutely certain our
self-awareness is accurate and exhaustive, then we probably have some
significant deficits. It is extremely difficult to measure self-awareness,
mainly because there are few objective ways to get a reliable comparative
assessment. We would have to be expert readers of other people's
honesty as well as experts in introspection to know for certain that we
have an accurate picture of ourselves. There are some formalized ways
to assess certain aspects of our personality, emotional intelligence,
physical ability, analytical reasoning and so forth, but such external
instruments tend to share the same intrinsic flaw, no matter how
comprehensive their methodology or advanced their technology. They
cannot take into account the intersubjective realities that generate human
experience, and those are what really determine the functional
perceptions, exchanges and outcomes that shape who and how we are
from moment to moment. For instance, it doesn't matter that my IQ is
any certain level or number, what matters is my intersubjective
intelligence. That is, how the people who rely on me can trust in my
intelligence, how I perceive my abilities relative to any given task, my
track record of applying my brain effectively in different situations, and
so forth. It is the synthesis of all such disparate perspectives that
determines the functional value of my intelligence. And the same goes
for my attractiveness, sense of humor, whether I am competent in a
specific skill, am emotionally intelligent and so on.

With this level of complexity, it is inherently challenging for us to
measure our level of self-awareness with precision. But there is one
reliable way to understand self, and that is through specific interior

disciplines. When we strengthen our innate introspective abilities, we gain an increasingly accurate picture of ourselves. Learning to listen to our intuition is one such avenue of exploration. Another is the non-judgmental introspection available through certain types of meditation. Certain forms of mystic activation, including the practice outlined at the end of Part I, are excellent avenues to accurate self-awareness. Just reflecting on our own thoughts and thought process through journaling or therapeutic dialogue will provide new insight into the workings of our being. As mentioned earlier in the emotional awareness section, one exercise I have encouraged students and clients to experiment with is simply turning their attention to where they feel different emotions in their body. Does the physical sensation of happiness occur lower in the belly or higher in the chest? What about anger? Anxiety? Sadness? Doubt? And so on. Each of these approaches provides a window into who we are and how we function, and over time they can help us build a solid and consistent sense of self.

But let's consider the bigger picture for a moment. How can we know if our self-assessments are accurate? How can we ascertain the exact shape and feel of our self-concept, self-efficacy or self-worth, even with careful and persistent interior discipline? In a truly objective sense, we probably can't know for certain, but that doesn't matter, because the introspective process is valuable in itself – and this is more to the point. The one thing we can be reasonably sure of is that, if we continue to develop high-quality interior disciplines, we will come closer and closer to the authentic substance of who we are, peeling away many distortions and eye-watering distractions of our inner onion. The destination is ever-changing because our existence is constantly evolving, but the journey will always be enlightening. The question just shifts from "Am I getting at the bedrock of reality, here?" to "This is exciting! Do I have some tools to take the next step?" to "What is the wisest, most nourishing course of self-exploration for me in the current situation?" to the many other angles into our interior landscape. In that spirit, then, the most powerful tool in your journey of self-discovery is mystic activation. As part of a broader set of integral routines, you can be sure that the more you stimulate and rely upon spiritual insight, the deeper, broader and clearer your understanding of Self will be. And in terms of accurate and useful introspective awareness, that is really the best we can hope for.

Is there the danger of delusion and misconception using this approach? Of course, but once again such a process is a continuum, not a destination. The arrival at a static sense of who we are, how effective we can be, or our inherent value in the Universe cannot be finalized if we are still breathing, growing and changing. But if we invest in a way of seeing that illuminates these facets of self with a compassionate quality of light, then our ongoing discovery will become self-referentially valid no matter how faulty it may sometimes be. Why? Because we are made of that light, and that light is made of us – we are trying to see the wavelength of our existence on that wavelength, so although there can never be objectivity, there can be direct, unmitigated, experiential apprehension. That is, we can infer all that we need to know from the hints and clues that such interior processing provides, and, over time, those inferences will be validated or dismissed as we concretely experience each new horizon of understanding about our place and purpose in the Universe. We will explore and express ourselves fully, and thus come to know ourselves fully. Through mystic activation, we will encounter certainty through interactions with the Absolute within. By training our mind, heart and spirit to recognize and integrate this unique flavor of perception-cognition, we gain an intuitive appreciation for the Self we wish to comprehend. This type of self-awareness may sound abstract and unapproachable to the unpracticed, but it is an ability we all have – we just need a reminder to embrace it every now and again.

An advanced quality of interior listening is the objective of many different exercises throughout this book. Of course, there is a narrow range of optimal function in our self-awareness. If I become obsessed with the minutia of my internal processes, I will interfere with my natural healing and growth. If I ignore my inner workings altogether, I will be oblivious to the warning signs that I need to change something, and the rewards that encourage me down a more productive and expansive path. At a minimum, our baseline nourishment in this channel should consist of daily doses of non-judgmental introspection, with as much of a mystic activation component as we are comfortable including.

Self-Efficacy & Self-Worth

Self-efficacy and self-worth are closely related, and are part of our overall self-concept. Self-efficacy is the confidence we have in our abilities and the trust we can sustain in the quality of our intentions and effort. For instance, having healthy self-efficacy is to know in our heart of hearts that we can rely on ourselves for high-quality nourishment, and that despite past failures we are our own most loyal and reliable provider, advocate and ally. Self-worth, on the other hand, is the overall value we place on our own existence, and the quality of satisfaction and contentment we have with our own efforts and accomplishments. The following is a list of questions that can help evaluate self-efficacy and self-worth as a deepening of the previous self-concept exercise. These likewise relate to nourishment, tying into certain dimensions and revealing potential barriers to our overall well-being.

1) Am I a capable and competent person who can fully nourish myself?

2) Do I feel safe and secure most of the time, or do I feel vulnerable or afraid?

3) Have I fully individuated myself? Am I my own person, and do I dream the dream of my own life...or am I still in a power struggle with my parents, siblings or other people in my life, still striving to establish personal autonomy or my own sense of self?

4) Do I present the real me to the world in all my quirkiness, or do I hide behind social masks or insincere reactions I have created to conceal and protect myself?

5) Do I have any unresolved grief in my heart?

6) Do I have guilt over anything I have done in the past, or have I forgiven myself?

7) Do I believe I have a purpose in this life, and that I am fulfilling that purpose?

8) Am I always honest with those I love about everything I think and do?

9) Do I follow through on whatever I commit to doing?

10) Do I fully live my life according to the goals I promote and the values I express?

11) Do I have a genuine connection with my spiritual self?

12) Do I love myself? Do I really care about my own well-being?

13) Do I enjoy life to its fullest?

14) Am I surrounded by people who want the best for me, and who connect with my beliefs, interests and values?

15) Am I a talented lover? Am I good at sex?

16) Am I a playful person? Do I have a playful sense of humor?

17) As a result of all of my actions and interactions, will I leave a positive legacy for those I most care about if I vanished tomorrow?

18) Am I able to really relax and let go in stressful situations?

19) Do I have genuine affection for my own body? Do I believe my habits and attitudes have a positive influence on my body's overall health and appearance?

20) Am I a creative and imaginative person?

21) Do I keep my mind sharp and agile? Do I keep it fed with new and interesting information? Do I regularly stimulate my brain?

Some of these questions may be challenging to answer at first, but the answers are there within us, wanting to be known. Try the exercise below to invite them to rise to the surface. As for the impact these questions have on self-nourishment, we may lean towards one of two extremes here just as we did with self-awareness. We could become arrogant and egotistical, with an overly inflated sense of our own importance and the effectiveness of our abilities. Or we could lose our sense of confidence and self-assurance, certain that we have little value or contribution in this life; that we are destined to fail at everything se set out to do. Between these extremes, if our self-worth and self-efficacy are supportive, it is likely we will ground ourselves in humility while remaining confident we can achieve our goals – knowing that our contribution to society and value as an individual are at least as worthwhile as anyone else's. Like everything in our internal makeup, we have strengths in some areas and weaknesses in others, and will undoubtedly experience fluctuations in our self-efficacy and self-worth over time. That is something we can happily depend on, because such fluctuations provide the fertile conditions required for ongoing healing and growth.

> **Exercise: Efficacy and Worth** Spend some time meditating on each of the questions listed above. That is, sit comfortably with your eyes closed, breathing deeply and evenly, and hold each question, one at-a-time, lightly in your mind. Avoid writing anything down for now. Just continue breathing and resting your awareness in each successive question, allowing whatever response arises within you to occur unimpeded and unevaluated. When you have completed one pass of the list, go back to the beginning and start over again, this time spending a little more time resting in the answer to each question that arises within. When you have completed the second review of the questions, spend some time with your journal writing down some reflections and conclusions.

Integrating the Ugly or Unbelievable

In the course of our daily life, we may be expending a tremendous amount of energy trying to counter, deny, repress or otherwise reject parts of ourselves that we have yet to fully integrate. This self-rejection can manifest in many ways. Sometimes it manifests as a projection on someone else, investing them with our attributes so that we can distance ourselves from what we find unpleasant, idealized or unrecognizable in ourselves. Sometimes it becomes a dark cloud of free-floating anxiety that follows us around everywhere we go. Sometimes it weighs us down with sudden bouts of depression, agitation or anger. Sometimes it rides us so hard we try to escape through frantic busyness, obsessive compulsive behaviors or even desperate self-destructiveness. And until we face this pattern of self-rejection and begin to integrate those parts of ourselves that we find so difficult to embrace, we will unwittingly sabotage our self-nourishment in one or more dimensions.

What are some examples of the "ugly or unbelievable" that people resist integrating? What is interesting about these attributes is that we tend to feel either extremely positive or extremely negative about them, mainly because we fear the power, influence or potential for radical alterations in self-concept they represent in our lives. For instance:

- **The ugly** – What we view as an innate weakness or flaw in ourselves, such as personality traits that might cause social embarrassment, sexual desires that are outside the perceived norm, patterns of thought or behavior that could harm ourselves or others, or some other recurring theme in our lives that we fear will produce guilt, shame or pain once it is exposed to the light of day.

- **The unbelievable** – What we suspect is an innate strength or advantage that we don't wish to acknowledge. For example, a natural ability in some special area, a wealth of available resources, some powerful influence we may have over others, or an untested aspect of ourselves that could, if exposed, create new challenges or expectations in our lives.

These traits or attributes may be part of any dimensions of nourishment, and will interfere with that nourishment center if they remain unaddressed. They will, if we resist embracing them, become ever larger factors in our own dissatisfaction and reduced function. They can even result in serious illness or premature death – all because we are too fearful to accept them as part of ourselves. So how can we acknowledge them? How can we transform our fear into love and acceptance?

Stage One: Recognition & Enumeration

An often humorous irony regarding our un-integrated attributes is that they are constantly brought to our attention. They froth forth from our subconscious when we least expect it. Our close friends and relatives remind us we possess them. Our coworkers and acquaintances innocently observe them and report them to us. As examples, consider some of the reflexive responses that can4 issue from un-integrated attributes:

- **Frequent apologizing, frustration or anger about our own habits.** For instance, that we're running late, or said something we didn't mean, or forgot something someone we care about thought was important, or crossed some boundary we said we wouldn't cross, or broke a promise, or did something stupid or inconsiderate, or were irresponsible in some situation, or inadvertently embarrassed or harmed someone, etc.

- **Frequent resistance to observations about our strengths.** For instance, denying that we are skilled at something, being embarrassed about compliments or praise, avoiding responsibility or leadership in some area others observe we are good at, becoming upset with people when they describe some strength or advantage they believe we possess, etc.

- **Forceful denial of the obvious.** For instance, insisting that we are never wrong or never make mistakes, that we don't have a particular weakness or strength that others observe in us all the time, that we haven't accomplished anything noteworthy, that we can't be blamed for something that really is our fault or can't take credit for something that really is our accomplishment and so on. In other words, when we adamantly refuse to acknowledge a part of ourselves that is obvious to everyone around us.

- **Habitual projection of our own strengths or weaknesses on others.** This can manifest as classic "pot calling the kettle black" situations, where we become impatient, upset or chiding with someone because of patterns in their behavior that mirror parts of ourselves we haven't yet accepted. Or this can manifest as surrounding ourselves with people we feel have idealized attributes that we don't recognize in ourselves, but fervently wish we had. Or both.

If we ask those close to us to help make a list of any such reflexive reactions they may have witnessed over time, we will probably get to the core issues fairly quickly. If you take this approach, be sure to ask someone you are certain will be honest, gentle and tactful with you – or train yourself not to react too strongly to their observations if they lack gentleness and tact. You might also spend a week or so tracking your reactions over the course of each day and logging them in your journal. In some way, it will be important to acknowledge and capture this information so we can take the next step.

Stage Two: Acceptance

Acceptance comes through letting go, a little bit at a time, of all those self-protective reflexes. First, take the list you've compiled of your suspected un-integrated attributes, and order it so that what you feel are positive and negative attributes alternate each other. Start with a negative attribute, then a positive, then a negative, and truncate the list once you run out of equal pairs. Right now it's important to have a balance. Now turn the list into a series of questions such as. "Am I impatient with people a lot?" or "Do I have attractive eyes?" and so on. Then take your list to the nearest mirror and try the following:

1. Look yourself in the eye and ask the first question. Note the emotions that arise as you ask it. Based on those emotions, is it a valid observation?

2. If it feels valid, change the question to an affirmative statement, such as "yes, I am impatient with people a lot," or "yes, I do have attractive eyes," and repeat that statement aloud while looking into your own eyes again.

3. Continue asking, pausing for emotional sense after each question, and converting to an affirmation until you have finished the list.

4. Go back to the beginning and repeat the statements of affirmation, this time adding the phrase "and I'm okay with that," or "and I have accepted that" at the end of each statement. Pay attention to the emotions that arise as you do this.

If this exercise works for you, you've taken a step towards acceptance of the ugly or unbelievable in yourself. If this exercise seems forced or somehow leaves you feeling nonplused, try it as a meditation with your eyes closed and your attention directed inward, toward the center of your chest. Or you could try it with another person reading the questions to you, and you responding to them with affirming statements. Whatever your approach, encourage your heart to embrace the parts of yourself that have been trying to get your attention for so long. Welcome them home. Then, over the following weeks, observe your own reactions to situations that previously triggered your rejection reflexes. Some of those reactions may still arise from time to time, but you will be increasingly aware of them and able to manage them more effectively. If you try all of these approaches and there are still one or two outstanding issues to address, there are many other therapeutic methods available, so avail yourself of some professional help.

Stage Three: Love

Acceptance is the beginning of the journey to integrated wholeness. Somewhere along the way we need to not only become comfortable with all of our attributes, but develop a healthy, humble fondness for them as well. By healthy and humble, I mean a fondness that is neither self-aggrandizing nor self-minimizing or self-effacing, but one that is warm, compassionate, happy and includes a generous portion of humor. This will take time to master. For some traits or attributes it may take years. But the goal here is to fall completely in love with all that we are – warts, haloes and all. One way to begin this love affair is to practice deep-felt, genuine gratitude for each attribute on a daily basis. In Part III, All About Love, we will explore a gratitude practice that can be adapted to this process. However we achieve it, the baseline for nourishment in this channel is to fully embrace what we perceive to be our failings, quirks, foibles and strengths, and to at least entertain the idea that we could, at some point, love ourselves because of them rather than despite them.

What if there is something we really, deeply want to change about ourselves? What if it is so eccentric, challenging or antagonizing to our well-being that we simply can't imagine falling in love with it at all? Well, even if that seems to be the case, acceptance is still the first step to any self-transformation and compassion the beacon that guides our way. The more we deny, dissociate or struggle against who and how we are, the more alienated we become from the possibility of truly transformative nourishment. The more we embrace and care for every aspect of ourselves, the more inevitable the progressive unfolding of our innermost Self and the enduring evolution of our being.

11 - Satisfying Sexuality

All of us are sexual beings, and sexual appetites, feelings and reactions have a consistent influence on how we function from moment to moment. In many ways, the cultural stereotype of the hormone-driven adolescent struggling with their sexual identity and desires is really a projection of the thrall of sexuality we may experience at any age or stage of life from the cradle to the grave. Many attempts have been made in Western culture to soften or even remove some of the taboos surrounding sex, but no matter how liberated we may feel from cultural constraints, our own sexuality and the sexuality of those we love can still be a strange mix of mystery, unpredictability, confusion, excitement and delight.

Before we explore this topic, we first require a working definition of what *satisfying sexuality* means. As a nourishment dimension, satisfying sexuality is any condition or interaction that produces sexual excitement, pleasure or release, which is not injurious to any party involved, and which is not being relied upon as a substitution for another area of nourishment. So pleasurable, non-injurious, non-substitutive sexuality. That said, the full spectrum of what may be satisfying for someone is so broad and varied as to be well beyond the purview of this discussion. And yet it is important not to overlook this essential nourishment center, and to define a recommended baseline as completely as possible.

For instance, it is crucial to include intimacy in any discussion of sexuality. The physical intimacy of comforting contact and the emotional intimacy dependent on openness and trust are in some sense independent of basic sexual satisfaction, and yet all of these frequently become intertwined. For some, assuming that sex naturally leads to intimacy or that intimacy naturally leads to sex creates much confusion in relationships. For one person, emotional and physical intimacy are inextricably linked with sexual arousal and satisfaction; in fact, for them sexual arousal is dependent on feelings of love, physical trust and closeness. For another person, an expectation of such intimacy contrarily interferes with sexual arousal and satisfaction. And there is a continuum of variation to how intimacy and sex are interrelated – based on the nature of a relationship, the level of sexual need, the circumstances of an encounter, personal history and so on. In other words, there is no "normalcy" in the dynamics of sex and intimacy – not for gender or age group, not for established couples or newly hatched romances, not for heterosexuals, homosexuals or bisexuals…not for anyone. We may crave a convenient handle to manage this difficult topic, but the one reality years of absorbing clinical research, providing couples counseling, and discussion with other professionals has shown me is that there are very few common denominators for how sexual intimacy expresses itself in any given relationship or situation.

So what does this mean? It means that the only way to navigate the fog of sexuality is to educate ourselves about what is possible for us, experiment in order to discover what we find preferable, and communicate frequently and openly with our partner throughout the entire process. For those who are shy about their physicality, or who feel uncomfortable discussing sex with anyone, this can be a challenge. But given the right circumstances, with ample breathing room, compassion and patience from all parties, even the most reticent partner can willingly explore and share their experiences, preferences and needs. So, as is usual in any relationship, there is shared responsibility in all communication about this topic, just as there is with any other topic. Ideally, we will want to find partners whose expectations of intimacy in sexuality are similar to our own, so that confusion, incompatibility or inadvertent emotional hurt can be averted. Alternatively, we will have to strike a compromise in our expectations. Sometimes it can be helpful to involve a therapist in the process to create a neutral, safe environment to talk about sex. But the outcome of such therapy should be the open, frank and tactful exchange that lovers must cultivate with each other to succeed.

What does healthy sexual satisfaction look like? Although the details of each individual's experience will be different, the outcomes and evidences are nearly universal – at least in what will be markedly absent. There won't be anger or fights over sex. There won't be guilt or shame. There won't be sadness, isolation or alienation. There won't be boredom, disaffection or contempt. And, unless this is a brand new relationship or newly discovered experimentation, there won't be obsessive preoccupation either. Aside from these absences, very little is probable and nothing is guaranteed. And yet, if we have balance in all the other areas of nourishment, our sexuality is much more likely to express itself in the most healthy, satisfying and constructive ways – no matter how we approach it. This is true for all nourishment centers, but there seems a surprisingly pronounced interdependence between satisfying sexuality and our well-being in every other area of self.

To achieve a useful baseline in this nourishment center, begin by asking yourself: "What is my level of sexual satisfaction overall right now?" Are you content or frustrated? Are you routinely disinterested or do you have an appetite? Is there frequent, open and honest communication on this topic with your partner, have you shut communication down a bit, or does the absence of a partner inhibit your sexual self-expression? Be clear with yourself and your partner on this, while remembering to be patient, gentle and tactful. Once you determine how satisfied you are, you can decide whether to explore new sexual horizons or be joyful, grateful and content with what you have.

> **Resources:** This is such a culturally charged and bias-inducing issue I have yet to find any source I can whole-heartedly recommend. However, some helpful starting places are the Kinsey Institute reports on sex, the Hite reports on female sexuality, and perhaps *Sex in America* by Laumann, Michael and Kolata.

12 - Affirming Integrity

For anything in the Universe to fulfill its potential, it must function in integrity with itself. Every force, condition, phenomenon and spec of dust is held accountable to its own nature, role, responsibility and overall purpose vis-à-vis the natural laws that govern space, energy, matter and time. And yet human consciousness tends to create an exception for itself. Because it has freedom to modify the course of Nature, to imagine different outcomes than those governed by predictable laws, and to act contrary to harmonious and constructive responses, the human mind often mistakenly equates the privilege of this freedom with an entitlement to act on any and all of its conceptions. On the one hand, this has produced wondrous advancements in thought and language, great works of art, almost magical technological inventions, an increasingly global cultural exchange, the astounding ability of our species to adapt to almost any environment on Earth, and a vision of fulfilling our grandest dreams of utopia. On the other, it has led to sophisticated weaponry that can destroy human civilization several times over, artificial epidemics like Type II Diabetes that undermine the quality of human life, the eradication unto extinction of hundreds of species of plant and animal, an explosion of population and exploitation of natural resources that has begun straining the Earth's capacity to sustain human habitation, and the possibility of realizing our worst dystopian nightmare. Over millennia of effort, evolution and applied intelligence we have exchanged the dangers of violent predators, harsh environments and natural darkness for the threat of violence, harsh judgments and preternatural darkness within ourselves. To whatever degree we have subdued the wildness of the Earth to our own benefit, we have emboldened the wildness of our nature to become an equal or greater enemy to the very existence we have striven to perpetuate.

Of course, the same consciousness that challenges the perceived order of the Universe to birth such grand dichotomies is also the seat of profound compassion. What *Integral Lifework* proposes is that whenever the impulse to challenge the governing principles of life is moderated with compassionate affection, we thus ground ourselves in cohesion and harmony again, and reinvigorate our integrity with our own True Nature. I trust this process because I have come to believe, through experience and observation, that the heart of that True Nature is love. And so, when I commit to constructive action, I follow through not from guilt or compulsion or a sense of civic duty, but because I choose to be in love with the beneficiary of that action. When I respond to someone's request, I answer honestly from the heart, and, whenever possible, with an intention amplified by loving kindness. When I spontaneously give of my time, energy or resources, I do so not because it fulfills some moral code or satisfies some karmic obligation, but because it aligns me with my True Nature. This is what Affirming Integrity represents in my life from moment to moment, because as I affirm the compassionate core of my being, I have integrity in all my thoughts, words and actions.

Because Western culture promotes a primarily individualistic, self-serving type of consumerism, the currents that eat away at societal cohesion and harmony in the U.S. can be strong. The resulting lack of integrity is evident everywhere. In competition for parking spots at the mall, in shady business dealings that exploit the vulnerable or unsuspecting, in egotistical power plays in the workplace, in commuter road rage, in bullying attitudes or unkind words at home, in the disconnection and isolation within neighborhoods and families, in the hostility between political factions and belief systems – in other words, in a fracturing of our overall cohesion and accord. And yet we cannot counter the abject consumerism meme by promoting another product, fad, program or policy that repairs this rift from the outside. The rift cannot be repaired via external agents, and further investment in externalized solutions just reinforces the same disempowering meme. We must instead let go of hopes we project outside ourselves and return to the root of our being for answers. By pursuing Affirming Integrity, we reinforce the guidance of that internal compass and amplify its effect on our lives. The natural consequence of this is our valuing what is contributive, collaborative and mutually beneficial above what is self-serving and destructive to the greater good.

What does this look like in terms of baseline nourishment? In concert with nourishing all our other dimensions – in fact, this is really dependent on those coinciding energy exchanges – we can practice a few simple principles. Affirming Integrity is essentially about each nourishment center operating in concert with all others; when we have internal consonance between nourishment dimensions, we have full integrity. What unites our nourishing efforts, what transforms disparate wavelengths into a focused, coherent beam of Light, is the energizing glue of love. If every thought, emotion and action springs from that single source, then everything we accomplish within and without naturally synchronizes with the good of All. Through love, we both constrain and liberate our consciousness to operate in integrity with its own first principles.

One way to remind ourselves of this process is through affirmations, and a few are listed here for you to try. As a starting point you can begin each day by looking at yourself in the mirror and reciting them in sequence, with as much conviction as your current state of being allows:

- "Because I am devoted to my own well-being, I seek understanding in my soul."

- "As I come to know my soul, my heart brims to overflowing with compassionate affection."

- "Because this love overflows my heart, my mind seeks a way to share it with others and let it expand into everything around me."

- "Because my mind discerns the way, I express the boundless love of my heart and the deep understanding of my soul through every action."

- "Because I trust in these intentions without reservation, I let go of the importance of my own involvement."

- "Because I let go of my own importance, the effectiveness of my love is miraculous."

At the end of each day, just before you go to sleep, try reflecting back over your day and assess how these affirmations played out in your thoughts, feelings, actions and interactions. If there are any areas that present special challenges, spend the next day focusing your intentions on those. Remember that the engine behind this overlapping integrity – of soul with heart, heart with mind, mind with actions, actions with outcomes – is committed and diligent multidimensional self-care.

Because of our intention, attention and follow-through in all other nourishment centers, we have a well of loving energy within us to lavish upon the world. Over time, with humility and faith, the depth of that well approaches the Infinite.

How Do We Make Time & Energy to Nourish All Dimensions?

At some point in this chapter, you may have begun to wonder "Is it possible to fit all of this in?" With all those separate channels within each dimension, the prospect may at first seem daunting. But one of the chief characteristics of *Integral Lifework* is that there are certain combinations of practices that actually provide nourishment across all dimensions in extremely efficient ways – a practical alchemy of self-care. Simply by beginning in one or two areas – in dimensions with the greatest need of special attention – you will create an additive synthesis with other nourishment centers. And as you integrate that synthesis into your daily life, you will see that multidimensional nourishment is not as demanding as it may first appear. In Part VI, we will be covering this and other aspects of the self-nourishment learning process in more detail, but the first step is really to acknowledge the importance of each nourishment center. That is, to consecrate each dimension with compassionate intention. If I can evoke a sense within myself that my whole being and its interdependent aspects are deserving of sacred space, then I can create that sacred space in my life for every mode of energy exchange.

Then again, perhaps you already have incorporated much of the nourishment spectra available in each channel, and only need improvement in a handful of areas to achieve the baseline recommendations proposed here. If that is the case, now might be a good time to take a break from reading and outline how you would like to approach those areas. Remember that holistic self-nourishment represents skillful, compassionate affection in the eternal present. There is no separation between our capacity and ability to love and our capacity and ability to nurture ourselves. And as we achieve wholeness through these efforts, that wholeness allows us to amplify love everywhere around us, expanding the sacred into larger and larger arenas of inclusion. As within, so without.

PART III

ALL ABOUT LOVE

How We Learn to Love

After introducing so many integral ideas and disciplines, we can explore beyond those foundations to the primary energizer, facilitator and ultimate objective of integral practice: love. Does each of us have an innate facility to love from the moment we are born, or do we learn what love is from our environment as we develop? In *Integral Lifework* it is assumed that all personal attributes have seeds in our native being, but our environment shapes how those attributes are expressed as we mature. A child submerged in a fearful and angry home may have more of a challenge relaxing into loving relationships than a child who was supported by love and acceptance growing up, but the kernel of love is always present and waiting for an opportunity to spring forth. But what if we have never witnessed compassion that we believe to be both genuine and effective? What if we have never experienced the kind of affection that profoundly nourishes us, and helps us grow strong in our heart and spirit? Will our ignorance prevent us from ever offering or receiving that kind of love?

Love expresses itself in countless ways, and none is more complex than the love between parent and child. At any given moment in the relationship with our parents, from our earliest childhood to old age, we will observe and generate feelings we associate with love, and each experience will evoke countless other emotional associations. This is how most of us learn to imitate the unfolding of loving relationships in our lives. So how can we sort through the tangle of often conflicting intentions, impulses and emotions to distill the most loving responses? As much as we may sometimes wish, we cannot escape how the past has shaped our sense of self, or the importance of our past and present relationships with our family of origin. To better untangle this conundrum, let's look at a real life example.

Most of my clients seek me out because they are suffering. That suffering can be emotional, physical, mental, or even spiritual. It can range in intensity from something they want to address because of a New Year's resolution to an increasingly compelling rationale for committing suicide. The perceived source or flash point could be a difficult relationship, stress at work, resurfacing grief from past trauma, physical illness, or any number of other life conditions. Often they initially seek help to deal with this perceived source of pain, and so that is where integral exploration begins. But that is rarely where it ends, for a therapeutic rule in *Integral Lifework* is that, with very few exceptions, the actual source of our suffering exists in another arena entirely from that where our symptoms present; some area of our life where we are severely undernourished, and where aren't yet aware of the deprivation. One way to describe this is to say that some part of ourselves is no longer loved – and perhaps has never been loved at all. And without love, the foundation of all real nourishment, that part of us is shriveling into nonexistence.

Theresa's Journey

Theresa is in her mid-thirties, newly married and, in principle, looking forward to starting a family. But she is terrified. Every time she thinks of becoming pregnant she becomes physically ill. Often this manifests as an irritating rash over most of her body, accompanied by fatigue, irritable bowels, confusion, trouble sleeping, mood swings, food allergies, severe headaches and a host of other debilitating symptoms. At different times she has been diagnosed with hypothyroid, chronic fatigue syndrome and other illnesses relating to her immune system. She has tried a wide variety of traditional and alternative treatments, but nothing seems to resolve her discomfort for very long. Now she has sought out *Integral Lifework* in the hopes of arriving at a new perspective on her illness and to overcome her trepidations surrounding pregnancy.

After our first few sessions, it becomes clear that Theresa is depleted in several areas of self-nourishment. For the last two years – the first years of her marriage – she has avoided hobbies and activities she once enjoyed, especially those that are solitary or don't include her husband.

Everything that remains in her life has become part of an overarching plan: to create a safe, reliable environment for her future child. And Theresa has a core belief that such stability will depend on her banishing all activities and desires that she feels are self-indulgent or might compete with her child's needs being met. This same tendency is reflected in her marital relationship, where she rarely states her own desires or interests, but defaults to her husband's will. As a result, Theresa is exhausted and despairing, and her body is crying out for help.

In *Integral Lifework* vernacular, Theresa is experiencing barriers to self-nourishment, especially in the areas of creative self-expression and belief in her personal purpose. Simply trying to push back against these barriers by implementing new nourishment routines has not worked for her. In fact, this has backfired by inciting even more rebellion and chaos in an already conflicted matrix of drives and needs. So the barriers must first be identified, accepted and either overcome or effectively managed by Theresa. Only then can she begin nourishing herself completely again. For most of my clients, this is where the really difficult work begins, and Theresa takes this task on with courage and determination.

So what barriers does Theresa discover? So many, and in so many different channels, that at first it is a bit overwhelming for her. Here are just a few of the substantial barrier mechanisms we uncovered in her first few sessions:

- Unresolved grief about the death of a close family member. Though it happened years ago, this event was never fully processed or integrated. Her emotions surrounding this loss are still deep felt, raw and powerful.

- Guilt about physical impulses and intimate desires she had as a young girl. At the time, they seemed natural and brought her intense moments of joy. But as she grew older, she was conditioned to believe they were inappropriate and ugly.

- Anger and hurt over her mother's perceived abandonment of her at an early age. Feelings of loneliness, isolation and anxiety surrounding these repeated events in childhood.

- An unidentifiable darkness, dirtiness and suffocating bleakness that overwhelms her when she tries to touch certain aspects of her inner self or certain parts of her past. When she accesses this space, she feels depleted, empty and flat.

All of these discoveries really center around one kind of debilitating experience: the bitterly felt absence of love. The family member who died had never openly expressed their love for Theresa, nor had she ever been able to communicate her own loving feelings, and yet there had always been an affectionate connection between them. Because their love was never openly expressed or honored, the grief is as much a loss of opportunity to communicate love openly as a loss of the connection itself. Consider also her guilt about physical desires which, at the time, were a natural and loving way to care for herself. Here, too, love was denied open and honest expression, for over time she was no longer allowed to honor her body's needs or allow herself the same carefree joy. Her mother's leaving withdrew a loving and supportive relationship at a critical time in Theresa's understanding of safety, trust and nourishment; how could she now believe that giving or receiving parental love could ever be reliable, or that she could provide a safe and stable environment for her own child? And finally there is the unknown darkness and taintedness that testifies to something deep within that her conscious mind cannot accept or process.

In all of these experiences and associations, love has been vanquished. In its place are other strong emotions that bury loving impulses and keep love from surfacing in all its natural strength. And this is the landscape in which Theresa wanted to bring new life into the world; these are the principles of incompleteness, instability, hurt, shame and woundedness that Theresa strongly associates with love. This is what she has learned love is. It should be no surprise that the undernourished parts of her rebelled and sabotaged her physical well-being. After all, with such deeply felt barriers as models for her future, how could Theresa believe that fully loving herself, her husband or her child could ever really be permitted in this life, or result in anything but more disappointment and pain? And as with all occurrences of undernourishment, the patterns Theresa was attempting to substitute for love (reflexively supporting her husband, working harder, denying her own interests, pushing herself to have a child, etc.) were creating ever more dissonance within.

So how will Theresa find her way back to fully loving and allowing love in her life? How will she heal and nourish those wounded parts of herself so that she can sustain the vision she has for her future? How will she grow in strength and purposefulness in the light of these weaknesses and impediments to joy? How will she unlearn the broken-hearted version of love that her life has taught her up till now? As with all transformations, the first steps are small ones. Our focus of the next couple of sessions is on reorienting Theresa's efforts from external to internal, to first have compassion for her own pain and care for the young girl who was so confused, abandoned and wounded. And as she begins to reach out to her younger self in comfort and support, the arrested grief and buried tears can finally flow. In Theresa's case, most of this work is in the form of guided meditation and imagery, where she can visualize her younger self and interact with that child in supportive ways. With each healing effort, Theresa gains more volitional influence over her own past. In other words, she is empowered to act as an adult on her younger self's behalf, whereas previously she carried all the helplessness of her childhood suffering around with her. And as we work through each painful experience together, Theresa finds the strength to project a more complete love and affection on a child who experienced the love of others in incomplete ways. In other words, she begins to love herself, rather than projecting that love energy outward into everything else in her life.

This is the onset of self-energizing that occurs when barriers are reduced through interior work. Theresa could then begin integrating different self-care practices with less resistance, and nourish herself in dimensions that had been neglected for years. And as she persists in those efforts, she gains ever more confidence that her decisions in other areas of her life will be self-sustaining rather than depleting. Over time, her anxiety about starting a family begins to ebb. Her chronic symptoms diminish, and her mood, sense of life direction and overall well-being stabilize. There are still some self-sabotaging impulses she has to manage, but she now has new skills and fortifications she can call upon. I believe there is still something large and scary in her past that she has not yet confronted, but as with any healing process the journey progresses in stages. In this stage, Theresa has learned what healthy love looks like by beginning to love herself and care for her childhood pain, and that is all she needs for now to find a way forward.

So this is one example of how we can relearn love and self-care in contrast to our childhood experiences. Not everyone is as courageous as Theresa in mining their depths for sources of pain and malnourishment. The desire to relieve suffering through external means, through some sort of quick, cathartic fix that does not involve self-examination or ongoing effort, is strongly reinforced by American culture and many traditional approaches. If I can take a pill or a weekend seminar that relieves my anxiety, why should I bother with all this work? If I can consume a solution, why should I produce a solution from my own effort? The answer is, of course, that unless an intervention is needed to avert a life-threatening condition, all a short-term fix can do is muffle the cries of our own being, like putting a wailing baby in a sound-proof room. The cries will continue whether we hear them or not, and unless we address the underlying cause, our being will become ever more depleted and ill. Consuming solutions will always be an inadequate substitution for producing them ourselves.

Intimacy with the Spiritual Self and the Ground of Being

As we begin to address barriers to self-care that have woven themselves into our life, there is another concurrent effort we can cultivate for love to become fully formed within and fully expressed without. We can come to know and unconditionally embrace our innermost Self, as well as the ground of being from which that Self emanates. Another way to say this is that we must fall in love with an evolving soul as it is expressed individually in us and collectively in All That Is. Language fails a bit here, because this kind of intimate embrace must be experienced to be fully understood – and perhaps even to be believed. The mystic activation exercise at the end of Part I aims us in the direction of eventual emersion in an all-inclusive Absolute, but what allows us to wholly inhabit our own essence and the essence of the Universe itself is once again love. So we must love ever more deeply in order to arrive at each new stage of spiritual intimacy and acquiescence. Spiritual connection introduces us to a vaster sea of compassionate affection, and the energy we draw upon to swim through that ocean is also love. In other words, without nourishment in the dimension of Authentic Spirit, we will rarely be able to connect fully or skillfully in other levels of relationship. Just as the dimension of Supportive Community provides opportunity to develop loving connections, the intensity with which we care for our own spiritual well-being solidifies those connections on ever-advancing levels.

It is easy to generalize that without complete nourishment in all of our dimensions we will be less able to love others effectively. If we are not fully charged as a whole person, we will quickly run out of the internal resources necessary to share that energy with others. But more often than with any other, the spiritual dimension of our lives tends to be substituted with other nourishment in the rush and tumble of modern life. Once that happens, we become like Sisyphus, forever bearing the burdens of the world up a mountain with extraordinary effort, only to eventually lose our grip on things just as we arrive at tranquility and true compassion.

In my work with clients and students from many different backgrounds, I have frequently encountered the same kinds of resistance to spiritual nourishment. There are countless and elaborate reasons available to excuse us from a spiritual connection. The anger and pain surrounding past experiences with organized religion, for instance, or a disbelief in the substance of our own spiritual being. I often hear recounting of research that proves the ineffectiveness of prayer, or complaints that observed suffering in the world and any form of spiritual belief are somehow incompatible. Sometimes it's just a vague incredulity about the whole "spirituality thing." At the other extreme, there are the confident assertions about personal spiritual achievements, the importance of careful adherence to certain religious systems, or the impossibility or danger of real spiritual connection in the context of certain self-limiting beliefs. Altogether, this can add up to a huge amount of interference.

Most of the time, however, such excuses do not represent failed efforts at genuine spirituality. Instead, they represent other failures. A failure to relinquish self-protective ego and acquiesce to a broader, more inclusive and transpersonal sense of self. A failure to differentiate between religious dogma and spiritual connection. A failure to heal from past hurts and move on to more jubilant living. A failure to supplant fear with love. A failure to embrace doubt and insecurity in the face of the vast, unknowable breadth of our existence. Harshly judging such failures does not avail us much, but recognizing them and working through them to a higher plane of compassionate awareness is a self-justifying effort. In the same vein, I would never assert that atheists or secular humanists are fragmented souls in need of spiritual healing, but I would insist that all beings have a spiritual dimension that requires care and feeding – there is simply a need to work through semantic differences to make that dimension accessible to everyone. Otherwise, the more we deny nourishment to that part of ourselves or any other, the more we cripple our ability to love effectively.

A Child's Eyes Are Opened

Most of us share many of the same developmental landmarks on our journey to adulthood. We cry to get fed and receive attention. We compete with siblings for the approval of our parents. We test the limits of our power with kids in our neighborhood and at school to determine the local pecking order and win appreciation and status among our peers. We try to understand ourselves in the context of community and society at large. We explore sexuality and romantic feelings amid hormonal confusion and emotional insecurity. And of course I went through all of this as well, and it is challenging – to the say the least – to clearly appreciate compassionate affection in this developmental context. It is, in fact, an extremely rare event. But there are moments along the way, which, if they are shaped by the broader understanding of the human condition, offer insights into how to love, and how to love effectively.

I received a great deal of loving kindness throughout my early life, but I could not recognize it for what it was, mainly because my primary examples of caring were wounded and debilitated in their own capacity to love. My parents divorced when I was two and struggled for years to regain their equilibrium. My mother suffered from intense mood swings and auditory hallucinations that she experienced as demeaning and accusatory; as a result, she became enraged, violent and abusive on a daily basis with very little provocation. My father was distant and dismissive, medicating his own pain with nicotine and alcohol, and parenting with a harsh, authoritarian style. Neither found much happiness or contentment during the years I lived with them, and neither was able to experience healthy, satisfying relationships within their family or in subsequent romantic involvements. My natural grandparents on both sides were either distant or controlling, and with the exception of an aunt and uncle on my father's side, I really had no examples of what introspection, encouragement or relaxed joyfulness looked like within my own family. It became clear to me at an early age that physical, sexual and psychological abuse, codependent reactions, emotional pain and loss were the baseline of all intimate relationships. So even when I was confronted with sincere compassion, I tended to mistrust it as manipulative maneuvering.

My mom's boyfriends sometimes tried to befriend me, but I didn't trust their intentions either. My dad's girlfriends tried to be supportive, but I was equally skeptical of their efforts. Despite my resistance, I did receive a lot of encouragement and caring from these quarters, but like most children I was always looking to my parents for clues to my own identity and worthiness. At different times in my early childhood I had a step-sister who was kind to me and fiercely protective, a school counselor who patiently helped me understand myself despite my outrageous misbehavior, and even a foster family who showed me what unhinged humor, gentle forbearance, clear emotional boundaries and integrity looked like. That was a revelation, but I couldn't trust it to extend beyond the walls of their home, could I? I had childhood friends who cared deeply for me and whose families accepted me into their home without hesitation. I even had a girlfriend or two who accepted me and cared for me in my damaged condition. Then came a new set of step-grandparents, from my father's third wife, who engaged me with clear reasoning, sharp wit and selfless generosity. At the same time, I was immersed in high school environment that welcomed and inspired me, with one teacher in particular who took genuine and extensive interest in my well-being. I also found new peers who reinforced friendship and sharing without any agendas. Could it be that the world was a friendlier place than I had imagined, and that I could not only become lovable but perhaps even love others without either of us being harmed...?

Not in a brilliant flash, but in a gradual, painstaking process of unfolding I began to believe in the possibility of love and let go of my childhood pain. My eyes were slowly being pried open with each constructive experience. Still, when I felt cornered, I could only respond in the ways I had learned to express connection: to criticize, lash out, placate, command, test, accuse…and so on. But as I began to relax into more supportive exchanges I saw the ineffectiveness of those antics. Still, I don't think I took the final leap of faith until, well, I took a leap of faith. At age eighteen, I was introduced to an authentically love-centered brand of Christianity. As much as I believed it to be a rational choice at the time, what really moved me to embrace that tradition was the love the folks of that church demonstrated toward each other – and toward me. This community was alive with an intensity of empathy and caring I had never experienced; there seemed to be no exhaustion of support and affection. Something was working powerfully in and through these believers, and I had to know what that was. They were connected to each other and to something greater than themselves that really did lead to joy. What could it be?

Although I caught glimpses of the answer, my process of discovery was tested in an unfortunate marriage and preoccupation with material security, followed by painful divorce and a concurrent disillusionment with my spiritual community. Although I learned much about myself and the nature of relationship and community from these adventures, my journey into healing was derailed for a time. Instead, I began to seek out substitutions. I threw myself into destructive romantic relationships. I engaged in hobbies with a high degree of risk, such riding my motorcycle fast and aggressively, skiing recklessly down a mountain side, or hiking alone in deep wilderness during extreme weather without adequate gear. And I isolated myself – rejecting or sabotaging long-term friendships and distancing myself both physically and emotionally from my family of origin. Of course, none of these satisfied my longing for love or helped me heal from the wounds of my past.

Over time, as my existence spun further out of control and my body began to communicate through illness and malfunction how out-of-balance I had become, I at first tried to treat symptoms superficially. Masking them, really – with entertainment, food, alcohol and drugs. I found that both urban culture and traditional Western medicine could skillfully oblige me in these engineered escapes. So I did that for a few years, and my various illnesses and conditions worsened to the point of seriously impeding my health and well-being. At last, when the pain and degradation of my quality of life became too great to ignore, I resolved to explore some causal factors through alternative therapies. And that was the first step in my surrender: realizing I needed help, that I wasn't caring for myself in constructive ways, and that my reliance on commoditized support systems wasn't helping at all.

We frequently hear stories of great epiphanies and cathartic peaks that have had a transformative effect on people. And, sometimes, both major and minor life events can trigger such realizations. But the realizations in themselves are not all that useful unless we follow through with some level of reformed or reconsidered action. The journey that begins with careful self-examination never ends, but leads to a natural unfolding of authentic Self. For that Self to emerge, however, there is a parallel process of letting go. Letting go of personas that interfere with that True Self's expression in day-to-day life. Letting go of habits that interfere with high quality nourishment. Letting go of attachments to specific goals or outcomes that run counter to our well-being. Letting go of all the compulsive wants that reinforce our ego. And letting go of both emotional pain and the past events that have caused it. And this recurring theme of letting go was perhaps the most important lesson I had to learn.

The following are some moments of healing, growth and transformation that occurred during my process of self-examination. I think of them as complimentary bookends to the traumas I experienced earlier in life.

- At 19, submitting to a spiritual discipline that stripped me of all my certainty, egoistic bluster and ardent cynicism, allowing me to absorb the true kindness and caring of strangers just as unconditionally as it was being offered. During this time I let go of what I had thought was most important for my own survival, and tried a different way of prioritizing and expressing my personal values for a time.

- At 21, under the guidance of a therapist named Rudi, learning to cry when I was in pain instead of becoming angry. Here I let go of anger as a first response to frustration or confusion. I also let go of some wrong-headedness about what being strong and assertive looked like.

- At 25, experiencing a divorce that brought all of my insecurity, fear and self-loathing to the surface. After initially running away from it, I began to examine some deeper turbulence, identifying early experiences that had introduced patterns of pain and grief, and letting go of those experiences one by one, primarily through forgiving those who had injured me and healing my relationship with them. This was facilitated by talk therapy and the gentle honesty and generous support of a few close friends immediately after my divorce.

- At 28, beginning to learn how to care for myself physically through better nutrition, regular exercise, and attenuation of long-term vices like sugar and caffeine. Here I began letting go of many things at once: habits that had brought comfort or distraction in the past; a deeply held belief that I didn't deserve to be well or whole; an egoistic conviction that I had boundless energy and was indestructible; and so on.

Such was the process of unfolding for the next several years, exploring different avenues of self-awareness and self-care until I cam face to face with the fundamental emotions, beliefs and behaviors that disrupted my nourishment and happiness. This is an essential part of the first stage of surrendering to love: becoming aware of what barriers exist and, slowly, coming to accept them. Both the awareness and the acceptance can come through similar means. Prayer, introspection, meditation, talk therapy, spiritual practices, certain physical disciplines, body-centered techniques designed to release buried or somatic memories – all of these can remove the veil to truths we hold within. But acceptance does not always follow naturally on the heels of awareness. Much more commonly, old habits press us to escape, avoid or deny them after an initial catharsis. For me, in some areas it took almost a decade to journey from a realization of the truth to my acceptance of that truth. During those years, I was gradually learning how to let go on mental, emotional, physical and spiritual levels. Then, once the reflex of letting go was imbedded as a mode of being in a particular area, acceptance could come rushing in to fill the void, thereby vanquishing the anger, grief, guilt, shame or resentment that had lingered for so long.

Jagged Stones

There was an old man with a sack of sharp, jagged stones
   which he carried with him everywhere
It was a large sack, and heavy, so he had to hold it
   with both hands
     and he could not carry anything else
In fact, it was so stuffed with stones
   he could barely see over the top
    its weight bent him over like a wilting plant
      and some of the pointy rocks poked through
        scratching him badly as he stumbled along

One day, a young child asked "Why do you carry such a big bag of stones?"
   "They're important to me," the old man answered
    "I've spend my whole life collecting them, you see."
"Oh," said the child. "Why are they important?"
At just that moment, the old man stumbled again
  crying out in pain
   "Aaaaah! Another one!" he bellowed
As the child watched, the old man set the big sack down
   dug another sharp, jagged stone out of the dirt
    and tossed it into his lumpy, swollen sack
"You see?" he said, "Every single one that has ever caused me pain goes into my bag"
"Oh. Yes, I see," said the child
Then the old man was on his way again
   stopping every so often to pick up another rock
    while the child followed after

Just as the day was coming to an end
   the young child stumbled noisily and cried out, "Ouch!"
The old man stopped. "What's wrong?" he asked the child
"I just stepped on a sharp rock, too!" the child replied excitedly
The old man smiled
   "Then you'll have to get yourself a nice, big sack," he said
   "Because you can only hold a few sharp rocks
    with such tiny little hands."

Thus began my reformation. By finally embracing love as the guiding and energizing force in my life, all the scars and barriers from childhood – and those intervening rigors of suffering – began to melt away. There would be helpful therapy and new relationships that taught me more about the nature of affection and how to become more loving in my self-concept and interactions, and there would be new spiritual horizons that would deepen my exposure to the essence of compassion. There would be failures and recoveries, hopes dashed and rekindled, externally enforced changes and internally inspired ones. But given my beginnings and my failures along the way, I remain amazed that I found a lighted path to the home of my heart. It is that amazement and wonder that convinces me that everyone, no matter how mistreated or wounded by suffering they may be, can find their way out of personal darkness to the blazing fires of love.

We can of course be introduced to love through the examples of others, and our own exploration of different levels of affection through intimate relationships will pry our heart open wide, but it is my belief that the door to the high art of true love can only be opened through integral discipline. As we strengthen our being through exchanges at every level, we create new synergies and synchronicities that add layer upon layer of intensity and complexity to our subjective encounters with compassion and our ability to express it. As we explore and support each dimension of our being, we encounter and expand all dimensions of the Whole. Eventually, as every part of us amplifies and supports every other, a critical mass of affection sparks perpetual momentum. Without even realizing what has happened, we catch fire. And if we continue to tend that fire, fueling ourselves with integral practice, its warmth will sustain us through any calamity, and its light will create a beacon through all kinds of shadow and doubt.

The great adventure of life is the discovery of love as the center and substance of everything. As a friend recently quoted to me: *amo ergo sum* – I love therefore I am. That is the final horizon towards which we are summoned from our first breath, and the abyss into which we must willingly fall if we wish to comprehend the meaning of our existence.

Loving Skillfully, With Discernment

One of the most formidable challenges in loving ourselves, others and All that Is is learning how to reliably contribute to the most beneficial outcomes for everyone. In U.S. culture, there are many widely accepted practices that we are conditioned to believe represent love. These practices may even have highly charged expectations in our family, in the workplace, among friends or in our support communities, and in society at large. However, in reality they may not be all that loving, instead creating barriers to true love, even to the point of counterproductive harm. Consider the following examples:

- An older man I meet on the street, whom I presume to be homeless and down on his luck, asks for money for food. Out of a sincere desire to help, I give him ten dollars. The next day, I meet him again on the street and he thanks me for the bottle of whiskey he bought with the money. His knuckles are torn and bloody and he has bruises all over his face. When I asked what happened, he says he got really drunk off the whiskey he bought and then fought with a friend. They are still so angry with each other he doesn't know if they will ever speak again.

- A young woman and her new boyfriend are about to have sex for the first time. They have already agreed to use a condom, but at the last minute, her boyfriend asks if they can continue without one. "I love you," he says. "Everything will be okay." The young woman, feeling very much in love, lost in the moment, and wanting to make her boyfriend happy, acquiesces. Unfortunately, her boyfriend unknowingly transmitted an STD to her in this way...so things were not all that okay between them after that.

- A wife complains to her husband that she is having bad cramps in her legs. He suggests that she go see their doctor, but she's too busy to go. The next day the cramps are worse, and the husband insists that she see someone, but the wife says he's being overly dramatic, and further that if he really loved her, he would offer to rub her legs to alleviate the pain. Out of guilt and concern, the husband agrees to massage her legs. The next morning, the husband finds that his beloved wife has died during the night. It is discovered that she in fact had large blood clots in both her legs, and that when the muscles were massaged, the clots broke free and migrated to her lungs and brain.

- A manager comes across one of her employees who is falling asleep at his cubicle. She is surprised, and asks what is going on. He's tired, he explains, because he's been working so many long hours. She encourages him to take more breaks, and to leave work on time, and he agrees to do so. At the same time, she knows he is one of the most productive employees she has, so she doesn't want to push to hard for him to work less hours. But a few days later in a department meeting, he nods off again. After the meeting, she again explains to him that he can't be falling asleep during work. He promises to change his habits, but over the next few weeks it becomes clear that he is a workaholic and can't make these changes without help. So the manager ignores the situation, knowing she can't easily replace his level of productivity, which benefits her whole team. Slowly but surely, morale begins to dip in her department. Other employees are taking long lunches or coming in late. When the manager confronts them about it, they declare, "Hey, you let him sleep at his desk and straight through most of our meetings!" Not too long after that, the higher-ups notice a pronounced drop in overall productivity for her team. And not long after that, the rumors about "the manager's favorite narcoleptic" filter up to higher management as well. Under increasing pressure, the manager is forced to fire the workaholic, and for the next few months she is fighting for her own job as she tries to pull the shattered bits of her team back together.

- A young boy tells his father that his stomach aches and he doesn't want to go to school. The father sees that his son is in real discomfort, but he wants his son to grow up strong. He knows what will happen if people think his boy is weak, because of what happened to him when he was young. "It's a tough world out there. You're going to have to face up to that some day." And he sends his son trudging off through a wintry morning to school. But the boy never gets there. He has acute appendicitis and his appendix bursts. When his father gets the call that his son never arrived at school, he rushes out to find him. But by the time he does, it's too late.

- A middle-aged woman has a dog that cannot swim, but she has just moved into a new home with a large, deep swimming pool. Out of concern for her dog, she arranges to have a fence installed around the pool, and resolves to keep her dog inside until the fence is in. But her dog is not used to being inside so much. He whines and begs to be let out, and then won't even come back inside when she calls him. To the dog's credit, he at least seems to stay away from the pool while he is outside. Out of sympathy for her dog's desire to be outdoors, the woman lets him stay in the back yard all day while she is at work. When she comes home, she finds that her dog has somehow fallen into the pool and drowned.

- After a stressful day at work I feel a strong desire to escape that stress or just collapse into a puddle. So that's what I do. First a little TV. Then maybe a beer or a glass of wine. Then some junk food. And I coast right on through till bedtime in a foggy glob of self-medicated numbness. When I try to sleep, I toss and turn all night as the stress from my day resurfaces. I awake groggy and irritated, resisting the day and all the new stresses is promises. I am sure that I am the victim and my only course of action is to endure long enough through my working hours to escape once more into TV, alcohol and simple carbohydrates.

There is a not-so-subtle pattern among these responses. First of all, these are not irresponsible or thoughtless people. They believe they are doing something considerate and caring. But in choosing what may seem an easier path, a path in which an expressed or implied want is expediently met, underlying needs are really being neglected. How often have we chosen fulfilling a superficial want rather than discerning the underlying, sometimes critical need? This is a common affliction of our species when authentic, skillful love is absent. So what would it look like if the mode of love in each of these examples had been authentic and skillful? Here is what might have happened:

- When the homeless man asked me for money, we talked for a little bit and I offered to buy him a sandwich. He thanked me but said no, what he really wanted was a drink. I said I couldn't do that for him, but that I would be coming back by tomorrow and the sandwich offer would still stand. He nodded and looked away, irritated. Then, after a moment, he turned to meet my eyes and offered me his hand. It was a very dirty hand, but I took it and held it. "I'll see you tomorrow," I said. When I noticed the tears in his eyes, I was surprised...and moved. He smiled and said, "Nobody's really looked at me for a long time. You know, really looked at me as a person. Thank you for that."

- The young woman smiled at her lover and said softly, "You know I want you like that, but it's too soon for me...without protection. I guess we could both go and get tested, you know, for STDs, and then we'll know it's safe." Her boyfriend was upset by this at first, but when he calmed down he agreed it was a good idea. They went to a community clinic the very next day and both got tested for free.

- For the first time in a long while, the husband decided to be stubborn with his wife. "You know I love you, so I don't think that's a fair thing to say. If you want me to rub your legs, please just ask. But whatever this pain is, it came out of nowhere and is getting worse, so I think it would be wise to drive you to the doctor's right now so we can find out what's wrong. Or you can just keep dealing with the pain yourself. Let me know what you want to do...."

- Once she realized that her workaholic employee wasn't going to change his behavior without help, the manager scheduled a disciplinary meeting with him. They reviewed a written summary of the problem together, and brainstormed ways to remedy it within a specific timeline. He agreed that if he was unable to make the necessary changes in the agreed upon amount of time, he would see a therapist about managing his impulse to overwork. Soon afterward it became evident that he wasn't making progress on his own. So he began working with a counselor. Within a few weeks, he was far less stressed about his job and, to everyone's surprise, even more productive than he was before. Not only was the rest of the team impressed with how the manager handled this, but the higher ups noticed the spike in productivity as well. At her annual review, the manager felt quite justified in asking for raises for all the members of her team.

- When his son told him his stomach hurt, the father decided it was time for a lesson in toughness. "I'll let you stay home from school, but you're going to have to do some work for me around the house." And despite the boy's many protests, he was put to work sweeping snow off the front sidewalk. In a short while, however, the father could see his son was doubled over in real pain. He looked pretty sick as well. So the father trundled his son into the car, and off they went to the Emergency Room, which ended up saving his life.

- After she had taken him on his morning walk, when her dog kept trying to paw through the door to get outside, she ignored him. Just as he had done the previous few days, he whined and barked and looked longingly out to the back yard, but she hardened her resolve. She made coffee and toast, listened to the radio, all the while avoiding eye contact with her dog. Eventually, he stopped whining and lay down on the floor. "Good boy!" she said, and promptly gave him a treat. After a few days, he stopped whining after his walk, and although he peed on the kitchen floor once or twice, she was glad she kept him inside until the pool fence was installed.

- After a stressful day at work I feel the strong urge to escape that stress or just collapse into a puddle, but I know from experience what will help manage that stress much better. I should go for a long walk outside, stretching my muscles and my whole being, allowing it to expand into the world around me. After a day of being protectively closed up tight to the onslaughts of a demanding work environment, I let go and open up. I breathe. I introduce some positive feelings, hormones and energies into my mind, heart, body and spirit. I give myself time and space to be myself, perhaps I stop to chat with a neighbor along the way, or smell some flowers in the public garden down the street, or play with the neighborhood dogs and cats. And when my walk is done, I feel refreshed and energized, so when the day comes to an end I sleep soundly and long. When I awake refreshed and content in the morning, I even harbor some hope that I can make a difference in that stressful and sometimes antagonistic workplace.

Aside from the difference in immediate outcomes, how do these two sets of examples differ qualitatively? There are some clear differences here. In the first set of unskillful examples, the caring intent is not backed up with disciplined effort. Instead, the easier and less confrontational path is taken. In the very first example, I feel sorry for the homeless person, so to quickly assuage my guilt I give money without really understanding the human wants or needs I am addressing. But if I truly take the time to understand the need behind the want, and then genuinely engage the situation and concretely contribute to a remedy or positive outcome, I invite a real connection with another human being. This means decelerating into emotional spacetime, being energetically present to the demands of an immediate situation, ready to offer what I can with compassion and discernment. I think this is a great working definition for blessing someone with love. Of course these same principles apply to meeting our own innermost needs as well. By paying attention to what nourishes and sustains me and creating space, time and self-discipline for those needs to be met, I bless myself. And when we examine the contrasting sets of examples, a pattern emerges for unskillful loving as well. In the unskillful responses, the initial spark of concern or affection is diluted by the hurried and reflexive habits that appear on the surface to be loving, but aren't. In such situations we can excuse ourselves from sincere effort by defaulting to what is expedient. Ironically, the negative consequences of unskillful loving can require much more effort to mend than taking time to meet the initial need.

Why do we often take such short-cuts in loving ourselves and others? This is where things get interesting, because it reveals underlying dynamics and the sources of various barriers to love inhabiting daily life. Often, our impulse to nurture others without discerning real needs or using effective methods stems from one or more of the following conditions:

- **We are afraid of being embarrassed, caught in some fault, or ridiculed.** Public shame is a powerful deterrent. Our self-protective ego does not want to reveal any vulnerabilities or shortcomings to the world around us, and when we are in its thrall we will do almost anything to avoid exposure. We have all seen three-year-olds who vehemently deny having made a mess in the kitchen, teenagers who swear they aren't really hanging out with the strange new kid at school, parents who can't admit to their family that they are about to lose their job, elders who forcefully reject observations that their lifelong abilities are failing. Avoiding embarrassment can lead anyone at any time of life down long, circuitous paths of misdirected effort.

- **We are confused or unsure about the best course of action.** Not knowing what to do but feeling compelled to do something – perhaps too quickly – can lead us into some stormy waters. And sometimes, to compensate for our feelings of inadequacy or incompetence, we may even forge ahead more forcefully, rejecting guidance or warnings because we feel we should know and are ultimately responsible for outcomes. I remember counseling one acquaintance about his extraordinary efforts to sacrifice his own well-being for the perceived benefit of loved ones. He was injuring and endangering himself in order to satisfy the unexpressed wants of others, certain that it was his responsibility to compensate for, and protect them from, their fears and worries. But nothing seemed to calm the storm. When I brought this pattern to his attention, he responded with anger. "I think I know what's best for my family!" he declared. Of course, not only was it clear he had lost his way with regard to effectively loving others, he had also sabotaged his own well-being in the process, all because he didn't know what to do, while feeling compelled to do something.

- **We are attached to being nice.** Have you ever felt euphoria when someone you cared about praised you for doing something thoughtful and loving? Or become elated when you were generous or caring towards someone without their even knowing it. These are normal responses to efforts at niceness. But what if we can't stand the thought of someone thinking we are *not* a nice person? What if failing to be considered nice makes us worried, upset, anxious or depressed? What if being perceived as being nice is more important to us than actually doing what is most compassionate or caring for someone else? Or what if generating those feelings of joy and euphoria on a regular basis becomes part of our identity or our sense of well-being, and we are loath to sacrifice those feelings for a difficult or confrontational interaction? These are signs that a normal outpouring of love has morphed into an addiction to being nice. It's a subtle thing, but it's pretty easy to observe in others. It's also to easy to recognize in ourselves if we find our own happiness has become dependent either on the happiness of others, or on their praise, appreciation or positive perception of who we are.

- **We are nervous about becoming responsible or accountable.** This is one of many characteristics of what appears to be a growing trend in American culture – what I refer to as *living in arrested adolescence* – and it is perhaps the most pronounced and easy to recognize of such traits. It is rooted in the simple desire to avoid growing up; to reject the mantle of adult responsibility and find comfort in escaping from societal expectations of roles, personal contributions and so forth. With all the pressures, rapid change and contradicting demands of modern society, this isn't a surprising reaction. To avoid personal responsibility, default to reflexive and superficial acts of kindness, and to rebel against cooperative effort, mutual connection and intimacy are appealing to the Peter Pan in all of us, especially if we haven't had inspiring or attractive role models. I believe another reason for this trend is that many people feel their childhood was too rushed, managed or contained. They never had a chance to "be a kid" when they were young, so they feel compelled to act out their fantasy of what childhood means when they leave home. But if I am trapped in arrested adolescence, I am simply too insecure to love myself or others in an effective or responsible way.

- **We feel overwhelmed, depressed or depleted.** This is generally about thresholds for enduring stress and or an inability to generate emotional energy, and is not always a matter of choice. Many types of anxiety and depressive disorders are physiological in nature – a structural barrier to love we may have dealt with all our lives. Or we may not realize that our particular physiology requires more of a certain nutrient than other people. Or we might have an undiagnosed chronic illness that is constantly draining or constricting our energy. The same symptoms might also be the result of unconscious habits that have depleted us over time.

- **We enjoy our position of being needed and relied upon.** If we are truly effective in blessing someone with love, they may become self-sufficient. But if our identity is wrapped up in helping people, this can make us feel less important – or even as if we are somehow failing. This can happen between parent and child, teacher and student, manager and employee, therapist and client and so on. It's been a great litmus test for my own integral counseling. For instance, I have observed that the biggest leaps in a client's awareness and their acquisition of new tools usually happen within four or five sessions. After that, it is highly likely that ongoing, regular meetings will interfere with their ability to heal, grow and self-nourish. Sometimes I forget this and my clients must remind me, and sometimes my clients need a little nudge out of the nest. In either case, it is a lesson for both of us in letting go, taking flight, and becoming healthily self-reliant.

- **We are afraid of losing love.** This is such a deeply rooted fear that we can often be deep denial over it. In terms of holistic nourishment, however, this fear can be disastrous. At one end of the spectrum, fear of losing love causes us to cling to unhealthy relationships, or overextend ourselves in meeting the expectations of others, or lose our identity in becoming what we believe others want us to be, or even accept unhappiness as a way of life. At the other extreme, this fear induces attempts control everyone and everything around us as we strive to plug potential leaks in our little bowl of love. In both cases, we are denying fundamental freedoms in how love can be expressed or accepted, because some part of us is sure that without such confinements love will escape our grasp. In reality, we are just putting love in cage and squeezing all the life out of it.

- **We have become inured to the destructive but familiar.** Simply through repeated exposure to abuse, pain, disappointment, anger, doubt or anxiety we can become numb to their damaging effects. Nowhere is this more prevalent than in an abusive household, where mistreated parties continue to deny anything is amiss, not even discussing the abuse amongst themselves. This capacity for accepting and even excusing brutality is astounding, and that such abuse is perpetuated not only for decades between members of a family, but also from one generation to the next, is truly devastating. And yet it is one of the most common forms of loveless suffering on Earth.

- **We are addicted to chaos or negative attention.** Chaos and negativity can be energizing. They get the heart pounding, the brain whirring, and release lots of exciting chemicals into our bloodstream. It can become such a physiological addiction that when external chaos ceases, we suddenly become depressed and moody. So we create a little more disruption within or without to feel better again; we sabotage authentic love so that we can continue to feel engaged or needed in superficial ways. If you ever want to see this cycle illustrated very quickly, hang out with some of the more intelligent varieties of parrots when they become bored. In a short amount of time, they will manipulate their immediate environment to maximize a highly destructive and chaotic effect. And boy-howdy are they happy once this is accomplished (especially if anyone nearby becomes really upset about it).

- **We are afraid of becoming happy, content or successful.** There are many reasons why people come to fear their own thriving. We might have mistaken beliefs about our own self-worth, or guilt over past experiences. We might not have the skills, willingness or ability to integrate new blessings into our old habits. Or we might harbor self-limiting beliefs about how living a just, compassionate or non-destructive life precludes success on a material or intimate relationship level. For instance, in my own journey it took years for me to differentiate between the deleterious effects of unassailable social privilege and a simple abundance of resources. I had seen too often how affluenza turned the guileless and humble into the arrogant and intolerant, the reclusive and iconoclastic, or both; I feared that every step I took towards successful living threatened to catapult me into one of these categories. Eventually it became clear that an abundance of resources need not lead to self-justifying attitudes of affluence, elitism or cultural superiority. In fact, such wealth can instead provide new avenues to achieve our purpose and promulgate compassionate action in ever-widening arenas – if it is a means rather than an end.

- **We are wounded, angry or in emotional pain, and are lashing out because of it.** Anyone who has tried to help an injured animal is familiar with this phenomenon. Pain and fear will cause them to lash out at anyone who comes too close or touches a sensitive area. Sometimes this self-protective response inflicts more damage than the animal's own injury. And we humans are not much different in this regard, except that our pain-response is not only provoked by physical touch, but also by circumstances, by the wrong words at the wrong time, by a misunderstood look from across the room, etc. And although love is the strongest force in the universe, it can be obscured for brief periods by these negative attitudes and emotions.

There are many more reasons we might choose less skillful short-cuts when caring for ourselves and others, but imagine if just two or three of the patterns above are present in your life. Can you see how they could interfere with your ability to love freely and effectively? We will be addressing these and other barriers to love in Part IV. For now, take a moment to reflect on any proclivities that might be interfering with your ability to love effectively.

> **Exercise: Love-Disrupting Patterns** One helpful exercise is to sit somewhere quiet where you won't be disturbed and review each of your interpersonal and interior relationships (i.e. your relationships with each dimension of essential nourishment) and ask yourself if any of the patterns listed here are present. With inward-directed focus, ask yourself: "Am I doing anything in this relationship that indicates I am afraid of losing the love between us?" Or "Do I enjoy my position of being relied upon in this relationship?" Or "Do I tend to create conflict or chaos when things start going smoothly?" And so on.

In the earlier contrasting examples, there are some obvious, short term benefits to loving more skillfully. But consider the impact on all our relationships over time for both models. Years of enabling someone's alcoholism versus confronting them and encouraging treatment. Decades of being quiet and nice versus holding a loved one accountable for their inappropriate actions. A lifetime of passively accepting abuse versus actively helping the abuser and ourselves heal from those wounds. In each case, we are not loving ourselves or others effectively when we avoid actively healing an antagonistic, dysfunctional or destructive relationship.

Characteristics of Authentic Love

It is almost impossible to describe the spectrum of love with words alone, for more than a feeling, or a set of responses, or a mode of being, love is a force of life. Think of all the phrases or words that refer to some sort of love in the English language: affection; compassion; caring; warmth; kindness; making someone's heart pitter-patter; desiring to please; wanting only the best for someone; devotion; protective feelings; fawning over someone; falling in love; sick with love...the list is virtually endless. And of course we can't really know love or describe love until we have experienced it firsthand. I recall a discussion two of my own spiritual influences had over the qualities of spiritual love, with one insisting its main characteristics were passion and devotion, while the other asserted a sober sense of duty and obligation. But if we see love as a large spectrum with many gradations, nuances and modes of expression, all of these descriptions can fit. So when I refer to love in general, I am referring to that all-inclusive spectrum. However, when I invoke the term *authentic love*, I mean something very specific.

Authentic love leads us to ourselves and leads the world to wholeness. It conditions responses that are healing and helpful, and encourages spiritually healthy emotional states. It nourishes and replenishes, facilitating growth and transformation in us, in others and in the environments around us. Why is it "authentic?" Because I believe anything that is authentic – that is true to itself – is just a little bit closer to the mysterious source from which life itself emanates. And in our impulse to draw nearer to that source, we are often eager to cling to substitutions that are either at a less productive or growth-oriented end of the spectrum, or are not love at all. We are quick to suckle at the nearest teat, often as a result of impatience, a lack of discernment, or because we are so externally fixated that we can't see the love within ourselves. What follow are some of the more definable characteristics of authentic love. Through evaluating such characteristics, my hope is that we can refine that inner compass a bit and find our way back to the pure center, the mysterious source that gifts us with life and purpose, and which gently goads the Universe itself to evolve into ever more spectacular expressions of being.

To make this list a bit more engaging, I like to describe love as if describing a person or spirit; a personification of life force. Why? Because then it is a little easier for me to relate to love and imagine myself manifesting its characteristics in myself, and in my relationship with everything and everyone around me.

- **Authentic love is honest.** If you ask love a question, it will always share its thoughts openly, even if you don't appreciate its answers at the time. Love has no guile, no capacity for deception, no means of distorting the truth.

- **Authentic love is courageous.** Love doesn't back down before fear or anger, or bow before anything but the deepest wisdom.

- **Authentic love is humble.** Even when it has the power to change everything in an instant, it still honors the autonomy of human will.

- **Authentic love is patient.** It bides its time, shining a beacon for wayward travelers gallivanting about in the wilderness, hoping and waiting for them to circle back toward home.

- **Authentic love is reliable.** True love won't ever let you down.

- **Authentic love is indefatigable, always able to care for and replenish itself.** The more demanding an effort that is inspired and guided by love, the more energy love makes available.

- **Authentic love is a free spirit.** It cannot be corralled, caged or cornered, and it cannot be bound to any purpose other than propagating itself. Authentic love has no hidden agendas. It does not want to convert anyone's beliefs, or maintain a status quo, or sell any products, or promote one outcome over another. It is of course willing to go along for the ride – but look out! Any hidden agendas will quickly be exposed and transformed as they yield to love's preeminent authority.

- **Authentic love lets go.** It does not hold on to guilt, resentment or anger, but quickly forgives. In fact, it has trouble even remembering what it was upset about just a few moments ago.

- **Authentic love is strong.** It is the molten lava in the bones of the Earth, the great currents of the sea, the endless winds that circle the globe, the countless rays of sunlight reaching out into the dark. Much stronger than doubt, hate, fear, fury or violence…which are only broken bits of cooling ash before love's fierce infinitude.

- **Authentic love is generous.** It shares itself and all that it loves magnanimously and unequivocally. It does not demand sureties or conditions, but blazes forth in unrestrained glory. That is why it is never jealous, because it knows there is more than enough to go around. And that is why, when it runs out of other things to give, it offers its own life in exchange for the well-being of others.

- **Authentic love is irresistible.** Like bright smiles, joyful laughter or a deep, loud yawn, love jumps lightly from one person to the next.

- **Authentic love knows how to have fun.** It is playful and giggly like hide-and-seek in the woods. Sometimes it seems to run away or disappear, but all the while it is rubbing its hands together in gleeful anticipation of being found.

- **Authentic love has a great sense of humor.** About itself, about human beings, about the wonders of the Earth and stars. Sometimes we don't understand the joke it is sharing with us, but it is impossible not to laugh along with love anyway.

- **Authentic love is just.** It intuits right from wrong and is happy to mediate between disputing parties. Whenever a bully or tyrant raises a hand to strike, love is there to turn the blow aside and explain a better way. Love is never ashamed to befriend those who have done wrong, or to remind those in power to cultivate humility, or to stand in joyful support of every human soul. True love does not need to choose sides, but always facilitates healing, wholeness and transformation.

- **Authentic love is equitable.** It falls in love with everyone and everything. There are no favorites, and the love available to everyone is equally boundless. However, whenever someone has surrendered completely to love, it may appear that their share is somehow greater, or that love flows more freely through them. But that is like saying the sun dims itself when we walk into a cave. Love always shines with equal brightness, we have only to open ourselves to its Light.

- **Authentic love is active.** It reaches out, lifts up, nourishes and protects. It endlessly and tirelessly creates and propagates itself. Love unaccompanied by action is not authentic love.

- **Authentic love encourages self-sufficiency.** It does not need to feel important or depended upon, but offers itself as a resource. It gently nudges, advises and explains rather than forcefully controlling outcomes or deceptively manipulating others. It allows people to make mistakes so they can discover their boundaries and learn wisdom. Authentic love demands nothing, but rejoices when others find their own way.

- **Authentic love seeks understanding.** It watches and listens, from the heart, in order to comprehend others as fully as possible. It remembers and acknowledges what is important to each person.

- **Authentic love is discerning and skillful.** It senses which inner thoughts and feelings will be most encouraging and helpful; it fashions just the right words to say and the right time to say them; it knows what actions will be most effective and when. Authentic love anticipates the beneficial outcomes of its expression and works steadfastly toward fulfillment.

- **Authentic love is mysterious.** There is something indefinable about true love that inspires and energizes us. It invites us to explore that mystery without ever promising to reveal itself fully. Without becoming coy or aloof, love tantalizes our being, lifting itself just beyond reach until, all at once in a delightful surprise, we are completely consumed by it.

- **Authentic love does not objectify.** It does not have affection for the special characteristics of its object or the object's state or stage of being, but rather for beingness itself – unadorned, unqualified and unconditional. True love's expression becomes perfect when the object of affection is embraced as having been perfect all along.

- **Authentic love is spacious.** There are limitless possibilities within true love, and ever-expanding room for many points of view, many ways of being, and many different beliefs and convictions. Love accepts all circumstances and all possibilities with unwavering equanimity. It embraces the whole, even though we cannot always perceive what the whole looks like or make any sense of it.

> **Exercise: Love Affirmations**   Try rephrasing the statements above as personal affirmations or meditations. For example: "Because of the love within me, I seek understanding. I watch and listen, from the heart, in order to comprehend others as fully as possible." Choose just one to recite in the morning before you start your day, and then reflect silently on its meaning for a few minutes. As with other affirmations, you could try using a mirror and offer them to yourself eye-to-eye. At the end of the day, just before you go to bed, consider how your thoughts and actions aligned with what you recited in the morning. Did you manifest any attributes of authentic love? There is no need to attach moral judgments to what you discover…just allow what has happened to unfold quietly in your awareness against the backdrop of your affirmations. The next day, try to reshape another phrase so that it inspires you to loving action.

Emotional States

Another way to look at authentic love is to examine the emotional states it evokes and promotes. The following chart is an expanded version of one found in my earlier writings. Here we see not only descriptions of emotional states but also factors and areas of nourishment that impact the health of our emotions. At first glance, this a high-altitude overview of emotional well-being; by evaluating our own emotional states and targeting growth in our weakest areas, the chart can be a powerful tool of self-transformation. Consider that all of the spiritually healthy emotional states listed here are really inspired by, founded on and expanded in authentic love.

Spiritually Healthy Emotional State (Evidence of True Love)	Spiritually Unhealthy Emotional State (Impedance to True Love)	Common Nourishment Barriers that Contribute to Unhealthy States
Hope and faith in a positive outcome	Despair and pessimism: presuming doom	• Survival persona • Inability to self-nourish
Courage to defend the well-being of self and others, with patience and forbearance	Indignant, self-righteous rage, which is easily provoked and unconcerned about the damage it inflicts	• Inability to manage emotions • Unhealed emotional trauma • Survival persona
Compassionate desire to nourish others with wisdom and kindness, while at the same time sustaining our own well-being	Compulsive need to rescue others without considering our own well-being, or what is truly best for those being "rescued"	• Chaotic, unsupportive or unloving childhood environments • Low self-worth • Unresolved grief or pain involving family of origin • Survival persona • Substitution behavior
Love that has no conditions or expectations attached to it, and that patiently accepts another's shortcomings	A desire to control disguised as attention and devotion, but that impatiently demands specific reciprocation	• Inability to take responsibility for own well-being • Low self-worth • Fear-based reasoning • Substitution behavior
Self-controlled ordering of effort according to what is most important (via spiritual discernment and intuitive insight)	Impulsive submission to every urgent or self-indulgent whim without a thought for what is important	• Confusion or ignorance about authentic love • Inability to self-nourish • Substitution behavior

Patience for, and an attempt to understand, those who oppose or antagonize us	Fear, paranoia and hatred of things we do not understand	• Fear-based reasoning • Lower moral valuation stratum
Gratitude and forgiveness	Resentment and divisiveness	• Unhealed emotional trauma
Acceptance and flexibility with whatever comes our way	Resistance to change, and panic when things seem out of control	• Chaotic, unsupportive or unloving childhood environments • Inability to self-nourish
Honesty and openness	Avoidance, denial and deception	• Survival persona • Fear-based reasoning
Peaceful and supportive internal dialogues	Chaotic and demeaning internal dialogues	• Low self-worth • Unresolved grief or pain involving family of origin
Admiration and encouragement	Jealousy and criticism	• Low self-worth • Inability to self-nourish
Contentment in any situation, rich or poor, because our focus is on human relationships and developing a wealth of spiritual understanding	Greed and avarice: a compelling desire to possess material power and wealth	• Fear-based reasoning • Survival persona • Lower moral valuation stratum • Substitution behavior
Guilt and shame, which resolves into humility and a renewed commitment to growth and maturity	Perpetual, unresolved guilt and shame, which injures self-worth and cripples any ability to change	• Unresolved grief or pain involving family of origin • Unhealed emotional trauma
Vulnerable and joyful sharing of sexual intimacy in the context of responsible relationships	Wanton lust: an immersion in carnality without considering emotional or spiritual consequences	• Unhealed emotional trauma • Substitution behavior
Mutual inspiration to greater achievement through fair-spirited competition – or better yet, cooperation	Egotistical competitiveness, which craves victory at any cost	• Substitution behavior • Lower moral valuation stratum • Survival persona
Confidence with humility	Self-aggrandizing arrogance	• Low self-worth
Taking pleasure in the success of others	Taking pleasure in the suffering of others	• Lower moral valuation stratum

Exercise: Tracking Your Emotions Try tracking your emotional states throughout the day, from when you rise in the morning until when you go to bed at night. Just jot them down as they happen. You don't have to be detailed; that is, there is no need to capture the specific content of your thoughts...just record the essence of the emotions you feel. For instance "Angry at driver who cut me off," "Laughed at Jerry's joke," "Sad to hear about

Maria's sick cat," "Bored to tears in afternoon meeting." Then, at the end of the week, look over your notes and note how your feelings mapped out over time. What were the dominant emotions? Were they mostly healthy or unhealthy? What emotional patterns do you notice, and which would you like to transform?

Nurturing Models

Where can we look for models of loving skillfully across all sorts of relationships and in many different contexts? There are countless possibilities. Many works on the subject of love focus on its romantic aspects, but there are also works on charitable giving, living according to a particular belief system's concept of compassion, or some other specific area of interpersonal application. What we are looking for here is a broader intention and methodology for loving all-inclusively and effectually across many different types of interaction – because that is what supports high quality nourishment. But can skillful loving be generalized in this way? I believe it can. And, more specifically, there are four fields of study that inform an approach particularly well. The first is parenting. I suspect that many authors of works on parenting don't immediately recognize the breadth of their insights, but a close look at healthy parenting models reveals that they are, in fact, applicable in one way or another to every kind of relationship. The second field of study is romantic partnerships, and since so much is available in this subject area, the real challenge is narrowing our focus to a few good examples. The third field is therapeutic models; that is, how to be an effective healing resource for people in need. And finally there is spiritual love, which provides us with additional principles that compliment what we find in the other three. We will briefly sample all four of these in the following section.

Parenting Styles

A friend of mine who is a parent once commented, "If you begin talking to people about parenting styles, be sure to clarify that you don't know a darn thing about it -- after all, you don't have any kids!" I think this has merit, in much the same way that someone who has never experienced a harmonious long-term romantic relationship probably isn't the best resource for couples counseling. And actually I have clearly drawn this line in my own therapeutic practice, as I do not offer family counseling or enter into formal therapeutic relationships with young people. Many of my friends have commented on the quality of my interaction with children – how happily I enter their realm of imagination, silliness and play; how easily I seem to understand and communicate with kids. But among those same friends, when one parent observes to their partner "Hey, he's really great with kids!" the other inevitably replies, "Of course, that's because he doesn't have any!" I think they believe my ability to joyfully engage with children would likely be short-lived if I had some of my own. In this sense, I am probably more like a child than a parent. So there, on behalf of my parental friends, is my caveat.

Parenting models can be applied to all sorts of relationships. That is, they are really *nurturing* models. In several parenting studies over the last twenty years, some notable correlations have been drawn between distinct styles of parenting and the resulting behavior of children. First, here is a quick overview of styles whose definitions build on the work of developmental psychologist Dr. Diana Baumrind and the many researchers who followed in her footsteps:

- **Authoritarian & Controlling** – Expectation that children should comply with rigid rules and boundaries without question and without clear reasoning or justification, often with sever consequences (harsh, disproportionate punishments or volatile reactions) if they do not comply. Authoritarian parents demand respect and even fear from their children, but above all they demand obedience. A child's individuation (independence of thought, volition and emotional state from their parent's) is severely restricted. Nourishment is present, but constrained to limited areas and dependent on obligatory compliance, suppressing internal motivations in favor of external rewards.

- **Permissive & Indulgent** – Expectation that children should be free to do whatever they want, without clear or consistent boundaries, rules or consequences, and a desire on the parent's part to be liked rather than respected or feared. A permissive parent is more concerned with not upsetting their child than with conveying specific values. Individuation is less important than a child knowing they can do whatever they want (including remaining dependent on their parent and never developing intrinsic motivation). Nourishment occurs on many levels, but without clear emphasis, priority or consistency.

- **Authoritative & Egalitarian–** Expectation that children operate with boundaries that are clearly communicated, explained and justified, with consequences that are consistent and proportionate. An authoritative parent's objective is to encourage independent thought, volition and emotional reaction in their child, while at the same time conveying specific values to guide a child's gradual individuation. Nourishment is available and responsively demonstrated on many levels, but self-sufficient nourishment is encouraged at the same time, so that internal motivation takes precedence over external rewards.

- **Uninvolved & Neglectful** – Expectation that children care for themselves without much parental involvement. Boundaries, values, consequences and nourishment are left unexpressed and undefined. An uninvolved parent often forces individuation suddenly and inexplicably, leaving a child to cast about on their own for understanding of pretty much everything. Nourishment occurs haphazardly, without guidance or appropriate reinforcement, so that self-nourishment and intrinsic motivation become confusing and contradictory mysteries.

What an increasing body of work has shown is that three of these styles result in clear deficits in children's ability to thrive personally and socially, while only one provides a clear advantage in a child's overall development.[2] As of this writing, a publications search on child development and parenting styles referenced data to support similar conclusions across different social strata, ethnic groups and living environments.[3] As you might suppose, the style with the most measurably positive outcome is the *authoritative and egalitarian* parenting style. The other three parenting styles tend to result in a higher occurrence of behavioral problems, more instances of depression and low self-worth, a lesser ability to think independently or cooperatively, and greater difficulty in decision-making and self-management. Why is this so? I think it is because the *authoritative and egalitarian* style represents a narrow range of optimal function for parental engagement in its level of demonstrated respect and affection, its responsiveness to a child's nourishment needs, and its balanced exertion of power over a child.

How do parenting styles relate to authentic love? I think the parallels are clear. Authoritative and egalitarian parenting demands all of the essential characteristics of authentic love and demonstrates their practical application. It also illuminates a principle of authentic love that is very difficult to communicate and exemplify: nurturing another's independent will (for example, the ability to sufficiently nourish oneself) while at the same time communicating a concrete set of values that channel that will in constructive ways. This is quite a tight-rope walk, and I do not know if there is another force available to humanity that can engineer this particular accomplishment other than authentic love. Within a love broadened and deepened by holistic self-nourishment, we can arrive at this balance of direction, guidance and free will much more easily.

Another way to describe authoritative and egalitarian parenting is that it honors a child's sovereignty. That is, recognizing that a child has the freedom to find their own way in the world, and, more than that, that they should confidently feel as if they are thus empowered. In Myla and Jon Kabat-Zinn's book *Everyday Blessings*, they expand on this idea as honoring a child's intrinsic endowment of – and aptitude for – self-determination, while at the same time encouraging a deeper understanding and experience of an equal sovereignty in others. This seems a decidedly Buddhist way of looking at interdependent relationships, and it lends us some very useful language for our discourse about love in support of the authoritative and egalitarian model. To become a mindful parent (or friend, or lover), we must recognize the importance of empathy and unconditional acceptance, and then remain fully present to what is happening in each moment – especially as it is affecting those we care about. This is unquestionably one way of describing the central aspects of true love, and adds more facets to the gem of skillful compassion. And of course it applies equally to all sorts of relationships; it is more about inclusive and collaborative nurturing than parenting alone. So I believe the more we can define and exemplify what constitutes mindful, compassionate, authoritative nurturing, the more we can understand the breadth of its applications to every aspect of life.

But there is an important principle hovering around all of these words, and the more it remains unspoken, the more we may come to believe it is possible to learn love simply through rote, by checking off a list of to-dos that look and sound like compassion, mindfulness, collaboration or authoritativeness. That principle, woven through our thoughts and volition, is that to be authentic in our love for anyone or anything, the love must be deeply felt, right down to the central axis of our being. More than a conviction or commitment, more than any convention of appropriate words, insightful thinking, or skillful deeds, love-in-action is an overflowing of heart and spirit. And children are excellent detectors of saccharin affection and false enthusiasm. Whenever I reach the end of my energies when interacting with kids, I quickly recognize my own misstep when I force myself to be jolly or silly without really feeling it. Younger children especially will immediately look at me questioningly, become less playful, or disengage completely when my excitement becomes inauthentic. One just can't fool them for long. And really, the same is true of lovers, life partners, coworkers, friends, relatives, animals and perhaps even plants – our inauthentic effort is not always consciously recognized, but it is unconsciously felt. When we try to spontaneously manufacture something we don't really feel, our audience's sixth sense is put on alert. Slowly, if the condition persists, it will erode our connection with our own inner life, along with everyone and everything around us.

Of course, some people are excellent fakers, and there are times when social convention expects us to mask our true feelings and perform insincerely out of a sense of duty or professional decorum. I have witnessed motivational speakers, health care providers, well-meaning business managers, spiritual teachers and close friends fall into this trap. And, of course, I have perpetrated this ruse myself more than once. But I believe the absence of felt caring and compassion occurs for a reason: it indicates nourishment depletion that requires our attention. It is time to take a break, recharge, realign and rediscover. It is time to care for self and remember our integral practice. The love is still there within us, waiting to spring forth, but it is asking for the right conditions. Conditions predicated on our own healthy, full-spectrum nourishment. Of course there are times when our routine becomes imbalanced, and parents are quick to remind me that children often can't respect adult boundaries – just as lovers, friends, siblings and our own parents also may not on occasion. And yet those boundaries are necessary for our own sustenance. We must find ways to replenish our dimensions of self when we become depleted. We must find ways to curb the interference of even those we most love and care for, or, really, we will have nothing left to give.

Why the other styles of parenting are as harmful as they are seems less fully understood, but there is a growing body of literature that discusses it either directly or indirectly. For example, in his book *Punished by Rewards*, Alfie Kohn makes an excellent case for why conditional rewards (which we can associate with either bargaining in a permissive parenting style or punishment in an authoritarian parenting style) undermine a child's healthy and necessary autonomy. In essence, such rewards condition a child to become dependent on extrinsic motivation instead of encouraging intrinsic motivation; they induce children to abandon their sense of sovereignty and their own discernment when making a choice. Here again, there is helpful language in Kohn's rejection of Skinnerian behaviorism and the facilitation and support of someone's power to choose – regardless of whether it is a child or employee, student or team member. The broader theme of nurturing is evident here as well. In *Integral Lifework*, the rewards issue is a classic example of how we can come to rely on externals to guide our lives rather than trusting our internal resources, which in turn discourages us from cultivating self-sufficiency in all dimensions of essential nourishment. Without that self-sufficiency – without that autonomy, sovereignty and a sense of collaboration as equals – we can never be fully nourished, and we will never become whole.

When I have encouraged clients to apply these nurturing principles to other types of relationships, I sometimes encounter resistance. It may seem inappropriate at first glance to consider anyone except our own children as someone to be nurtured. In society at large, many parents might resent the application of such a model with their own children by teachers or family friends, considering it potential interference with their primary parenting authority, and they certainly wouldn't want strangers to nurture their children in this way. And adult strangers interacting with other adult strangers…well, modeling a parent-child dynamic is understandably challenging to embrace in this context as well. Reactions usually run along these lines: it's demeaning and condescending to treat adults like children; it interferes with other people's parenting priorities to interact with their children this way; it's arrogant to assume we should nurture anyone but ourselves or our own children; and so forth.

At the root of this resistance is, I believe, a fundamental mistrust of the power relationship often present in parent-child dynamics. That is, it is usually someone's own negative experience of being poorly parented that leads to rejecting a parenting style model for interactions. And, by delving a little deeper into this with someone, we usually discover these reactions are in fact rooted in their experience of one or more of the unhealthy styles: authoritarian, indulgent or neglectful. So by living with an unskillful parent, we learn to equate parenting with lording it over someone, dominating them, and "treating them like a child" (i.e. authoritarian and controlling style). Or it equates becoming a doormat, "letting them walk all over you," or being otherwise disrespected (i.e. permissive and indulgent style). Or it means disengaging to an ineffectual distance, so as to appear aloof or uncaring altogether (i.e. uninvolved and neglectful style). But again, these are merely reflections of unhealthy nurturing styles. If instead we draw upon the authoritative and egalitarian model, the relationships blossom in mutual respect, appreciation and interdependence. We might even call it co-nurturing, for that is in fact what occurs over time.

So in this nurturing model I initiate a relationship with someone of equal worth and potential, with an expectation of mutual discovery, collaboration, self-sufficiency and shared contribution to positive outcomes. I may be a teacher in this moment, but I fully expect my student will become my teacher in the next moment. I may be knowledgeable or experienced in some area of interest right now, but at any moment I anticipate being surprised by something new, interesting and alive that this person introduces to me. No matter what the perceived power dynamic, the conviction I hold at the forefront of my consciousness is that this other being and I are really one and the same;

that is, we share the same essence, the same interdependence and the same non-hierarchical place in the Universe.

Let me provide an example that reminded me of this equality in a powerful way. At one time in my practice I decided it would be helpful to gently nudge a client out of mental spacetime for a while and avoid any more talk-therapy. In this instance, I thought Reiki might be an appropriate way to help her shift consciousness away from intellect and into her body. To be honest, I was pretty self-satisfied with my assessment, and probably saw myself as a problem-solver or gentle teacher in that moment. She agreed and I commenced with the Usui hand positions. At some point in the process, something inside of me cracked open. Suddenly I felt as if the flow of energy between us was mingling or perhaps reversing, and I began receiving deep instruction on several levels at once. It was as if – and I don't really have the language to adequately describe it – her body was relieving me of a vast ignorance. From my beginning in smugness, I was suddenly a complete novice, in worshipful awe of the being gently snoring on the table before me. Like a flash of lightening through my heart, I was brought to tears of humility, gratitude and wonder. I was the student here, and she was the teacher. Even unconsciously prone before me, she was showing me more in a few minutes than I had learned in months of solitary practice. For me, this is a fine illustration of an enduring truth: it embodies the unshakable reality of the inherent, egalitarian mutuality of all relationships. I am not the healer or teacher for anyone but myself, and the experience and wisdom of my practice only allows me to help awaken the healer and teacher in someone else – to remind of them of their own power and wisdom.

To be authentically realized in each of our interactions, this mutual recognition and empowerment must of course be anchored in love. The moment I cross the line into controlling, authoritarian attitudes and behavior is the moment I begin to annihilate the very qualities I value so highly, namely each individual's extensive ability to govern and nourish self and contribute to the good of the whole. But because this autonomous, mutually respectful experience is a relatively rare event in most people's lives, there remains an understandably deep-seated mistrust of the power dynamics implied by any mention of parenting – or even nurturing. To those whose understanding of loving relationships leans more toward control behavior, non-involvement or the permissive and indulgent, the proposition of "authoritative and egalitarian love" smacks more of anathema than blessing. So perhaps this dynamic requires new language. So far we have used terms like authentic love and love-consciousness to hint at how this mode of being pervades a life committed to integral, transformative practice. Perhaps "a transformative exchange of co-nurturing" is a good approximation. These terms have been used before and are borrowed here because they come close to the mark. But the concept being proposed here is really is subtly different than all of these, while at the same time being no more extraordinary than a spontaneous smile.

What, then, is the lesson we can learn from the parenting model about our own effective loving? Here is how I would summarize it:

1) All healthy relationships are authoritarian and egalitarian, respecting the sovereignty, wisdom and transformational capacity of every individual, while at the same time asserting clear roles, responsibilities and boundaries for interaction.

2) Relationships based on reward systems undermine our intrinsic capacity to love freely and unconditionally, and interfere with self-sufficiency in nourishment.

3) Relationships that veer into other nurturing styles invariably sabotage the relationship itself and the ability of each party to love themselves or others effectively.

Romantic Partnerships

Another resource we can draw upon to understand nurturing models is the vast body of work on romantic relationships. There are an endless variety of approaches to this topic, as perusal of any bookstore's offerings will reveal. Of all the literature I have read on romance, there are two books that stand out for me. One is *Conscious Loving* by Gay and Kathlyn Hendricks, and the other is *The Seven Principles for Making Marriage Work* by John M. Gottman and Nan Silver. I recommend anyone who wishes to heal and strengthen their romantic partnerships read these two books – and, of course, work caringly through the exercises in each one.

Let's glean a few helpful principles from their pages that apply to love and nurturing in any context. Consider first the following ideas rephrased from *Conscious Loving* and how they might apply to any relationship in your life:

1) If we do not learn how to love consciously, we will repeat the patterns of unconscious loving we learned in our childhood. This often involves attempts in the present to heal wounds we suffered in the past, using our current relationship as a crucible for resolving old resentments, angers, pains and hurts. This is inevitable because the intimacy of love brings all of our emotional history to the surface. So part of our responsibility in being whole and available to love in the present is to work through those issues and find healing and completion for past experiences of pain.

2) All parties take full responsibility for their contribution to the success or failure of all communication and interaction in a relationship. There can never be an apportionment of blame. Taken one step further, we must also take full responsibility for creating our own lives and the quality of all of our relationships. The objective here is to empower ourselves and others, and release any vestiges of victimhood in our self-concept.

3) We commit both to being close to and vulnerable with those we love, and to maintaining a healthy separateness and self-sufficiency at the same time. This helps us avoid slipping into codependent modes of interaction, where we are governed either by controlling or approval-seeking behaviors.

4) We maintain integrity and honesty in our communication and commitments. When we love consciously, we express the truth of our heart – how we feel in this moment – "without fear of punishment or expectation of reward." In other words, we share our most intimate selves without any justification for doing so other than the inherent value of the act itself. And we share that honesty with both immediacy and tact. In the same vein, when we also keep the

agreements we make with those we love, once again for the self-justifying purpose of keeping them, and of maintaining our integrity as part of loving interaction, rather than because of any positive or negative consequences.

I think you can quickly appreciate how these principles apply to all manner of mutual nurturing. The conscious efforts of healing, integrity, vulnerability, honesty, responsibility, commitment – these are the building blocks of all intimacy. Without them we are forever cast adrift on a choppy sea of emotional upheavals, blown about by the chilling winds of unconscious patterns and past failures. So the Hendricks have offered us some solid contributions to a template for all manner of affection. We can see in these principles the common threads in caring for ourselves, for loved ones, for strangers in need, for society as a whole, the Earth and every other arena of loving kindness. Just as with the healthy parenting model, we need not confine these attributes to one type of relationship but can uncover a range of optimal function within which all relationships thrive.

Now let's see what Gottman and Silver have to offer. Here are a few paraphrased morsels extracted from their *Seven Principles*:

1) When we pay close and compassionate attention to someone else's life – to all the details and minutia that occupy their thoughts and prioritize their efforts – we demonstrate caring and strengthen that relationship. Through paying attention to the worries, aspirations, events and changes in a loved one's world (in *Seven Principles* these are called *love maps*), we are really coming to fully know and appreciate them in all their complexity. And in knowing them fully, we can support them fully – and they can have more trust in us to do so. How does this happen in a practical sense? We check in with them regularly, we listen attentively to what they share and respond to it supportively, we actively engage with them and encourage our loved ones to engage with us with enough frequency to maintain and expand a mutually supportive connection.

2) When we feel deep admiration for all the qualities and experiences someone brings to a relationship, the relationship flourishes. And if this is true, we will regularly demonstrate that admiration by

allowing that person to influence our decisions or help us with our problems. We actively share power with them in the relationship. But when admiration descends through indifference to dismissive scorn, our relationship is headed for disaster. Over time, if we instead maintain a positive view of someone, our fondness for them remains constant. As we look back over our shared history, we can either focus on the victories and joy, or the pain and disappointment; how we sustain our fondness and process our relationship's past is certain to determine its future.

3) In all of our communication, we try to deescalate negativity and antagonism however it may manifest. Gottman and Silver narrow the field of grave communication offenders to *criticism, contempt, defensiveness* and *stonewalling;* when any of these persist, they say, the relationship is in danger. Instead, when things don't go smoothly or there is discord, we can remain calm, make attempts to repair the situation and convey the honor and respect we have for someone, opening up a space for them to reciprocate. We don't do this merely to placate or avoid conflict, but because we sincerely wish to mend a rift. We try to remain open instead of closing ourselves down, boxing others in, or fencing ourselves off with willful barbed wire and emotional landmines. So instead of griping, resisting or avoiding we demonstrate acceptance of another's faults and imperfections, and try to resolve problems through genuine compromise.

Here again there is ample overlap between what works well in romantic partnerships and what benefits any relationship or exchange. If we allow these ideas to percolate for a while, patterns of effective loving begin to emerge that we can apply to every situation in our lives. According to these two works on relationships, how can we be the most nurturing? Let's count the ways:

1) Becoming healed and whole as individuals, carrying the responsibility for our well-being ourselves, rather than resting it on the shoulders of those we love.

2) Taking full and unequivocal responsibility for the quality and success of any relationship.

3) Consciously creating new loving habits that displace old, unconscious patterns of relating.

4) Remaining open, present, attentive, genuine and available to those we love, demonstrating our admiration and respect by:

    a) Paying attention to all the details of their lives...and remembering them;

    b) Letting go of past wrongs;

    c) Being thoroughly and proactively honest in all of our communication;

    d) Actively including our loved ones in our decisions and following through on the commitments we make to them; and

    e) Softening and resolving conflict or ongoing challenges by accepting another's faults and imperfections, repairing negative escalations and ferreting out real and lasting compromise.

I would like contribute a couple of nuggets from my own experience counseling couples. First, realizing at some juncture that we may have made a poor choice of partner does not preclude us having a successful long-term relationship with them. Any two people, as long as both remain willing, can invent and constantly reinvent the healthy dynamics necessary to remain together over time. With persistence and some mutually supportive skills, even the most wounded and broken relationships can return from stormy seas to the warm meadows of terra firma. However, it is also important to evaluate whether a relationship is worth maintaining and why, and it can be difficult to be honest with ourselves about this.

At the root of this evaluation is understanding the nature of our commitment. Are we committed to a partnership because we share common goals and dreams and want to support each other in realizing them? Are we committed because the well-being of our children is best facilitated by that commitment? Are we committed because we enjoy our partner so much, we just can't imagine life without them? Both parties really do not need to be committed for exactly the same reasons in order for the relationship to flourish, but each person must discover the uncompromising truth about the value they place on continuing. And, sometimes, what becomes clear through self-examination is that our commitment does not stem from the fulfillment of dreams, the welfare of children, the joy of friendship or any other healthy valuations, but because we are afraid. Afraid to feel the pain of loss or inflict that pain on someone else. Afraid to be alone. Afraid of what our friends and family will think. Afraid of admitting failure to ourselves or our children. Afraid of losing a comfortable lifestyle or gaining new financial burdens. And if our commitment stems from such fears more than from any other quarter, then these alone are not sufficient reasons to continue an intimate connection. Instead, it is probably time to face those fears and begin planning how to reveal our feelings to our partner – after all, that would be in keeping with the principles we have just outlined.

I include this here because, sometimes, the kindest, most loving thing we can do in a relationship is let go of it. This requires courage, and wherever true love is present, courage is also present. Does this translate more broadly into other exchanges? Absolutely. Whether a friendship, business partnership, membership in an affinity group or other type of connection, we can apply the same criteria for evaluation to the relationship. And we should do so frequently. It is easy to end up on autopilot, relying on the momentum of decisions or commitments made years ago to carry us forward. But if we cannot fully recommit in the present moment, each and every day, then something is amiss and we need to pause, take a breath, and think and feel it through. Really, this is a question of authenticity. Is my love for someone or something authentic if it is motivated by fear? If it is inauthentic, why am I perpetuating a charade? Whom does it benefit? Are there other choices that would benefit all parties more? These are the difficult questions a caring heart asks of every relationship.

Therapeutic Models

Having read this far, it should come as no surprise that *Integral Lifework* promotes a therapeutic model grounded in love, and what that love looks like is influenced by many different modalities. Here is a sampling of the theory and practice that not only informs the broader discussion of true love, but also the particulars of my own approach as an *Integral Lifework Practitioner.*

Psychotherapy

The person-centered psychotherapeutic model of Carl Rogers – and the many others since who have built on his principles – defines in large degree the nature of a caring and empathic therapeutic relationship. Rogers' fundamental assumption is that people already have within them the desire and facility to self-actualize. There is no need, therefore, for a therapist to be directive or manipulative – no need for them to forcibly take control or fix what is wrong. In fact, person-centered therapy emphasizes trying to understand things from the client's point-of-view, to listen attentively, with great respect and empathy, and provide a supportive space for clients to process things on their own. In order to achieve this mode of interaction, it is incumbent on the therapist to develop themselves, to mature enough to be able to let go of power relationships and controlling modes of interaction, and instead focus their attention on the client's experience and process. In other words, to exemplify a mode of being that is open, transparent, self-aware, genuine and above all compassionate. This person-centered approach is founded less on specific techniques, and more on creating constructive intimacy between therapist and client.

Another therapist and researcher whose focus is a compassionate therapeutic relationship is Ron Kurtz. In Kurtz's Hakomi method, the therapist encourages a client to access and express their felt experience in the present, carefully creating a safe and inviting space for them to do so. The emphasis is on helping people learn (through the therapist's modeling and specific supportive techniques) a compassionate, non-judgmental mode of interaction with their innermost processes. A mindful introspection. In so doing, the client can begin to work through the core material that is causing them pain, impeding progress, evoking certain patterns of thought or emotion and so on. Reminiscent of Rogers' premise, Kurtz emphasizes that a client isn't presenting problems to be solved, brokenness to be fixed, or pathology to be healed, but "an experience that wants to happen." In Hakomi, people govern their own outcomes, and the therapist becomes a trusted, non-destructive facilitator of that self-empowering process.

One particularly potent supportive technique in Hakomi is called *taking over*. In an irony of therapeutic language, this sounds like some sort of forceful manipulation, but it is really the opposite. This method supports a client in whatever they are feeling or thinking by honoring it with external, complimentary effort. For instance, one of my clients was experiencing severe anxiety over a past romantic relationship and how her feelings were interfering with a present relationship. Every time she described what she felt, she would lean forward and touch the flat of her hand to her breastbone, often using the words "I just can't stop loving him!" to express her upset. To *take over*, I asked if she would lean forward, pressing her breastbone into the flat of my hand with her full weight, while I said, "You just can't stop loving him..." in a calm, non-judgmental, matter-of-fact way. In other words, I *took over* these outward expressions of her inner turmoil. When I did this she experienced a strong emotional release; her tension and distress around the ended romance became much less prominent and insistent, and her ability to clearly see what was really behind her distress became easier. By experiencing some simple physical support, she could finally relax enough to work through some underlying assumptions that interfered with her well-being. This technique is one of the things that makes Hakomi a body-centered flavor of psychotherapy. There are many variations to this approach, but one thing Kurtz emphasizes is that when adapting this technique in new situations, the client always remains in the driver's seat; it is their process, and relies upon their readiness and willingness to explore.

With all this being said about honoring a client's self-empowering effort, I feel it important to admit I have fallen off the non-directive wagon many times over the years in my own therapeutic relationships. I might offer a suggestion or insight that the client just isn't ready to hear, which inevitably takes them out of their own process, distracting them from unfolding realizations and interrupting self-actualization. If this happens frequently, it can introduce instability, mistrust and doubt into a therapeutic relationship – or it can create unhelpful dependency on the therapist. So why does this happen from time to time? I think because therapists with years of experience and/or a well-developed intuitive knack can often spot the endpoint of a client's unfolding or the causal factors behind some pattern fairly rapidly, and can become excited about sharing these observations for the client's benefit. And, sometimes, if a therapist offers such insights when they occur, the client can make great leaps of their own because they now have a handle for what they have already intuited themselves; they have a name to wrap around what had only been a vague sense for them before.

When such conditions coincide, a therapist's jumping the gun on the conclusions in a client's process can sometimes be helpful. But only sometimes – enough so that the partial reinforcement of past successes might encourage therapists to take that risk. I have experienced this sort of supportive revelation when I was a client myself, and it was extremely beneficial. But if conditions aren't right, if a person is still struggling with a concept or is unwilling to explore the next step in their process, then any such offerings can feel like added pressure to hurriedly integrate ideas that are not yet fully understood, and end up introducing a barrier instead of support. So discerning when to take this risk and when to let things unfold more organically is, I feel, a skill learned over the course of lengthy experience and prodigious self-reflection.

For another approach, a friend of mine who is a social worker introduced me to *Motivation Interviewing* by William R. Miller and Stephan Rollnick. This approach likewise relies on the client's perceptions, internal resources and motivation to bring about positive change, placing the therapist in a collaborative and supportive role that continually honors the self-directedness of the client. What sets this approach apart is that it holds to these fundamental principles even when interacting with clients who may not be entirely clear about the destructiveness of certain habits or outcomes; for instance, the impacts of substance abuse or other addictive patterns. By encouraging the client to reflect and dialogue about their most deeply held values and goals, the therapists helps the client recognize discrepancy between what they desire out of life and how they are currently living it. Once again, the therapist avoids confrontation over these issues, and instead cultivates a trusting, empathetic interaction that selectively reflects back to the client their own observations and conclusions about desirable change. This process continues through successive phases, increasing awareness and optimism about taking a new direction in life, then reducing the inevitable ambivalence people feel about both the need for change and the planning and follow-through required to achieve enduring results. What reigns at the heart of Motivational Interviewing is the respectful, attentive, caring, supportive, relationship-driven dynamic between therapist and client. In other words, the same person-centered approach that is woven through the other two counseling approaches we have just reviewed.

In the final assessment, the appropriateness of any technique must be weighed against criteria that emphasize empowerment of the client in a facilitative process, rather than the importance or expertise of the facilitator. Those criteria can be explored with questions such as these:

- Do I care about this client and empathize with their perspective? Is this effort a reflection of that caring and empathy?

- Does this create a safe and supportive environment for the client's unfolding process?

- Is my intention in sharing something to facilitate the client's self-directed journey, or to increase their dependence on my skills and insights?

- Is the client ready for this?

- Am I adequately mature, developed and prepared to offer this to my client?

- Is the client invested in or excited about a particular outcome as much as I am?

- Have I patiently sought the client's permission to proceed in this direction, or am I impatiently forcing my will on them?

And so on along those lines. The common theme that spans these questions is a deeply held belief in the sovereignty of the client to determine their own path to healing, the intrinsic wisdom they possess to develop that path, and the power they hold within themselves to heal and become whole. What these counseling approaches encourage echoes the nurturing models we found in parenting and romance: to truly love someone is to trust them, encourage them and empower them to fully love themselves.

Reiki

There are many different streams of Reiki coursing through U.S. Culture. Many more, it seems, than there are in Japan where the practice originated. I think we like to do that in America -- tweaking things, rethinking them or rebranding them. Sometimes these alterations lead to improvements, and sometimes they don't. Reiki has seemed particularly susceptible to this phenomenon, and there remains much controversy over what is original or authentic, what has been corrupted or distorted and so on. Whatever course it took to reach me, the training I received from the Usui method (Usui Shiki Ryoho) has aided my work and contributed in surprising ways to the *Integral Lifework* therapeutic model. For those unfamiliar with Reiki, it is healing practice that Mikao Usui introduced in Japan in the early 1900s. In its simplest form it involves the practitioner applying a series of precise hand positions on the client's body that are intended to channel and amplify a specific form of healing energy. Along with those hand positions, Reiki training also includes principles about the right relationships between Reiki, the practitioner and a client. Here are a few of them from my training:

1) Always ask permission before offering Reiki.

2) Reiki energy is universal life energy, and so anyone can become a channel for it.

3) Reiki has the intelligence to know where it is most needed.

4) A practitioner's foremost responsibility is to regularly practice on themselves.

Further, Reiki practitioners are encouraged to recite and live by the following precepts:

Just for today:

- Don't get angry
- Don't worry
- Be grateful
- Work hard (spiritual practice)
- Be kind to others.

As a therapeutic model, then, Reiki is very simple and straightforward, yet it offers us powerful lessons about the healing and nurturing relationship. To ask permission honors a person's sovereignty; trusting Reiki's ability to heal likewise softens our ego's involvement in the process; practicing on ourselves first and following self-regulating precepts reinforces the idea that healing ourselves precedes and enables helping others. And, although it does not explicitly propagate any traditional religious belief system, Reiki presumes there is a spiritual component to healing that cannot be ignored.

The Other Side of the Coin:
The Client's Responsibility in Therapeutic Relationships

A clear and concise exploration of a client's proposed orientation to therapy can be found in Mirka Knaster's book *Discovering the Body's Widsom*. In this useful guide Knaster enumerates the plethora of modalities that focus on the mind-body relationship (she calls these *bodyways*). In one chapter, Choosing and Working with a Practitioner, she elaborates with honesty and directness that it is the responsibility of every client not to become passive, or expect to be rescued, or in any other way turn their wellness process over to someone else. Instead, the quality and content of the client's healing experience depends on their active participation in the process, their receptivity to healing, and their commitment to ongoing wellness. This orientation is really the starting point of healing for anyone. Most people who seek out help have not been ordered by the courts or an exasperated family member to do so, but there may still be natural resistance, skepticism or fear about a particular modality or their ability to heal or become whole. So the nurturing impulse resides in all parties involved, and the model for that nurturing is the same for everyone.

Knaster goes on to discuss client/therapist psychodynamics, the vulnerabilities in therapeutic relationships and the resulting necessity of a transparent ethical framework, and then the desirable qualities in a therapist. What she does with this chapter is place equal responsibility for effective and appropriate care in the hands of the consumers of that care. In a culture that promotes a quick sell, sensational promises, snap decisions and one-up/one-down power relationships in interactions with most professionals, this is a mandatory reorientation in any self-care model. It is the flipside of Rogers' person-centered approach and all of the other models we have discussed thus far. And it is the unguarded secret to our first steps in all healing, growth or transformation.

Similar sentiments can be found throughout literature on wellness and alternative therapies. The seminal works of Carolyn Mees and Jon Kabat-Zinn – instrumental in my own journey – devote considerable effort to empowering people to retake control of their healing process. They stress the importance of taking ownership of our own attitudes, intentions and relationships in language very similar to what we find in works on healthy romantic partnerships. Without naming it as such, they are really discussing a person's departure from the passive, codependent standard of victim-identity to an active, self-nourishing standard of healer-identity. As Kabat-Zinn writes in *Full Catastrophe Living*: "The price of wholeness is nothing less than total commitment to being whole and an unswerving belief in your capacity to embody it in any moment."

Conclusions

In all of these models we can see the same nurturing principles found in other fields of study. The acknowledgement of a person's sovereignty in self-direction and responsibility; the necessity of personal authenticity and honesty; the prerequisite of seeking wholeness for ourselves before presuming we can create a supportive relationship; and so on. Perhaps all these disciplines have unconsciously borrowed from each other or intentionally cross-pollinated within the postmodern culture they proliferate. For whatever reason, all the pieces fit neatly together. These ideas are components of the same overarching meme, a meme captive to a central belief that healing, wholeness and transformation are innate capacities of every being, constantly pushing at the surface of our thoughts, emotions and perceptions, exhilarated at the prospect of springing forth into complete and robust manifestation – like an energetic canine companion waiting for a stick to be thrown. All of us hold that stick. We may stare at it a while, wondering what it is for. Perhaps we use it to poke around in the fertile dirt of our desires, or try to pry loose some huge boulders of anger, frustration or pain. Maybe we hit ourselves with it a few times, just to see what that feels like. All the while the loyal dog of our infinite potential bunches her muscles in wild expectation of bursting free in gleeful fulfillment. As seekers of love, healing and nurturing we must first come to acknowledge that we alone hold the stick – it cannot be given to us by anyone, nor can anyone take it away from us. The therapist likewise becomes just another person with potential to love, heal and grow; they are holding onto a stick of their own. And by holding that stick a certain way – without prodding or poking each other with it – the therapist and client demonstrate in concert how that stick can be loosed: through humility, patience, kindness, genuineness and empathy; through careful attention, intention and follow-through. Through authentic love.

Transpersonal Ideals of Transformative Love

How do spiritual and cultural traditions define love that is expressed in supportive and nurturing actions?   What we are searching for here is language that describes a love that compels us to think and act in nourishing and transformative ways, while at the same time inspiring the wisdom, discernment and effectual means of creating that transformation.   With the conventional caution that we cannot fully comprehend the language of other cultures until we have immersed ourselves in their traditions, it seems prudent to search through that language for helpful concepts.   Here, then, is a smattering of love-in-action memes from various spiritual and cultural vocabularies:

- **Seva** – Selfless service; compassion in action; being available when the need arises.

- **Prajna-Karuna** – Wisdom with compassion and compassion with wisdom; insight with responsive loving kindness.

- **Bhakti** – Devotional love towards Krishna that seeks expression through worshipful service in every aspect of living.

- **Maitri** – The unconditional friendship with self that leads to compassion towards others.

- **Upaya** – A skillful means or method; practical wisdom.

- **Mudita** – Celebrating another's joy regardless of our own circumstances.

- **Agape** – Unconditional loving kindness; God's parental love for humanity; divine love.

- **Mitzvah** – An act of human kindness; fulfilling divine commandments.

- **Chesed** – Kindness as action that is its own cause, that intrinsically justifies itself.

- **Ishq-e Haqīqi** – Passionate love of Allah, and of all things as they are a reflection of Allah.

- **Diakonia** – Committed and impartial love resulting in charitable service to others.

- **Amity** – Peaceful harmony, friendship and mutual understanding.

- **Altruism** – Unselfish concern for the welfare of others.

- **Amate** – The imperative to love.

This is but a fraction of terms describing actions that result from wise and compassionate insight, and which implicitly or expressly include skillful kindness as a key component. Both as concepts and actions, they are understood to have a supportive and nourishing impact on all parties involved. Through distinct cultural, spiritual and linguistic lenses, such terms depict ways to relieve suffering, introduce harmony and healing, and facilitating liberation from uncaring self-absorption. As guidelines for constructive effort, they expand the focus of beneficent intention beyond the boundaries of self, sometimes advocating a moral imperative for doing so or, as is more often the case, hinting that any felt imperatives to act are the natural consequence of a state of being. As the *Tao te Ching* explains: "Someone who is truly good isn't aware of their own goodness....The greatest virtue is to act without a sense of self; the greatest kindness is to give unconditionally; the greatest justice is to see without prejudice." In other words, what we find in most wisdom traditions is that compassionate action is a consequence of compassionately being; loving kindness is the fruit of an indwelling spirit of love. We cannot separate our devotion to God, our compassion for self, our intimacy with the essence of reality or any other form of spiritual self-realization from actions that benefit the Whole. In an absolute sense, the fundaments of love, insight and wisdom are not evident until they are expressed in beneficial ways through action.

We can learn much from studying such love-in-action memes. First, that we can only comprehend the depths of true love through personal growth and self-discipline; it is not something bestowed on us from without, it springs from within as a result of focused effort that seeks to harmonize with spiritually being. Second, that the propagation of love occurs mainly through action; as wise and compassionate affection takes root within us, it will evidence through skillful interactions and reinforce itself, and we will recognize its presence in our lives. And third, as a spiritual principle, love is either an explanation of how and why we came into being, or the pinnacle of our consciousness, or the natural response to the miracle of our existence, or evidence our divine nature has percolated to the surface...or all of these things. It is both the source and the object of itself; it both self-justifying and self-reinforcing. Ultimately, what the world's great wisdom traditions teach is that there can be no separation of our spiritual faith or philosophical orientation and our love-in-action.

All of these principles align neatly with every other principle we have encountered in this brief survey of approaches to nurturing. Regardless of perspective, love never looks like hate, anger, brutality or any other deleterious impulse. It can be clearly defined through a specific orientation of consciousness, a spectrum of awareness and an expression of beneficial action. Love is the nourishment we give to ourselves and share with those we care about, and it always has the same effects – its ultimate result is to support, nurture, encourage, connect, strengthen, heal, transform, transcend. It replicates itself in a strong and self-sufficient child; in an open, honest and affectionate lover; in a client who courageously chooses to be whole; in a spiritual aspirant who falls in love with Life and Light and devotes themselves to the promulgation of the divine.

Authentic love is infinite in its manifestations, but finite in its focus to sustain, enrich and enlarge the joy of living. It is the most noble and refined effort of our consciousness, and the most radical and self-justifying purpose for our species. No matter what other dichotomies are present in our relationships, love is always there at the center, anchoring every exchange in the most powerfully unifying force in the Universe. In every great wisdom tradition, it is the center of gravity around which everything we ever seek to understand or achieve must of necessity orbit. True love is the fulfillment of our dearest wish, lavishing our existence with purpose and meaning and our hearts with enduring contentment. Whether Buddhist, Jainist, Hindu, Christian, Muslim, Jew, Bahai, Wiccan or the devotee of any other religion, love is always our most worthwhile destination.

| Resources: | For a wonderful sampling of love insights from the world's monotheistic traditions, I recommend Daniel Ladinsky's *Love Poems from God* and his various renderings of Hafiz. Coleman Barks' translations of Rumi are also helpful, as are the New American Standard Bible version of *Psalms, Proverbs, Ecclesiastes* and the *Gospel of John*. For a Hindu perspective, explore Eaknath Easwaran's translations of the *Bhagavad Gita* and the *Upanishads*. You might also enjoy Robert Henricks' translation of *Lao-Tzu Te-Tao Ching*. To understand Buddhist ideas about spiritual love, try a web search on maitri or metta. In fact, try searching each of the terms listed above to better

understand any of them. For a broad survey about the various concepts of love in humanity's wisdom traditions, check out the *Encyclopedia of Love in World Religions* by Yudit Kornberg Greenberg.

Falling in Love Again & Again

If we discover that we have spent much of our lives operating from distorted or incomplete love principles, it can be challenging to believe there is another way and take the first steps toward true love. If we decide we want to expand and deepen our love-consciousness from the solid and healthy foundation we have already experienced, there will be less resistance to taking that plunge. If we are already well-advanced incorporating compassionate affection into all our thoughts and actions, there will be a natural yearning to grow and intensify the love in our being. Yet in each case the process of initiating forward momentum is very similar. In a sense we must begin again, stepping out of our old habits and into a new childhood where wonder, possibility and magick greet us in every moment. In another way we must also take very adult responsibility for our choices and actions. Where can we find a natural union of such joyful abandon and mature carefulness? By letting ourselves fall in love again. By surrendering every molecule of our being to the greatest love affair of our lives, and never looking back. By giving up and giving in: giving up all the craziness and woundedness and hurtful cycling of our willfulness, and giving in to love.

You may have noticed that I have not been very diligent about differentiating various kinds of love up until now. That is because I believe there is a breathtakingly broad spectrum of love, with many gradations and qualities of expression within each band of the spectrum, with all of it emanating from the same source. What we perceive on the surface as different kinds of love are much more closely related than Western culture's Cartesian and Baconian prejudices tend to permit. But the love of family, tribe and nation are varying degrees of the same devotion. Love that is romantic is really no different than love that is platonic, it just allows additional avenues of affection, depending on the social morays and boundaries of the times. Ultimately the love we have for others is a reflection of the love we have for ourselves, and external relationships in fact succeed or fail based on how complete and unconditional our interior relationships have become. As my heart loves my soul, my intimacy with others is ever more complete. As my mind loves my body, my connection to the world around me strengthens. As my spirit loves my mind, I am lifted up into the very center of divinity's fire. And so on into ever broadening circles of experience. For how can we say we love the Earth, or the Universe, or Deity as we understand them, if that love is not proven through how we honor ourselves and those around us?

It does not matter what our belief system is – or our cultural conditioning, or the programming we received from our familial relationships, or the failures we have accumulated in the past. The door to love always remains open to us, and both the impulse and strength to love fully and deeply are intrinsic to the fabric of our being. It does not matter how much loss, pain, tragedy and grief we have sustained over the course of our existence. The remedy to a broken heart is truly universal: by allowing ourselves to become even more broken, but this time with a purpose. To hurl ourselves off of a mountain built on ego, avarice, willfulness and pain, and fall helplessly into the arms of love. As poetic as that may sound, it is really an essentially practical solution. The only meaningful question that remains is how to most effectively go about this.

Surrender & Renewal

Awareness, acceptance and letting go are really catchalls for an array of stages in resolving personal barriers and deepening our experience of love. In some ways, this process can only be seen clearly in retrospect. Can we ever know what falling in love feels like before it happens? Although the experience is unique for everyone, with each stage occurring at a different rate or sequence, there are some common milestones we tend to encounter along the way. In the following chart, we will see some parallels between the stages of surrender a general sense, and the progressions of grief resolution and intimate relationships (both romantic and platonic) more specifically.

The surrender of falling in love and the surrender that overcomes personal barriers to nourishment and well-being are one and the same. It can be a little odd at first to think of the phrases "falling in love" and "resolving barriers to wholeness" as being synonymous, but understanding this coincidence is a key to lasting joy, contentment, and living an effective and purposeful life. One by one, every aspect of our being must surrender to love in order to resolve impedances to holistic self-care. Our judgments, our presumed inadequacies, our fears, our hopes, our dreams, our coping mechanisms...everything. And once we have given up and given in, once we have entirely let go of who we think we are and let love consume our patterns of consciousness and our sense of self, then we can truly be reborn. Love's renewal is therefore a focused and specific process in the overall healing of our being that is interconnected with every other process in the human experience.

As with the many other charts and diagrams among these pages, I encourage you to take a few brief moments to absorb the overall flow of these ideas rather than working through them in detail, then return later to explore them more fully.

FALLING IN LOVE AS SURRENDER & RENEWAL				
← Stages	Barrier Management	Common Events & Emotions	[1] Grief Resolution	[2] Intimate Relationship
Ignorance	Suffering without knowing why.	Sadness, depression, sickness, despair, nourishment substitution.	Initial shock and denial, often with self-isolation.	Loneliness, disconnection and isolation.
[4] Awakening	Acknowledging that patterns, relationships or conditions exist that impede nourishment, love, joy and happiness.	Anger, hurt, blaming, guilt, shame.	Volatile reactions such as anger, panic, despair, and acting out.	Acknowledgement of mutual interest, excitement, anticipation.

Discovery	First glimpse of causal relationships between nourishment barriers and our unconscious behaviors, between barriers and underlying associations, and between these associations and events in our past.	Surprise, confusion, curiosity, fascination, anxiety, fear.	Casting about for reactions and coping mechanisms; mood swings, neediness, substitutions, medication, desperation.	Mutual curiosity, exploration, self-consciousness, anxiety, experimentation and initial exchanges.
Resistance	Denying the impact of past life events on current behavior, avoiding further discovery, or resisting correlations of nourishment depletion with current challenges or symptoms.	Rebellious-ness, self-destructive substitutions, escapist thoughts and behaviors.	Bargaining or denial that delays or suspends grief resolution.	Fear of intimacy, involvement or commitment.
Depression	Erosion of resistance to acknowledged impact of life events, and resulting depression, despondence and grief over those events. [Beginning of **Grief Resolution**[1] process for each barrier]	Depression, sadness, grief, pain, anxiety, despond-ence.	Depression, disorganization and hopelessness.	Longing for emotional connection and exchange.
Acceptance	Acceptance of nourishment barrier's existence and willingness to mitigate its impact.	Relief, release, emotional catharsis, letting go.	Acceptance of loss.	Acceptance of love.
[3] Conviction	Commitment to take action that heals wounds and manages their impact on nourishment through revised patterns of thought and behavior.	Sense of conviction and resolve; first inklings of hope for positive change.	Decision to begin living life without self-identifying with the loss.	Decision to take action that deepens connection and exchange.
Integration	Ongoing disciplined follow-through with real progress in management of barriers and increase of nourishment – especially in depleted areas – as achieved through integral practice.	Sense of hard work, challenging effort and the first taste of positive results.	Through consistent effort, resolution of intense grief and reorganization of values and priorities.	Committed effort that results in elevation of Circle of Intimacy, Level of Acknowledgment and Level of Commitment (See "Relationship Matrix")

Gratitude	Honoring and celebration of well-being and balanced nourishment.	Sense of wellness, wholeness, gratitude, joy and contentment.	Contentment with memory of what was lost, with gratitude for that memory and honoring of its continued importance.	Honoring and celebration of a special relationship.
Inebriation	An overwhelming fullness and expansion of self, especially in areas that were previously depleted or blocked.	Goofiness, silliness, happiness, playfulness.	First real sense of satisfaction, nourishment in area of loss, and enjoyment of life after loss.	Limmerance phase; a classic feeling of being "in love" or "drunk with love."
Courtship	An expression of that fullness and wholeness in an overflowing of affectionate compassion for others – even those whose actions reinforced our barriers – with genuine concern for their well-being and a desire to alleviate their suffering.	Forgiveness, compassion, affection, generosity, caring, kindness, empathy.	Openness to expansion and vulnerability of self in area of loss. [For example, allowing prospect of new **Intimate Relationship[2]**]	Courtship, wooing, expressions of interest and affection; impressive displays of resources, talents and abilities; prioritization of exchanges.
Devotion	Blossoming of love-consciousness and an enduring conviction that commitment to a life of compassionate affection for self and others is the only viable expression of our state of being.	Sense of purpose, directedness, duty, endurance, accomplish-ment.	Where barriers are concerned, a commitment to their management in order to achieve holistic self-nourishment. [Returning to the **Conviction[3]** stage under **Barrier Management**]	Formalization of relationship and public acknowledgment of mutual devotion.
Positioning	Egoistic interference that insists exercising control over events or others is the only way to prevent recurrence of barrier causation or ensure healing, nourishing and loving outcomes.	Fearfulness, anxiety, distress, compulsiven ess, jealousy, self-righteous-ness.		Power struggle over roles and responsibilities in relationship.

Acquiescence	Relaxation into a trust that appropriate attention, intention and follow-through grounded in love will produce the best outcomes regardless of the situation, and that supporting the sovereignty of every individual to find love and fulfillment is more important than controlling their actions.	Joyfulness, gratitude, hope, trust.		Resolution of power struggle into distinct roles and balanced mutual nourishment (as contrasted with enmeshment or codependence).
Authentic Intimacy	The fruits of love-consciousness: harmonized interaction with everyone and everything around us – even those that have led to barriers in our lives.	A sense of closeness, synchronicity harmony, being "in the flow."		Relaxation into genuine, easy closeness, affection and mutually supportive exchanges.
Sustained Commitment	Sustained commitment to the process of acceptance, forgiveness, gratitude and integration with respect to all barriers and all dimensions of nourishment.	Confidence, persistence and an undistracted clarity of purpose.		Deepening commitment to continued importance of the relationship.
Sustained Contentment	More fruits of continued love-consciousness: deepening contentment and satisfaction in every dimension of our being.	Equanimity in almost any situation.		Deepening contentment and satisfaction with the relationship.
Challenges	Challenges to our equanimity and persistence: hurdles and hiccups, alienation, faltering trust, incomplete communication, irritations and brokenness.	Humility, new insight, surprise, chagrin, humor.		Hurdles and hiccups, alienation, faltering trust, incomplete communication, irritations, brokenness.

Growth & Maturation	Repeating the cycle of barrier management for each new challenge, and integrating those experiences into our ever-expanding love-consciousness.	A sense of cycles, seasons, revisiting past lessons, rediscovery, wisdom.		Recognition that effort is required to heal broken aspects of the relationship. [Initiating an **Awakening** [4] stage under **Barrier Management**]
Skillfulness	Skillfully, effectively and powerfully supporting and propagating love-consciousness in the world around us.	Unselfconscious actualization, manifestation, being.		A skillfully loving intimate relationship.

What is perhaps most essential to our progressive well-being, especially in those areas where we are most wounded or depleted, is to realize that unless we learn how to love in healthy ways, we will always revert to the old, unhealthy habits. Along with that, learning how to love in one area does not guarantee we will love effectively in another. Each dimension of nourishment, and each set of internal barriers, present unique opportunities to learn more about love. For example, I may have developed a healthy love in my close friendships, but that does not ensure the same level of skillful caring in my romantic relationships. Just because I can lovingly nourish my mind does not mean I can lovingly nourish my body with the same level of skillfulness. I may have a wonderful relationship with one parent or sibling, only to struggle with anger or resentment with other members of my family. That said, learning how to love effectively in one area will at least demonstrate to us that it is possible to do so, and encourage our confidence to begin love affairs in other, depleted areas once we uncover them.

So how does this process work in real life? How do we "fall in love" with our various aspects of self? In essence, by passing through the stages outlined in the chart in each dimension of nourishment, as well as for each barrier we encounter along the way. Returning to Theresa's example, in some areas we will find the progression of love relatively fluid. In others, quite challenging. For instance, using some simple techniques, Theresa's resentment towards her mother (part of her Supportive Community dimension) resolved itself fairly quickly, and in just a few days she could sense *integration* occurring and even had glimpses of the *gratitude* phase. Regarding the guilt over her physical desires at a young age (part of her Healthy Body dimension), Theresa found herself stuck in the *resistance* phase, needing more time and space to work through the underlying beliefs and assumptions that led her into that guilt. With respect to the grief over a lost family member, she passed from *awakening* through *discovery* and *resistance* in a few weeks, while the *depression* phase lingered for months. At times, she felt she had reached *acceptance*, but then she would encounter the loss again during some component of integral practice, and sadness would set in once more for a day or two. And this illustrates and important principle in our healing process: none of this can be forced. We can bring conscious awareness to our interior transformations, but they will unfold at their own pace and in their own unpredictable way. In other words, they evolve sequentially through each of our processing centers (mental spacetime, emotional spacetime, etc.) until they are eventually embedded in who and how we are.

Love-Consciousness

The ultimate goal of falling in love with each and every aspect of self is to achieve continual love-consciousness. Love consciousness is a state of heart, a state of mind, a spiritual state and a way of being. There are some hallmark patterns of emotion and ideation involved – gratitude, contentment, compassion, devotion, affection, kindness and so on – but these thoughts and feelings are only facets of a complexity. One way to describe love-consciousness is a loving impulse without an object; the felt experience of affectionate compassion without a defined recipient or expression. Another is to say we are in love with everything and everyone all of the time. Still another is a caring response to the world around us that is not dependent on expectations, outcomes, reciprocation or attachments. And another is to observe that loving action springs from the center of our being, rather than from conscious effort; it has become an unconditional response that is not self-conscious, needy or insistent, but accepts whatever has happened, is happening or ever will happen. A love that has let go of egotistical concerns and let go of itself. Love-consciousness operates in the highest strata of moral valuation, but does not measure itself in this way. Surprisingly, entering into this state of being does not require extraordinary act of will power; in fact it often requires a complete relinquishment of personal volition.

Over time, if we persist in nourishing all essential dimensions from a place grounded in compassionate affection, we will arrive at love-consciousness spontaneously and effortlessly. There are, however, practices that can accelerate our journey into all-consuming love. It is possible to experience this state in a concentrated processing space – if we are willing to take that risk and exercise discipline. And there's the rub: for it does sometimes require exceptional effort to initially pass through the door to authentic love if we have only experienced imperfect representations in the past. The force behind the door – an upwelling of devoted and tender fervor – will effortlessly and rapidly propagate itself once the door is opened. But, like a captive who has been locked away in a dark room for a long time, we may emerge confused and disoriented; we may not know how to express or apply what we have encountered there. And so a secondary benefit of disciplined practice is creating a channel for that newly released energy; a means of riding the wave as it surges forth, then guiding its living wildness in helpful and sustainable directions. Perhaps just setting love free within ourselves seems a sufficient justification – and certainly some traditional approaches claim this as their major achievement – but as we will see later on, creating a capable, confident and discerning vehicle for love energy is equally important.

As we have discussed before, when encountering the infinite and ineffable, what nearly all approaches share is an emphasis on experiential learning. This is a critical distinction. To practice arriving at the door is to arrive at the door prepared, but the door itself – the sudden awakening to love – cannot be entered other than through willingness, openness, doing and being. So I encourage you to try the exercises that follow, and to keep trying them until one of them speaks to you in a powerful way. If you are drawn to one style of practice, and are initially uncomfortable exploring another, I suggest you start with the uncomfortable ones first. It is a natural response to resist change because we have a false sense of security in the familiar. But change happens whether we want it to or not, and the familiar slips away no matter how ardently we grasp after it. Discomfort and avoidance are certainly parts of self that deserve love and respect, and they may require thoughtful listening and gentle negotiation along the way. Like everything else within us, internal resistance will evoke important lessons and provide tools for our journey. However, in order to begin a personal transformative practice, we must gently set a boundary for that resistance, however it manifests, requesting its cooperation and promising our full attention to its concerns at a later time – after our new, invigorating exploration has begun.

Encouraging Love-Consciousness

There are many ways to allow love to permeate our being and guide our consciousness. One way is to develop a practice of gratitude throughout our daily routine. It works something like this: as our consistent gratitude for All that Is deepens through renewed awareness, our sense of joy and contentment also deepens. As our joy and contentment deepen, our vitality flourishes. We experience a fullness of life and are unconsciously nourished in countless ways. And as this dynamic of gratitude, joy, nourishment and vitality is amplified over time, something mysterious happens. We spontaneously begin to feel more love – for everything and everyone. This feeling begins to infect everything we think, say and do. And then it is no longer only a feeling, but an inherent facet of our being, a current that runs through all phenomena within and without. Then, gradually, a shift occurs in our consciousness. We begin to see the world differently. We understand appropriate nourishment differently. The best ways to love ourselves and others becomes clearer and easier to carry out. To assert that love-consciousness then leads to an effortless way of loving effectively is no overstatement. And then, of course, we still have much to be grateful for, and the cycle of transformation reinforces itself.

Pretty cool, huh? So for starters, what does a "gratitude practice" look like? Once again, it can be different for everyone, but there are some common characteristics. For one, this is a heart-centered practice, not a head-centered one. The head may be involved initially in ferreting out those first few things to be grateful for, but it is the heart's felt sense of thanksgiving that is activated, and it is emotional spacetime in which the processing takes place. Another characteristic is that the trigger than opens our heart to gratitude can't be too complicated or abstract, or we will remain in our heads. For instance, one person may find prayer an instant avenue to feelings of gratitude and thankfulness, while another finds prayer confusing and distracting. For me, when I first began applying Reiki to myself I found new founts of gratitude waiting to surge forth. For Theresa, learning a self-care meditation awoke a sense of gratitude she had never experienced. For other *Integral Lifework* clients, simply entering into meditative stillness evokes feelings of peace, contentment and gratitude. There is also a gratitude meditation I have taught in classes that seems to work well for many people, and I have included that below. But notice that, like love-consciousness, the field of gratitude need not be connected to any object, nor directed toward anyone. It just *is*, in an all-consuming way.

Exercise: Gratitude Meditation

1) Objective: Between 15 and 75 minutes of continuous meditation each day. If you can, insulate this with a buffer of five minutes before and after so it never feels rushed, and so you have time to reflect on your experiences.

2) Find a quiet place to sit and relax, and begin your meditation with an inner commitment to the golden intention, i.e. "May this be for the good of All."

3) Relax every part of your body. Start with your hands and feet – perhaps moving them or shaking them a little to release tension – then your arms and legs, then your torso, head and neck.

4) Breathe deeply and evenly deep into your stomach, preferably in through the nose and out through the mouth, so that your shoulders remain still but your stomach "inflates." Practice this until you are comfortable with it.

5) In the middle of your chest, just above and behind your sternum, gradually fill your heart with gratitude. It need not be directed at anything or anyone, but you could shape this as an offering to the Source of Life, or Nature, or Deity, or simply to the present moment.

6) Begin with a small point of feeling, and allow it to slowly spread with each breath until it fills your whole being. For some, it may be helpful to visualize this spreading gratitude as light or warmth emanating from a point in the center of the chest. For others, repeating the mantra "thank you" over and over again can assist with mental focus. Maintain this state for as long as you can.

7) As other images, sensations, feelings, or thoughts arise, let them go and return to your focus of gratitude.

8) If you become disquieted, uncomfortable, jittery, or severely disoriented, try to relax through it. If the sensations persist or become extreme, cease all meditation for the day.

9) Give yourself space after your meditation to process what you have experienced. Just *be* with what has happened without judgment or a sense of conclusion.

Remembrance Practice

Many spiritual traditions teach that invoking a worshipful gratitude during certain times of the day or during certain activities aligns us with our spiritual source and directs us more purposefully throughout our various routines. This is usually accomplished through specific rituals that remind us of that alignment and help us remember an intended nature of our relationships with community, spirit, divinity and so on – however it is defined within that tradition. At the heart of those relationships is of course transcendent love, and so inherent to such rituals are both an acknowledgement of love and a heart-felt response in kind. In such moments we are deeply grateful for and humbled by the love we have experienced, and passionately willing to propagate love in and through ourselves. Of course, anyone who has taken part in personal or communal rituals of remembrance knows that there are many traps in these routines that can undermine authentic love. Ritualistic habit may be conformed to out of fear, for example. Or it may become empty of felt meaning after endless repetition. Or it can be so strict and confined that any minor deviation robs it of its intended value.

Or it can become associated with a belief system we no longer adhere to, or perhaps even find distasteful. And so forth. So rather than adopting a conformist, stringent or dogmatic regimen of remembrance, I suggest you invent something on your own; something you can feel deeply each time you practice it.

Here are some personal examples of my own remembrance practice. I consider these the building blocks of my spiritual rhythm throughout the day. They set the tone and resonance for my heart, mind, spirit and body, so that subsequent thoughts, actions and reactions are sketched against a frequency of consciousness patterned in loving gratitude.

- **Morning Worship.** When I go for a walk early each day, I notice with wonder and gratitude all of the miracles around me. The smells, sights, sounds and textures of this amazing place called Earth. What mood does the sky offer today? What texture are the clouds? How deep is the blue? What flowers are the bees and humming birds choosing to visit? What do those blossoms smell like? What images do the water droplets on this leaf hold? How does the air taste? What sound do my footsteps make as I walk? How does the bark on this tree feel against my palm? All of these wonders bring a smile to my heart, if I create room inside myself for them to speak to me. And I can then turn that smile into a sort of prayer of the heart, offering gratitude and celebration with all my being to the Great Spirit, the Goddess, the Creator or whatever name I am comfortable choosing for the source of all this beauty and variation. And once initiated, I consciously offer this prayer of the heart throughout the rest of my walk, until it becomes a sort of song woven into each breath, each step, each thought. And later, when my thoughts wander into all the tasks before me, the song continues somewhere within, so that even when I am distracted or irritated by the inevitable but unexpected twists and turns of my day, a part of me still remembers those more important qualities of my relationship with the Universe.

- **Before Each Meal.** Perhaps you recall the famous Norman Rockwell painting entitled "Saying Grace," where an older woman gives thanks with a young boy while others in the restaurant look on. It depicts many aspects of ritualized remembrance. The potential social awkwardness of personal spiritual practice, for example. The earnestness of faith. Perhaps the painting suggests the provenance of such faith is the old and the young, where those in the prime of life might only respond with curiosity, skepticism, surprise or a vaguely nagging guilt. But what a practice like this means for you personally is of course all that matters. Although I do sometimes forget, I try to pause and bow my head before each and every meal. What I do during that pause has shifted dramatically over time, but I still use the ritual to awaken my heart and revive my awareness of spiritual relationship. I think of the effort of those who prepared the food and am grateful to them for it. I think of the animals that gave their life for my sustenance, and I send my heartfelt thanks to them. I think of the plants, the water and the soil without which I would not have life. I offer intimate gratitude to the living Earth for the flavors, textures, smells and overall pleasure of the meal I am about to enjoy – remembering both the long evolutionary miracle that lead me to this moment, and the wonder and delight of my own senses, thanking my own body and the forces that brought it into existence. And whenever I am with friends or family, I acknowledge our connection and togetherness in that moment as well and am deeply grateful for it. As a continual offering, I rest in awe of a Universe that evolved all of these wonderful things into this moment. Once again, this is a prayer of the heart, and it is wordlessly felt more than it is thought.

- **At Bedtime.** In the moments before I fall asleep, I reflect upon the events of my day and try to be grateful for each one. I also sometimes perform Reiki self-care, which evokes a general sense of gratitude. Sometimes I will look out the window at the moon and stars, and offer them joy and thanksgiving from the depths of my being. Does it matter which deity I remember at these times? Perhaps, though likely not for the reasons we are persuaded to believe. What matters much more is the act of remembering itself.

There are many other ways to develop love-consciousness. As we saw reflected in the Surrender & Renewal chart, healing from grief, learning to manage our barriers and creating intimate relationships all contribute to the foundations of love-consciousness. Mystic activation and other practices in the Authentic Spirit dimension will lead us into deepening love-consciousness as we practice them over time. In fact, you may wonder why the gratitude and remembrance practices weren't referenced earlier when we explored baseline nurturing for all twelve dimensions. Mainly this is because these practices invoke a more advanced level of nourishment – nudging us towards the transformative end of our optimal range – and in fact are dependent on a well-established integral practice as their foundation. How can we consistently feel deep gratitude if we are depleted in other areas? How can we honor All that Is if we neglect our own being? If we cannot remember to take care of ourselves, remembering the Source of Life will avail us little. Our relationships with each nourishment center are, after all, the laboratories in which we perfect high quality exchanges. As we deepen those relationships and the compassionate affection we exercise within, we create a bridge of consciousness between the ground of being and all the realities we perceive around us. This bridge supports the lifelong arc of personal evolution, where love-consciousness becomes our constant companion.

Some form of gratitude practice, therefore, becomes our primary access to this next level of self-nurturing, and the best overall method of establishing an enduring, awakened mode of being. If we nourish every dimension of self with gratitude, then love-consciousness will naturally spring forth from us, permeating everything we think, feel, do and are.

WHAT LOVE ISN'T

Although the following principles are woven throughout other chapters, it seems helpful to zero in on what isn't love, if only to provide additional contrast and food for thought. Because there is such widespread confusion about the nature of love in Western culture, it is fairly easy to slip into harmful substitutions. What is portrayed as love in films or pop songs, sold as love by advertising firms, exemplified as love by well-meaning but misinformed role models, or preached as love by religious enthusiasts are often distant relatives of the real thing. A reliable litmus test for authentic love is that it rarely has any additional agendas other than propagating itself. However, it is sometimes difficult to discern (in ourselves as well as others) what unconscious agendas may be present. Here are some things to look out for that often either masquerade as love or inappropriately justify themselves in the name of love:

- **Obsession and narcissism.** These are really two sides of the same coin, because they both place something or someone at the center of the Universe. Narcissism insists that they only person who matters is me; obsession insists that the object of the obsession is the only thing that matters. Authentic love, in contrast, offers our energy, resources and attention without such comparison or insistence. In mature love-consciousness, everyone and everything are equally lovable and deserving of our compassionate affection, because love-consciousness naturally evolves us into higher and higher strata of moral valuation and an all-inclusive personal identity. Of course we begin with smaller arenas of affection, and at first we must of necessity prioritize our own self-nourishment above the wants of others so that we can be healed, whole, and able to give of ourselves. But that does not mean we relate all events, energies and resources around us to our own well-being or cultivate all relationships to exclusively serve our own needs. Really, such behaviors tend to be rooted in fear rather than love; fear of not being nourished, fear of not being loved and so forth. And those same fears tend to drive obsessive thoughts and behaviors as well. Because some undernourished part of us believes that it will continue to be undernourished, we obsess over externalized pseudo-nourishment to ease our fears, and thus try to control the flow of affection by confining and singularizing its focus.

- **Possessiveness and control behavior.** To possess a thing implies that its value is somehow dependent on a one-up, one-down relationship. Something that belongs to me is subordinate to me; I can own it because its intrinsic value is not as great is my own. I am greater and it is lesser, and the greatest worth this object has is in how it amplifies my own sense of worth. So by possessing something I not only devalue it, but devalue myself my externalizing my own worth, making my value dependent on the things that I possess. This cycle of acquisitiveness will of course never end, because we can never own enough things to liberate ourselves from the sense that what we own is not enough to be valuable, worthy or...lovable. So possessiveness demeans the possessor as much as it demeans the objects of possession. And if those objects are people, well, you can see where this is leading.

Control behavior is just another variation on possessiveness. By controlling a person or a situation, I place myself in a higher echelon than whatever is being controlled. Whatever my justification, by undermining the sovereignty of those around me through controlling attitudes and behaviors I interfere with their ability to self-nourish and love. Those who become teachers, therapists, mentors, parents, bosses or someone who has otherwise taken on the role of conveying skills, information or wisdom have special challenge in this regard; they have, after all, taken on the mantel of increased responsibility for environments and individuals. But increased responsibility is not the same thing as lording over. That responsibility should be shared, to whatever degree is possible, with each student, client, disciple, child or employee. The responsibility of any leader is to further empower those being led, not to further empower themselves.

- **Codependence.** As we touched upon earlier, codependence abdicates responsibility for our own well-being, externalizing it by focusing on the wants of others, which are all too often substitution behaviors and not real nourishment. In a codependent relationship, each person is dependent on the other for their sense of safety, wholeness and love. By tacit agreement, no party involved in a codependent dynamic is allowed to fully nourish themselves. That would, after all, liberate them from their dependency. Although overt possessiveness and control behaviors are often present in codependent relationships, the mutual dependency can be much more subtle. For instance, it can be as simple as my not being able to feel happy unless someone else feels happy, or an insistence that someone else's well-being is more important than our own, or a sense that I cannot be whole or fully nourished unless I am in a certain kind of relationship. By making our well-being dependent on how important we are to others, or how skillfully we can help someone else feel whole, or how much someone else demonstrates love for us, we enslave everyone involved in a crippling and depleting process. People in codependent relationships resist both necessary individuation and healthy interdependence by insisting that each party remain helpless, needy and dependent in some way. That is what love looks like to them, and embracing truly loving concepts like sovereignty or self-sufficiency can be quite frightening.

- **Empathy without remedy.** To witness the suffering of another human being without feeling anything for them or their situation certainly indicates a paucity of love. But what if we do empathize and choose not to act? Sometimes, if a suffering person has willfully brought their situation upon themselves, or has mitigating resources they refuse to utilize, then non-action can be both loving and instructive. But if we have the means or insight to help and they do not, what would prevent us from offering what we can? What would prevent us from taking action to remedy suffering? It might be arrogance that prevents us, or fear, or ignorance, or preoccupation with our own priorities...but it is never love. Love always empathizes with suffering, then seeks to remedy it. Always. Even if that remedy involves forbearance, boundaries or non-action, love responds to all pain with deliberate and persistent healing effort.

- **Action without empathy or compassion.** As the poem by Yeats describes in *The Second Coming*, "The best lack conviction, given some time to think, and the worst are full of passion without mercy." When action is empty of either empathy or compassion, it is backed by more destructive energies. The absence of love does not equate neutrality. Whether we are conscious of those darker forces or not, they will rush to fill the void created when love is forgotten or misplaced. Why does this happen? Because love is always present in everything living, it is the most pervasive influence in the Universe, and in order for love to appear vanquished it must be displaced or hidden by lesser impulses. Anger, indifference, hatred, guilt, fear, sadness, doubt…any of these might become stand-ins for love when we compel ourselves to act without empathy or compassion. This is the danger of perpetuating empty habits that were once grounded in love, or doing something because we think it is socially expected, or acting out of situational expedience, without first checking in with our heart of hearts. If actions initiated by love are no longer a felt experience of compassionate affection, it is time to recharge our batteries by nourishing depleted dimensions of self.

- **Loving others without fully loving ourselves.** One of the most common misconceptions about love is the belief that love must first and foremost be directed outward – toward family, toward society, toward tribe, toward Deity, toward anything other than ourselves. But that is a recipe for self-depletion, and once we become exhausted how can we fully give of ourselves to those we care about? By first focusing on feeding the nourishment centers within us, we will naturally engage in loving relationship with others. But the emphasis remains on fortifying our own being throughout that process, not on slaughtering that being on the altar of self-sacrifice. This is the difference between effective altruism and wasteful martyrdom. In the former we generate bountiful reserves of compassionate affection that are carefully amplified through discerning interaction; in the latter we rapidly expend our own substance in support of an idealized or romantic vision of true love. The fundamental idea here is that our essence is holy and good, and by nourishing that essence and allowing it to overflow through every thought, feeling and action, we will gift the world with our inner light of love. By focusing our energies on external representations of love, we deprive ourselves of the nourishment necessary to amplify that light. We must first focus on what is within, so that it can fully manifest without.

In the next section, we will explore some of the common barriers to holistic nourishment, healing and wholeness. Along the way, we will encounter more examples of how our natural ability to love can be thwarted. In fact, simply be reviewing the twelve dimensions of nourishment and how developed they are in your own life, you will discover what parts of self require more love. Through that process, some of the substitutes for authentic love that you have relied upon to nourish yourself will become more evident. And such realizations will continue no matter how far down the road we travel in our integral practice. *Integral Lifework* is designed to continually question our assumptions about what love is and isn't, mainly because cultural programming continues to exert such a strong influence on our conceptions of love. We will do well to remember that a major component of that programming is to discourage all self-examination.

PART IV

*UNDERSTANDING & MANAGING
BARRIERS TO WHOLENESS*

What Are Barriers?

Overcoming barriers to nourishment, healing and wholeness is a core function of all integral practice. But what do these different barriers look like? And how are different barriers addressed with love-consciousness? There are countless vocabularies to describe these barriers, each one rooted in a specific worldview or values prioritization. And there are just as many propositions for resolving them. In actuality, different language and techniques for barrier resolution may be a fundamental necessity of the human condition, for just as one philosophy, religious tradition or organization of values appeals to one person more than another, so too barrier resolution techniques tend to be more successful for someone who has an affinity with the underlying beliefs that authored those techniques. For one person, any terms that sound religious may be alienating. For another, psychoanalytic lingo sends a chill down their spine. For others, the language of their personal religion or mainstream Western medicine are more comforting than echoes of Eastern philosophy, New Age thought or Chinese medicine. Of course, there is such a rich conceptual vocabulary among the many healing modalities available to us, it seems a pity to exclude any of it. So I will try not to do exclude, though I may redefine some familiar terms to be more inclusive. But it remains important to recognize that what is a wonderful "aha" for one person may be a grating antagonism for another, depending on the vocabulary used. With that in mind, let's examine the nature of some of our most common barriers and how we can go about managing them.

In *Integral Lifework*, barriers are the natural consequences of an array of specific influences. Those influences are listed below. You will notice that some definitions include the terms *functional* or *structural* to differentiate type of influence. A structural barrier is defined as an inherent component of our physical, mental, emotional or spiritual makeup – or an immutable aspect of our surrounding environment. Functional barriers are learned components within our makeup, or environmental barriers we have created. As an example, a person having blue or brown eyes is a structural component of their physical makeup, but a person having a rapid return-to-rest heart rate is (generally) a functional component of their physical makeup. One is the result of DNA, and the other is the result of regular exercise. Functional barriers are patterns of thought, emotion and behavior that are, simply put, more superficial and easier to manage. Pushing ourselves to stay up late in order to watch a favorite TV show, and therefore not getting enough sleep, is a functional barrier. Another might be answering the phone no matter who is calling or when they call. Or not chewing our food because we never give ourselves enough time to eat.   Or not communicating our needs to loved ones in clear and understandable ways. You get the idea. If these habits are indeed just habits without some deeply held belief to support them, they are relatively easy to adjust.   Structural barriers are more challenging because they may indeed be genetic predispositions, or represent inescapable environmental constraints, or they may have deeply held beliefs attached to them such as "this is the way I've always been and the way I always will be." Sometimes, functional barriers become integrated as structural barriers through years of repetition. Here are some common examples of these types of barriers:

- **Cultural programming.**   The social expectations, morays, conventions and patterns that we integrate in order to be accepted and successful in our cultural environment; these begin as functional adaptations, and over time become structural components of our being.

- **Structural limitations and chained associations.**   This is an interrelated set of influences that include physical characteristics and natural impulses, as well as the connections we have created between certain past events and our most successful responses to those events. Depending on the scope of these influences and our sensitivity to them, all of them can result in structural advantages or disadvantages in any dimension of nourishment.

- **Substitutions.** When we perpetuate ineffective or destructive appetites to compensate for undernourished dimensions of self, we often choose substitutions that seem like nourishment but really aren't. These begin as functional barriers but can become more structural as our beliefs in a substitution's viability gain rigidity.

- **Alienation from our True Self.** When we avoid getting to know our own soul, we interfere with our healing and wholeness. This is mainly a functional barrier, unless chained associations turn it into a structural one.

- **Karmic barriers.** Our past has consequences that impact our ability to self-nourish; even if we are focused, loving and disciplined in our efforts, we may need to address karma before nurturing becomes effective. This can be either a functional or a structural barrier.

- **Egoism and willfulness.** If some part of us still believes we are more important than other people or are entitled to get our own way, this naturally disrupts nourishment to our being. In the case of serious mental health issues such as narcissistic personality disorder, this can be a structural barrier. Most of the time, however, it is purely functional.

- **Stress.** As lethal as stress can be, there are ways to transmute many types of stress into nourishment. Unless there are physiological or environmental factors entirely beyond our control, this is mainly a functional barrier.

- **Counterproductive desires and impulses.** Those desires and impulses – whether biological imperatives, part of our psychological makeup, the whim of an instant or whatever else – that somehow lead us into deep or tumultuous waters that interfere with our self-care. These can be both functional and structural in nature.

How these influences become barriers to our well-being is fairly straightforward. They either restrain or expand our ability to self-nourish based on how they shape our perceptions, assumptions, beliefs and abilities. Nearly every choice we make in each moment is dependent on our perceptions, assumptions and beliefs, as well as our natural abilities and those we develop over time. These impact our nourishment prerequisites as well – our fulfillment orientation, our level of discernment and our ability to sustain the golden intention are all facilitated by the perceptions, assumptions and beliefs that dominate our lives. So the question becomes how we can reshape our worldview and patterns of thought, emotion and action so that self-nurturing can occur more fluidly, and any obstructions to nourishment can be softened or eliminated altogether. For each barrier, then, we will discuss some of the ways we can transform non-nourishing patterns into nurturing ones.

Cultural Programming

Earlier we covered the importance of shifting from externally dependent motivations to more self-sufficient, intrinsic motivations; to rely on our internal compass rather than external pressures and events to guide our way. This reflects a broader principle about nourishment and one of the most common interferences to self-nurturing: placing a greater emphasis on what happens outside ourselves than what happens within, so much so that our well-being relies almost entirely on those externals. Am I blaming a friend for how angry I feel? Am I despairing because I lost my job? Am I overjoyed to have received a special gift? Have I fallen in love with someone because they have treated me with more respect than anyone else ever has? All of these indicate a form of externalization. And if we are convinced that we can only be happy when certain external conditions exist, or that our sadness or frustration is mainly the result of other external conditions, or that our sense of purposefulness or satisfaction can only result from external achievements, then we will always be blown hither and thither by the prevailing winds of our experiences – or, more precisely, by our dependency on those experiences.

In one way, externalization is really a learned interference with accurate self-awareness. Instead of separating out external conditions and events from our interior reactions, we identify them as one and the same. But of course they aren't. Although it may seem that our response to a situation is sometimes reflexive and uncontrollable, in reality our response is rooted in a set of beliefs and assumptions we have learned over time that simmer beneath the surface of conscious thought. When left unexamined, those beliefs and assumptions will guide us into continually repeating patterns, inducing thoughts and actions that reinforce our underlying beliefs and assumptions. When we become aware of such patterns in our lives, we can begin digging around below the surface to uncover our unconscious beliefs. To begin this process, we benefit immensely from interrupting our automatic responses to each situation by stepping back, taking a few calming breaths, and letting go of reflexive reactions. An approach we should revisit is conditioning ourselves to ask "why?" Why am I reacting to this with fear? Why do I believe this is what I need to do right now? Why am I insisting I be heard? Why do I find this situation irritating? Why do I find this person attractive? And so on. By asking why, we begin peering into the gaps between what is happening, what we perceive to be happening, and the most constructive ways we can respond.

Perhaps the most prevalent and harmful form of all disempowering and externalizing influences in our lives is the programming – the dominant cultural memes – we integrate from the culture that surrounds us. Because our every waking moment can be consumed in cultural interactions, this programming often has the greatest impact on our nourishment, while at the same time flying well below our self-awareness radar. Apart from a brief period of questioning, rebellion and experimentation during adolescence, most of us integrate cultural programming into our everyday function by the time we reach adulthood. We integrate it so thoroughly, in fact, that its functional impact will alter our physiological structures over time. As a result, it becomes increasingly difficult – though not impossible – to divorce ourselves from cultural influences.

Once we discover our nourishment is being impeded by such conditioning, how we can set ourselves free? We can begin our own liberation by challenging those tacit beliefs and relying on more consciously generated motivations to govern our choices. With practice, we can let go of self-limiting and externalizing enculturation and step forth with the inspiration and strength of a self-directed life. When we externalize our being, we become trapped in a meaningless ebb and flow of circumstance. When we let go of externalizations and invest our confidence in interior discipline, we energize our choices with wisdom and purpose that is innately part of us – that issues from our own essential substance. These habits have tremendous impact on what unfolds in our lives. Here we consciously create opportunity for energy exchanges, rather than unconsciously accepting barriers imposed on us from without.

Exiting the Flow of Enveloping Culture

We initially conform to societal expectations because we want to be nurtured. To belong, to have an emotionally supportive community, to feel safe and protected, to be part of a broader purpose...all of this feeds into our tendency to obey social guidelines. And yet conformance without question can inadvertently result in harm to us and those we love. If we have not reasoned through our decisions and actions, but are relying on the reasoning and conclusions of others, we are sacrificing intrinsic wisdom to mob rule. We are relinquishing free will and conscious choices in favor of mind-numbing autopilot. As a result, there are unintended consequences. Our conscience is quieted. We lose our ability to distinguish shades of gray, and tend to see everything in a polarized way, as high contrast extremes of black and white. We become defensive about this condition, either avoiding any situations where our beliefs might be questioned, or aggressively attacking anyone who opposes us. Because we have chosen not to reason through our decisions or consider them from alternate perspectives, we can't explain ourselves...even to ourselves. Ironically, by choosing conformism over consciousness, we risk sabotaging the very outcomes we cherish because we live in an uncritical, reflexive and reactive mode.

Human history has many examples of this phenomenon. One of the most striking was Nazi Germany. At that time the German population became mesmerized by the idea that giving up their personal freedoms and critical self-awareness for the sake of a shared idealism would somehow produce desired outcomes. But it didn't. Because when these otherwise good-hearted folks annihilated their own freedom of thought, will and action by subordinating unquestioningly to the Nazi agenda, they gave the leaders of that agenda too much power. As a friend of mine, Tomas Firle, said in his memoirs about Germany at that time: "Under a totalitarian regime, oppressed people just don't have many choices. There are significant limitations to civil rights. It is important not to step out of line, to remain invisible. You had better learn how the system does things...learn to watch your step, what you say, how to say it and to whom." And so what began as a desire for social cohesion and order resulted in the Holocaust.

Over and over again throughout recorded history we can observe the deleterious effects when conformist groupthink goes unchallenged. And although this tendency may be no more prevalent now than in previous times, I believe it is exacerbated by the overwhelming acceleration of change that technology has brought, by the deluge of contradictory information available to us from countless ideologically biased media sources, and by the equally dizzying array of choices we are presented with each day. As a result, we must navigate a storm of mainly subliminal invitations to conform.

With so many tumultuous input streams and the inherent difficulty of evaluating them, it is not surprising that many people today gravitate towards uncritical groupthink. An excellent example of this is the political election process in the U.S. If I am a loyal Republican or Democrat, I don't need to fully understand the issues, the intricacies of various initiatives on the ballot, or the candidate's specific experience or positions – I just need to know what my party recommends. From there I can exercise either avoidance behavior and steer clear of all debate and self-examination, or numb my conscience by hurtling into the fray and fiercely quoting borrowed rhetoric. In either case, if I identify strongly as a member of the Democrat or Republican tribe, I will defend that tribe and my membership in it with tooth, nail and little regard for the truth. We do this because conformance isn't about understanding, exchange or solving difficult problems, it's about belonging, loyalty, and justifying convictions through larger and larger numbers of adherents. And as in any other case where conformity takes precedence over so much else, the results are not constructive. What clearer evidence do we require than the gridlock and partisan polarization of U.S government at local, state and national levels?

Conformism can of course be more subtle. Consumerism in the U.S. is a pertinent example. Consider that pharmaceutical advertisements in prime time TV generate substantial, hugely profitable sales for drug companies, often to treat medical conditions that few had even heard of until the ad is aired. Do your legs feel cramped or uncomfortable on occasion? Then you must have Restless Leg Syndrome. Do you suffer from severe headaches? Then you need migraine medication. Have you ever sneezed? Then you need to treat those undiagnosed allergies with powerful chemicals. Is your stomach upset by rich foods? Then you need prescription strength antacids. Any pain in your muscles? There's a pill for that too. Why tolerate any discomfort at all when there are medications to mask our symptoms? Consumers respond to this pharmaceutical prompting in droves, insisting doctors prescribe them drugs for conditions they might or might not have. However, this reflexive response to advertising rarely improves people's physical health or any other aspect of their well-being.

Along the same lines, do most dieting fads really help people lose weight and remain healthy over time? Do popular clothes, accessories, perfumes and makeovers really provide us with the romantically satisfying relationships the ads promise us? Does the cool new car, gadget or golf club really deliver lasting contentment, greater sexual performance or higher social status? Of course not. No more than eating fast food creates happy families or the newest cell phone plan manages teen behavior – or any of the other fallacies touted by mainstream advertising. But when we are running on autopilot, accepting the false nourishment we are sold without questioning its efficacy, we begin a downward spiral of substitution and depletion, a maelstrom of malnourishment from which it is impossible to escape unharmed.

On the surface, it seems easier to conform to the norm. After all, this allows us to succeed in the moment, and perhaps even realize personal dreams that are acceptable to our cultural programming or immediate community. By suppressing our conscience, or the messages from our bodies, or our unique qualities or inclinations, or anything else that runs counter to the mainstream, we achieve a veneer of tranquility. In a commercialized, commoditized culture, all viable strengths and vision are simplistically defined by mass media and readily available for purchase. If we buy in, things will appear to run smoothly for us. If we can commit to being dutiful consumers who externalize our self-realization and emphasize only those traits that are facilitated by material exchanges, we might indeed thrive by the narrowest, most worldly definition. But by its nature this mode of operation cages our neglected facets of self, crippling our ability to actualize and nourish our being in its entirety. We become shells of our True Self, and our lives likewise become empty and meaningless. Unless the bona fide purpose of our existence is to consume or sell things we really don't need or want, our soul will slowly starve.

So what are some exit strategies? How can we stop this downward spiral? One escape plan involves a reactive rebelliousness akin to what many of us experience in adolescence. Here we search for environments and people that harmonize with subversive, countercultural proclivities. We invest in a lifestyle contrary to the mainstream as long as it improves our status among equally rebellious peers, and doesn't require too much energy or commitment. If our efforts are unsatisfying, we can always rebel again and move on. But in the meantime, we have a supportive subculture, a comforting substitution that is really just another version of conformance. If we aren't certain who we are, what our purpose is, or how to go about living our life, it is easy to fall into this self-deception.

Another variant of superficial escape is relocation therapy. Here we flit from one set of relationships to the next, one job to the next, or one living environment to the next, without ever putting down roots or committing to anyone or anything. We skip along the surface of life, keeping thing fresh and exciting with continual movement, thinking we are making progress without ever plumbing the depths of who we are. Whenever we encounter resistance or difficulty, it's time to move on. There are people who are born travelers or explorers, nourishing themselves and others through new relationships, cultural exchanges and the discovery of exotic vistas around the globe. But even born travelers learn that the most satisfying adventures occur in the ever-deepening connections, meaningful sacrifices and personal accountability of hearth and home. As big as the Universe appears, we can never escape from ourselves.

We could also choose another form of running away by creating a cocoon of imaginary segregation and isolation. If we protect ourselves from influences that antagonize us, won't we finally be free of destructive enculturation? Whether a sound-proof apartment, a gated and homogenous community, a religious commune, or a cabin in a pristine patch of wilderness, this perceived exit from the mainstream can be seductive. But the escape is an illusion. The more we sequester ourselves away from offending culture, the more we are really spreading the seeds of that culture into new, isolated environments. We still carry the dominant memes of society within us, and we will re-create the human condition with different veneers over the same patterns. No matter how many walls we erect to protect ourselves from cultural influences, we will eventually end up recreating the unhealthy choices of our cultural programming.

Is there a more effective solution? A significant principle of integral practice is that we honor and cherish what doesn't conform to the norm. That is, we emphasize nourishment to areas that society perceives as unimportant or weak. In a disciplined and focused way, we accept and integrate those aspects of self that do not conform to cultural expectations – or that haven't been ascribed a contributive advantage in society. We bring what we have hidden from others and ourselves out into the light, holding our heads high. We learn not only to accept those aspects of ourselves, but to fall in love with them. To honor and celebrate them with affection and joy. To see them not just as deficits, nagging irritants or teachers of patience and fortitude, but as part of our unique contribution and purpose in this life. And to incorporate all of our perceived weaknesses – even those that have brought us the most pain – into our integral practice. By doing this, we eventually become whole. And because this wholeness is distinctly individual in its construction, it naturally resists conformance. As we are guided by authentic love, we become unique contributors to the good of All through this uniqueness. So instead of isolation or avoidance, there is integration and engagement; instead of destructive conformance or nonconformance, there is constructive contribution.

This principle may be difficult to appreciate without experiencing it first-hand; here is a personal illustration. One of my own so-called weaknesses is a desire to create for creativity's sake. That is, to creatively express myself because I value that process and its outcomes. The culture that enveloped me in my childhood did not value this inclination the same way I did, and I was routinely discouraged from pursuing purely creative activities throughout my early life. Sitting by myself, silently playing with ideas, musical notions or mental images resulted in accusations of laziness and a few more chores to "keep me busy." Writing poems, taking photographs, drawing pictures and composing songs were likewise considered a childish waste of time by all but one or two of my relatives and friends. And, as I grew older, I saw the cultural validity of these assessments in terms of career choices. Most artists worked in some other field to support their art. The few who could tailor their creative impulses to established industries were able to make a living at it, but in most cases they had to significantly compromise their creative vision. For instance, a fine art painter who survives by painting pulp fiction book covers, a singer-songwriter who makes a living with advertising jingles, or a gifted actor whose only reliable revenue stream is derived from playing the same sitcom character over and over again. For the most part, I decided, very few people ever achieved material stability or success through a genuine expression of their creative passions.

But this realization did not keep me fry trying to win my culture's creative lottery. I put in the requisite 10,000 hours writing and performing music, attempting to get short stories published, marketing my photography skills, and launching a stage acting career. I tried to mold my self-expression to the marketplace while still remaining true to my muse. But the tension between these two demands became exhausting. There was a market for wedding photographers, performing rock standards in smoky bars, bit acting parts in community pageants, and either gruesome or pornographic fiction. But those things weren't me. I was a folk singer. I liked to photograph abstract patterns, candid shots of people, and the beauty of Nature. I wanted to play demanding parts in meaty plays. My fiction was more cerebral than visceral. So, after several years of unsuccessful efforts to reconcile these two extremes, I concluded that the odds were too great to find common ground, and threw in the towel.

At about the same time, I went through a similar struggle in my spiritual life, and ended up denying nourishment to both my Playful Heart and Authentic Spirit dimensions. Eventually, I hit rock bottom. I struggled with health problems, had bouts of depression, and felt a deepening sense of alienation, bitterness and loss. Parts of me seemed to be dying off and decaying, but it took me a while to recognize what was happening. At last, I was able to return to creative self-expression as well as reinitiate a spiritual practice. I gave up trying to conform my creative impulse to the capitalistic expectations of my culture, the joyful energy of my interest just kept expanding and enriching my life. Now I write, take pictures and make music for the joy of these things alone. I connect regularly with the ground of being. I honor and care for all of myself, and share what I create with those who can really appreciate it. I give to myself because I feel compassion for myself, and I give of myself because I feel compassion for others.

What happens when we achieve such equilibrium with our culturally perceived weaknesses is that we are stepping out of the river of enveloping culture without abandoning it altogether. We are empowering ourselves to the point where we can be truly free, allowing the water to lap at our feet without sweeping us downstream. Our perceived weakness becomes our strength – not the strength of society's valuations, but the strength of a being that is loving, passionate and whole. And when we have become sure of our own footing, we can even venture back out into the water and show others how to find their way. What begins as challenging our culturally programmed assumptions ends in offering our individual gifts back to society. And in the greatest of ironies, our offerings may in fact have a transformative influence on the culture that initially oppressed us.

All of this we accomplish not as a consequence of ego, or even because we think it is right, good, noble or true; we do this because we have infused ourselves with the meme of love-consciousness, recognizing that authentic love is a more effective door out of the harmful current of conformist impulses. In my view, this is the only way out that provides healing and wholeness. Every action then flows out of our steadfast commitment to compassionate affection – first for ourselves and then for others – manifesting as full-spectrum nourishment and then, eventually, as something that benefits the good of All.

The Meme of Personal Empowerment

Over the years many popular self-help techniques have encouraged finding our personal strengths and focusing on their development. If we do this, so the thinking goes, we will cultivate a more fluid and natural way of being and succeed at our endeavors with greater ease. We will also tend to be more enthusiastic and satisfied with our efforts. After all, why make life more difficult by struggling with the same inadequacies day after day because we continue to choose a path that relies upon those inadequacies or self-limiting thoughts? Along the same lines, there have been an equal number of widely embraced methods to acknowledge and embrace our strongest longings and dreams, and to actualize them in seemingly miraculous ways. In other words, there is a resurgent meme circulating through Western culture that if only we could find the right combination of self-awareness, strength of conviction and innate talents, our lives would sail powerfully and easily toward a paradise of personal fulfillment. This is the meme of personal empowerment.

This meme encourages and relies upon a series of deeply held beliefs. For instance, that this effortless unfolding of beneficial conditions is somehow a natural part of our reality, if only we could access it. That negative and self-limiting attitudes are all that stand between each individual and their greatest accomplishments. That unlimited personal potential is waiting to burst into our lives, if only we could find a key to the door of that level of consciousness. Somehow we have lost our way, and all we need to do is get back on the path for our lives to run smoothly. And so on. And because the meme of personal empowerment appeals so strongly to these underlying beliefs, it is very attractive. Because many of the techniques offered really do work on many levels, and because there are showy glints of truth in the idea of effortlessly being, some of the results of these methods can indeed feel powerful. But those results really aren't nourishing, because there is a fundamental flaw in the way this meme functions: it depends either upon our conformance to societal norms when framing our goals, or the cultural acceptance of our efforts.

Here are some examples of how this has played out in people's lives:

- After years of failed relationships and frustrated career aspirations, Joe was searching for a more peaceful way of living his life. After reading many books, taking many classes and attending seminars and retreats, Joe decided to live in an ashram in India for a year. There he learned interior self discipline through meditation and other transformative practices. He learned how to live simply and how to cease impatiently obsessing about having his every need met.

He also developed an enduring sense of detachment from the many concerns that had brought him so much grief in his life. He also found time to think a lot and write down his thoughts – two things he had never found time to do back in the States. And when his year in India came to an end, Joe returned to his life in the U.S. with a powerful set of tools to maintain a different array of personal priorities, a grounding mode of equanimity, and a fattening journal of philosophical musings. Very soon after his return, however, Joe began to experience disruptions to this new mode of being. When he began a new job, the stresses and demands of his workplace began to shift his priorities, leach away his equanimity and rob him of his thoughtful introspection; nevertheless, he knew he would need the job to buy a house. When he started driving a car again, some of the old impatience and frustration with other drivers began to surface; however, he needed the car for his new job. And, after a few months, when he found himself beginning a new romantic relationship, he was shocked to discover many of the same old insecurities and disappointments that had led him on his quest for peace in the first place were resurfacing; yet everyone seemed to expect him to get married and have kids, so he persisted. Now he had no time at all to pursue the self-enriching activities he had enjoyed in India. At the end of his first year back in America, it seemed as though he had undone all the progress of his personal evolution – or perhaps that the progress had somehow been an illusion all along.

- Tina loved animals. She adored the variety of wildlife she experienced around her home as a child – the birds, the squirrels, the raccoons, the frogs and insects and everything. She could sit and watch them for hours. In particular, though, she loved watching the horses that galloped through open pastures just down the road. One of her earliest memories was saving up all of her allowance so she could take horseback riding lessons, just so she could be around those horses. As soon as her parents allowed it, she would spend all of her free time at the local stables, grooming and mucking and doting on the ponies there. She was so devoted and so talented with the horses that the locals began calling her the "Barn Rat Princess." Eventually she purchased her first horse, a gelding Quarter Horse, training and riding every day. She loved that horse, most of all when she set him loose in the pasture. At the encouragement of other owners, she began competing in dressage, doing better and better each year. Then she purchased another horse, this time a Morgan mare, and began training with her for other events. She thought she was fulfilling her childhood dreams, but somehow she still wasn't happy. Something wasn't right. And she was spending so much time, energy and money on her horses, she had hardly any other life to speak of. Then one summer a friend invited her out to a ranch in Nevada, where for the first time she saw wild mustangs running free. It changed her life. Seeing horses gallop across the open plains cracked something loose inside her. Memories of those childhood days spent watching wild animals run around the yard and horses prancing in their pastures came rushing back, and she realized she had taken a wrong turn somewhere. Her own horses were confined to small barn stalls and paddocks most of the time. Her gelding would never prance proudly around his herd the way the Mustang stallion did. And when she saw what the ranchers did to gentle the wild Mustangs they roped, she was heartsick and ashamed.

• Andre was a natural athlete. As a young boy, he loved to run through the woods for hours, run over to visit his friends, even run all the way to school. When one day a football coach saw Andre running, he tracked him down later that day to ask if he had ever thought about playing football. If he joined the team, the coach promised, he could run all the time and maybe even get a scholarship to college. Andre said that sounded like a pretty good deal, so he joined up. He worked hard at football, learning and practicing and competing, and for the first time in his life he was really popular at school. He had such a busy social life, he didn't even have time to run through the woods anymore. He missed that, and didn't really enjoy the aggressive competitiveness of football as much as other boys did, but he kept thinking about girls and college and the possibility of a bright future in the NFL. Then, in the fall of his senior year of High School, Andre was running a Hail Mary to the end zone when a side tackle took him down hard. At first he thought he was fine, but when his teammates pulled him up, he couldn't walk. In fact, his knee began swelling into a melon. After two surgeries, months of a leg brace, and weeks of physical therapy,

Andre could finally walk again.   He would never run again,
however, at least not with the carefree abandon he had so enjoyed
earlier in his life.

What pattern can we see emerging in these examples?   I believe the
intention of each of these people was sincere, and that they followed the
same process that has brought success and happiness to many others,
but somehow they did not succeed.   Why?   Allow me to propose a
unifying reason for this failure, one that I have encountered over and
over again with my *Integral Lifework* clients: these individuals did not fit
the common mold for success in their culture; their strengths and talents
were not allowed to develop independently, but pressured to conform to
societal expectations; their innermost longings and dreams ran slightly
askew to the overwhelming flows of energy that surrounded them.   And
that is where the personal empowerment meme gets turned on its head.
Because if my strengths and dreams do not resonate with the culture or
subculture within which I reside, then no amount of personal
empowerment will allow me to flourish there with ease.   In fact, my
strengths and dreams will continue to be a hindrance to my own
fulfillment and happiness, because wherever they run counter to the
prevailing winds, they can interfere with my ability to nourish myself on
one or more levels.   They may, in fact, be perceived as deviance if I do
not conform.   Unfortunately, pursuing them in any fashion tends to lead
down a path of isolation, alienation and depletion.

In Joe's case, what if he had kept prioritizing those activities that had
brought him so much satisfaction and equanimity wile he was in India,
even after his return to the States?   What if he had decided he didn't
need a car, or a full-time job, or a romantic relationship as much as he
needed to meditate, reflect and write?   What if he had let go of those
other expectations and stuck with what helped him grow and change so
completely?   If Tina had been encouraged from a young age to follow
her bliss of watching wild animals at play, instead of conforming to
cultural norms of animal interaction, who knows where that would have
led her.   Perhaps she would have been a wildlife photographer, or
worked tirelessly to defend wild Mustang habitat, or educated people
about respecting and preserving wilderness, or otherwise focused her
passion into constructive, balanced and self-nourishing ends.   For Andre,
the choice to use his physical gift competitively made complete sense for

the social conventions of High School popularity and parental expectations of a college education. But what if Andre had been left alone to enjoy his gift without such conformist corralling? What if he had found his own way to contribute? Perhaps he could have raised money for charity with cross-country runs, or become an Olympic champion who inspired millions, or just lived a long and healthy life of incredible fitness. In all of these cases, the idea that people should empower themselves by conforming to specific, culturally viable goals undermined their well-being and effectively wasted their time and talent.

Where did this conformist self-empowerment meme originate, and why does it keep getting perpetuated? I believe the personal empowerment meme in the West is a distinctly commercialistic phenomenon. In capitalist culture, the human condition is of necessity pared down to its most saleable and consumable elements. What inspires and reinforces beliefs about success, wealth, freedom and an entitlement to personal possibility is its commercial viability. And every individual strength, talent or aspect of personal visioning that conforms to cultural norms of success is quickly absorbed into the dominant meme's marketing package. To think positively is to become affluent; to manipulate people's feelings is to become popular and accepted; to believe in a corporate mission or don the mantle of team player is to rise to an ever higher pay scale; to follow your commercially workable bliss is a potent measure of happiness. And so on. Anything that fits neatly within the modalities of mass production and consumption seems miraculously successful, reinforcing its own narrow truth, when really it's just another way to play the game within a system of inflexible values and exchanges. This is one reason why free market solutions will never solve all of the world's challenges; they will only solve problems where consumers with reliably acquisitive values meet producers with reliably saleable ideas. The beautiful diversity of human beings is not accounted for in market solutions, but is subsumed in a subtle variant of feudalism. The more we rely upon consumption-based models to solve humanity's problems, the more poverty of spirit we will experience as a whole.

So rather than playing to our strengths, the empowerment meme often leads us to play to our strongest weakness; that is, the weakest ability or desire that conforms most closely to what is acceptable and supported in the parent culture or surrounding subculture – the weakness that allows us to succeed in material terms, or which allows us to gain acceptance in our immediate social circles. To truly play to our strengths, we may need to abandon the promise of material rewards or social acceptance, and redefine what it means to flourish. In *Integral Lifework*, flourishing entails being fully nourished on all levels in every dimension. That is a place where contentment, peace and passionate enterprise are a natural unfolding of effortlessly being ourselves. It includes the support of a loving community and the fulfillment of all our basic needs, but assumes we actively create that community rather than conforming to our situational default. If financial security is an added benefit, then we can consider ourselves privileged and blessed. But "empowerment" in the context of *Integral Lifework* is more about the holistic satisfaction of our most intimate hungers, and our ability to share that satisfaction with those we love, broadcasting tranquility and joy into the world around us. As such, this is not something we can commoditize, market or trade in the commercial sense, because it emanates from unselfconsciously being rather than calculatedly doing. Otherwise, if we keep trying to conform, we will expend tremendous energies attempting to synthesize and sell an elixir of love rather than becoming love itself.

Now, with all that said, are there some offspring of the conformist empowerment meme that actually work? Are there sincere practitioners who are not merely playing to their weakest conformative strengths? Of course. There are always exceptions to any generalization. But consider that, in many self-empowerment models, affluence is a de facto prerequisite for broader, more holistic definitions of success. In these models, we must of necessity consume in order to self-actuate; we must rely upon externals in order to learn and grow. And the moment any system directs us outside ourselves for strength, insight, wisdom or a sense of purpose, that is surely the first sign of a disempowering commodity.

The River

I awoke to find myself adrift
   upon a quickly flowing river
   warm and comforting
   carrying me I knew not where

I shared this journey
    the swift current
        churning forward in a rush
    with a million million souls
Some competing to lead the way
Others struggling to stay afloat
And a few challenging the status quo
    clinging to rocks
    rallying against the forceful flow
    or pulling themselves out
        and up the distant, muddy banks

For a moment I thought:
"Why am I drifting here?
Where will this take me?"
And in my first questions
    something stirred:
A will to learn, to know
    to understand

Slowly, carefully
    I swam my way across the streaming throng
    pushing past faces just like mine
    some sleepy with contentment
    others purposefully driven
    many gazing about in bewilderment
    or troubled by my passing
        until at last I found a different course

The river's pull was strong
    invisible hands, strange and familiar
    clutching at my will or barring my digression
And though the banks were gouged and trenched
    where sodden refugees had tread
I could not find my footing
    but slipped and clawed and slipped
    crawling hopelessly amid the muddy wet
    for a lifetime, maybe more

Then, just as my energies were spent
I heaved beyond the river's reach
    beached myself
    caught my breath
    saw the current and its floating host

    all at once for what it was
    and terror stilled me

Some sorrows seek company to bear
Others crave the silence of solitude
This one cried out across the water
    a clarion for the brave
    a siren for the ignorant
    a raging grief of disbelief
        with each new bobbing head
        and flailing limb
        speeding toward oblivion

Then other questions rose
To drown the first:
    "What should I do?
    What can I do?" I cried
Despair a stronger tide
    threatening to wreck my mind
"Stand up," the answer came
    whispered in the leaves
    and lapping, bluish waves
"Show it can be done
    remember those who went before
    and find your own way home."

So I stood, stood firm, and beheld
    a thousand knowing smiles
    lighting the forest's edge
Here at last my feet craved dryer earth
my heart the weight of soaring on its own
and my soul the naked, chilling air
    of freedom

Resources: To explore constructive views of personal strengths, try Howard Gardner's *Multiple Intelligences: New Horizons in Theory and Practice*. To appreciate liberation from cultural influences, try J. Krishnamurti's *Freedom from the Known*.

Survival Personas

Aside from how we use our strengths or weaknesses, another aspect of cultural programming are the survival personas we cultivate over time. Personas are social masks we adopt to gain acceptance and approval from others – to integrate with our immediate environment – and to partially nourish ourselves in one or more dimensions. As such, they are basically protective personality traits, and are by their nature inauthentic representations of who we are to other people. Anyone who has spent time on an elementary school playground has seen this at work. Think of a child's impulse to laugh when a school yard bully makes fun of someone else – that is a survival reflex. If the child doesn't laugh, perhaps the bully will beat them up, or they'll be socially ostracized, etc. Survival personas grow out of this same preservation impulse, but become so deeply patterned in our day-to-day lives that we cease to consciously recognize them; sometimes we even modify our core beliefs to accommodate them. At first we laugh because everyone else is laughing, but maybe we feel guilty about it, or a bit sorry for the person being picked on, or even angry at the bully. If we suppress these contrary impulses, keeping emotions in check that might put us at risk, a persona begins to take root. Then, when our laughter has the desired result – that is, when we avoid getting picked on ourselves because we express support for the bully – the laughter may arise a bit more easily next time, with less of the guilt, anger or sympathy we initially experienced. If we don't challenge this pattern early on, and our environment continues to encourage it, the reflexive persona becomes something more. We begin to adopt or manufacture beliefs to support our survival behavior. Perhaps we start blaming the victim of the bully's abuse, incorporating malicious gossip about the victim into our newly forming notions of right and wrong. All of a sudden the bully is *entitled* to be angry, and the victim *deserves* all the abuse they receive. Besides, we are powerless to change the situation anyway, right? And, if this progression continues, maybe we even participate in bullying ourselves – after all, it makes people laugh. And thus a survival persona is born, solidifies, and grows in strength.

Early on in life, when we perceive ourselves as helpless and dependent, the personas we adopt seem like powerful allies. Where once we were at the mercy of our environment, suddenly we have some influence over it.

And as we grow, those personas may continue to aid us in combating fundamental insecurities. They may help us to survive in a challenging and even hostile world. But there is a cost. Those social masks are not really us. They belie our first impulses. They distort or change our core beliefs. They turn us into someone we may not even like. The more we wear them to protect ourselves, the more we become them, and the more conflict – the more cognitive dissonance – we feel within. Why? Because part of us remembers that these are just an act, they're just convenient behavioral fibs. Part of us knows that the more our personas dominate us, the more inauthentic our life becomes.

Let's take a look at some common survival personas, keeping in mind that there is no limit to how many may inhabit us over the course of time, always interacting and evolving. I like to categorize these according to various *identity types* influencing our choices. Identity types are the dominant archetypes of our surrounding culture (in this case Western culture). They are personifications of primal, perpetual forces of survival that have aided past generations; the deep metaphors that have enabled the success of our species at one time or another. These memes reside in a larger, collectively shared understanding simmering beneath the surface of day-to-day interactions – an unconsciousness awareness of what has traditionally facilitated humanity's existence. Of course no one can fully manifest these ideals; they are merely reference points we might strive for without consciously knowing it, and so we don't always recognize the survival personas derived from them, nor do we realize that a certain identity type may have become obsolete or irrelevant to the human condition in the present day.

Our individual personalities seem far too complex and diverse to categorize under absolute headings, and so identity types are expressed individually as unique survival personas, hybrids of those dominant influences. These in turn also interact, change and evolve; the dominant personas we developed when we were young might fade away entirely, merging with or replaced by other, more current personas, or morphing into something entirely new, but still rooted in a guiding identity type. You will get a taste for this variety but perusing the examples on the following chart.

Identity Type	Example Survival Personas	Common Behaviors	Possible Supportive Beliefs
Warrior	• Rebel without a Cause • Fighter • Agitator • Champion • Loose Cannon	Rigid, impulsive, combative, judgmental, defensive and self-righteous	Danger is imminent; nothing is safe; I must assert myself or I will be swept away
Conqueror	• Sexual Aggressor • Abuser • Destroyer • Winner at Any Cost	Serial relationships, jobs and interests; highly competitive	Nothing has any value until I conquer it; I prove my worth to myself through dominating others
Helpless Victim	• Noble Stoic • Perpetual Failure • Chronically Sick • Depressed Person • Orphan	Psychosomatic illness, self-sabotage, rejecting help, avoiding growth, always suffering	I can't cope; I have no power; I am helpless
Nurturer	• Always Nice • Rescuer/Enabler • Parent • Teacher	Premature agreement, premature intimacy, enabling behaviors	My self-worth is wrapped up in helping others; disagreeing with people is a bad idea; if I am liked, then I can like myself
Perfectionist	• Know-it-All • Critic • Master • Anal Retentive Person	Assertively competent, perpetually stressed, compulsive, dismissive	If I can control my environment, everything will be okay; if I am better at something than everyone else, that makes me a more valuable human being
Hermit	• Happier Alone • Lone Survivor • Painfully Shy • Grumpy Old Person	Self-isolation, rejection of society and social expectations; distrustful of other people	Relationships are too challenging; if I'm alone then I can't hurt anyone, and no one can hurt me
Adrift	• Happy-Go-Lucky • Peter Pan/Tinker Bell • Flower Child	Unreliable; can't commit or follow through; doesn't want to be responsible or accountable	I'd rather not be suffocated or oppressed by someone's expectations of me; I need to be free; I don't want to be judged
Responsible One	• Fiercely Loyal • The Boss • The Strong One • Social Organizer • Busybody	Always proving themselves; taking control; interfering with others' lives or offering unsolicited advice	No one else can be trusted to do it, so I'll do it myself; other people are incompetent; I need to be an important person

Adventurer	• Dare Devil • Adrenaline Junky • Risk Taker • Traveler	Always pushing the envelope and seeking new experiences	There is always something better around the next bend in the road; sitting still is boring
Social Emblem	• "I Am My Job" • "I Am My Family Role" • "I Am What Society Expects of Me"	Suppresses own needs and wants; loses own identity in the expectations of others	My self-worth is defined by my position in society; safety and security are result of how people perceive me
Unworthy	• Deviant • Bad Person • Criminal • Deceiver	Self-sabotaging, self-effacing, self-destructive	I am a bad person; I don't deserve to succeed; I can't be forgiven
Lost Soul	• Space Cadet • Airhead • Unable to Commit • Hopelessly Lost • Innocent	Naive, perpetually preoccupied or adrift; not present, shut down, unable to evolve	If I stay below the radar and avoid responsibility I'll be safe
Jester	• Class Clown • Black Sheep • Misfit • Drama Queen	Never serious; always exaggerating or joking around; often ending up the center of attention even when not trying to do so	If I act ridiculous, humorous or emotional, no one will expect anything important of me, but I can still express what I think and feel and get the attention I crave
Lover	• Heartsick Romantic • Passionate Lover • Codependent Person • Secret Lover	Exaggerated romantic self-expressions and expectations; extreme efforts to express romantic interest or gain affection	I must be "lost to love" to be happy; unless someone is in love with me, I have no self-worth; I must be sexually attractive to be loved
Wizard/ Shaman	• Visionary • Miracle Worker • Spiritual Leader • Healer • Sage Advisor • Genius	Rises quickly to a position of influence, leadership or decision-making; seeks to have large impact on the lives of others; demonstration of supernormal attributes	Only the incredible is interesting or worthy; only the exceptional deserves love; I must be exceptional for my life to have worth
Deceiver	• Seducer • Confidante • Charmer • Weasel	Won't take "no" for an answer; overconfident or arrogant; deceptive and persuasive; every word and action is driven by hidden agenda	If I can persuade or manipulate someone to trust me, then I have control over a situation, and that gives me power I wouldn't otherwise have

Truth Seeker	• Spiritual Aspirant • Investigator • Willing Disciple • Student of Life	Endless questioning and searching for answers; inability to accept things at face value; eagerness to learn special knowledge	The truth is more important than anything else; if I know what is true, I can feel confident about my decisions; without the truth, I'm lost
Skeptic	• Cynic • Scientist • Doubting Thomas • Hyper-rationalist	Disbelieving, dismissive, disinterested, analytical, condescending	Things aren't always what they seem; if I always question, I'll never be wrong; process is more important than outcome; other people accept things too readily
Sexless	• Virgin • Androgen • Sex-Averse	Avoiding physical intimacy, rejecting social or relational expectations (especially with respect to gender); ambivalent about sexual needs	Sexuality is base and repulsive; I don't agree with society's gender roles; sexual intimacy makes me too vulnerable; if I'm not sexual, people will leave me alone
Fearful	• Superstitious Person • Paranoid Person • Reactive Person	Irrational mistrust, fear-based reasoning and choices, unpredictable responses	The world is not a safe place, I am always at risk, and everyone I care about is always at risk
Righteous Authority	• Holier-than-Thou • Religious Zealot • Judgmental Person	Exaggerated importance of own role and responsibilities; over-emphasis of authority for own position; black-and-white reasoning	I have to be right to feel okay with the world; others have to be wrong for me to be right; there is only one way to view reality (i.e. mine)
Prosperous/ Successful	• Social Elite • Privileged Person • Miser	Perpetually striving for more wealth or social status, overly concerned about material security	The only way I can feel safe or successful is by accumulating material wealth; affluence is necessary power; money facilitates happiness
Destitute	• Poverty Stricken • Homeless Person • Beggar	Financially irresponsible, unable to support basic needs or contribute to society; off the grid	If I keep myself down, I have nothing more to lose; poverty is more noble, or more spiritual, or just easier, than affluence; no one should expect anything of me
Narcissist	• Self-Indulgent Person • Conspicuous Consumer • Self-Centered Person • Egoist	Egoistic self-absorption, viewing all interactions through lens of own wants and needs; lacking in empathy	Nothing matters but me; I am the center of the Universe; other people exist to serve my wants and needs

Exercise: Personas   As you review the chart, take a moment to
reflect on some of the corresponding behaviors and beliefs, and
see if any of them feel familiar to you. What survival personas
do you recognize when you examine the relationships, decisions
and nourishment patterns in your own life? If any of them are
recognizable, what dimensions of self do you think you are
nurturing or protecting with a given persona? Can you think of
ways to nourish yourself in those areas more consciously and
effectively?

Many of these personas have, at one time or another, been the cultural
ideal for how certain elements of society should behave in order to
maintain social stability, cohesion and predictability. In essence, they
have been embraced at one time or other as an efficient means of serving
our primary drives and fulfillment impulses. Even today, certain tacit
cultural expectations endure that are facilitated by these personas.
However, they rarely provide nourishment to individuals who rely on
them to navigate relationships, nor do they allow society to be
completely honest with itself. This results in impedances to personal
and societal healing, growth and evolution. As enduring and self-
protective as these forces are, is it possible to be free of them? Yes it is.
First, we must recognize which personas reside in us. This can be
accomplished through introspection, meditation, the forthright
observations of those friends who have themselves learned to be
genuine, or via a therapeutic relationship. Once identified, we can
challenge our personas, questioning whether we wish to represent
ourselves to the world through them. Do they align with our core values
or not? Do they facilitate the nourishment we desire or interfere with it?
Once we can clearly see the impedances to well-being that personas
create for us, we can begin to let them go and reshape our default
assumptions and responses. How? Once again, by getting to know the
True Self deep within, and allowing that Self to expand up to the surface
of our personality. There are focused methods to accelerate this process
– such as mystic activation – but really all that is required is consistent,
multidimensional nourishment. That's all. Once we nourish every
aspect of our being with affectionate compassion, our True Self – the Self
that is grounded in love and an awareness of its spiritual essence – will
rise to the surface, and we can sustain the energy, insight and courage to
be genuine in every moment.

In reality, of course, we all have a little of every identity type in us; this is part of the human condition and contributes formatively to our overall personality. When we are immersed in particular situations where we feel vulnerable or unprepared, we may even adopt a particular persona – even one we have never relied upon before – to cope with that situation. So our objective here is not to reject the existence of such coping mechanisms, or to harshly judge them in ourselves or others; personas are, after all, necessary for our survival early on in our development. However, our goal can be to realize what these reflexes are when they occur, and work steadily to lesson their interference with nourishment as we mature.

> **Resources:** Much of the world's literature is replete with identity types as they manifest in different cultures and environments. From the plays of ancient Greece to modern entertainment, familiar stereotypes and caricatures mirror the variety of survival personas within us. Carl Jung took this observation in a slightly different direction with his *archetypes* – insisting among other things that the persona archetype remained necessary and even healthy throughout adulthood – and his observations deserve careful exploration. Another intriguing resource is C. Robert Cloninger's character schema, which defines character types using *self-transcendent, cooperative* and *self-directed* dimensions; Cloninger's approach may offer insight into why certain personas take over at any given moment.

Structural Limitations and Chained Associations

Structural Limitations

Even when we resolve self-limiting beliefs, however, there will always be hard limits on certain areas of personal potential. In *Integral Lifework* these are called structural limitations. It's important to understand what these are – and how to deal with them – as they can become substantial barriers to nourishment. Structural limitations block access to certain kinds of nourishment, obscuring some passages through life's maze and influencing how we navigate others. They are insurmountable finites, and everyone has their own unique cluster of them.

For instance, here are some of my own structural limitations I have encountered over the years:

- My right and left hands can't quite operate independently enough to play complicated piano pieces, no matter how diligently I practice.

- Despite diverse treatments and approaches, my digestive system doesn't tolerate hard alcohol, caffeine, gluten or large amounts of animal fat.

- As I have gotten older, my capacity for memorization has waned. Where once I could read a passage once or twice and repeat nearly all of it intact, or rattle off the phone numbers of all my friends, or recall the details of a previous conversation word-for-word, those tasks are now relegated to my journals, day-timer and various scraps of paper strewn around my living space.

- The echoes of abuse I suffered early on in life have abated through much compassionate attention and interior work. Profound healing has reshaped the consequences of this abuse from a chaotic fear to a softer sadness. But that pain continues to be part of me, lingering quietly beneath the surface, and when I am tired or depleted it can sometimes surprise me by demanding my full attention once more.

- I cannot for the life of me perfect the art of astral projection! Although my perceptions have occasionally and spontaneously extended far outside my body, as well as into what I believe to be other realms of being, I have not been able to reliably project my subtle body across the material plane. Is this a hard limit?

Notice that there are all sorts of barriers and limitations in this list. Emotional, physical, mental and even spiritual. And structural limitations are not necessarily only the things we have been born into, they may also be the result of life experiences or the influences of our environment. When an event occurs that creates chained associations within us – that is, associations that are indelibly linked with strong emotions or physical sensations – then those associations stay with us indefinitely. Some folks may argue – because of their own personal victories, a deeply held belief in transcending such limitations, or generous goodwill – that these are only perceived limitations, and that if we could just inhabit the right frame of mind, all of them would fall away. And, in principle, I would agree with this, for I have experienced periods in my life where each of these hard limits has seemed to soften or dissipate for a time. I would also agree that it is important to discriminate between structural limitations and more conditional or functional limitations; for instance, recognizing that one or two uncomfortable encounters with ice cream does not constitute lactose intolerance, or that flunking Algebra does not mean all mathematical concepts are beyond reach, or that a mistrust of certain types of relationships may be rooted in beliefs we can change with a little loving effort, etc. Unless, of course, there are strong associations formed by these experiences that cause one type of response to become chained to one type of stimulus, so once again we must take care to differentiate. But of equal importance is accepting structural limitations for what they are...instead of beating our heads against the barrier and thus curtailing progress in other areas.

Structural barriers tend to be tied to deeply rooted patterns in our mind or body, and are usually more difficult to manage than functional barriers. For example, a traumatic event in childhood may have created a chained associations that guide much of our thinking, action and reaction. Returning to Theresa's case, her mother's emotional withdrawal persuaded Theresa that, among other things, love from others was unreliable and trusting people might not be safe. Since I was physically abused as a child, my body tends to react to stress in those areas that received the most abuse. And if someone is born with a genetic propensity for a certain type of illness, or their body is severely injured at some point during their life, these can also become structural barriers. And of course environmental influences – petrochemicals and other pollutants, the stress of living in a war zone, extreme climate conditions, lack of availability of nutritional food, etc. – can all contribute to our structural limitations. As yet I have not observed or experienced a complete reversal in structural barriers using any technique, integral or otherwise. However, if we can fall in love with these barriers and the patterns they have generated, nourishing them to whatever extent we can with affectionate compassion, then their negative impact on our ability to love and thrive will be substantially lessened.

So what are these limits all about? In the cultural vernacular in which I was raised, limitations are failings that somehow translate into a low valuation of self. To describe a limitation is to explain how "I am bad at that." What an unnecessary burden! I think we can actually be very grateful for our limitations. They teach us a whole host of lessons crucial to our own growth and effectiveness. Once recognized, they point the way ahead for us in blazing clarity. For starters, here's the short list of how structural limitations can contribute to our well-being:

- Helping us avoid repeating mistakes and pain.

- Helping us identify and appreciate our strengths and the paths of least resistance to our own well-being.

- Helping us clarify our priorities from day to day.

- Helping us prefect the art of opening up and letting go.

- Helping us learn how to be grateful.

- Inspiring us to love generously, with humility and without set expectations.

Who would have thought that failings could be so liberating? As we become aware of our structural limitations, they can guide us into a more appropriate focus for our energy and time. As we accept our limits and let go of the struggle to correct them, our lives can open up to new visions of fulfilling action and interaction. Really, this is the process of falling in love with our limitations, which may involve grieving about them as well; I suggest returning to the "Falling in Love as Surrender and Renewal" table to review this process. That is not to say we should assume certain limits prevent us from achieving goals available to others who don't experience the same barriers, but there is no reason we should assume our limitations exist solely to be overcome. In other words, our structural limitations should not become our identity. Instead, they are tools to help us navigate the maze of our existence. They are partial boundaries that contribute to our overall choices and course of action, but they are not our masters.

Chained Associations

One of the objectives of *Integral Lifework* is to restructure any fundamental beliefs that are self-limiting and depleting. Just as with the personas we adopt to interface with others, what we believe about ourselves and the world around us shapes how we process reality and every avenue of energy exchange we allow into our being. In fact, personas may originate from these underlying beliefs. So exploring our belief tree – the confluence of factors that resulted in our current set of beliefs – will lead us not only to the source of our personas, but to a direct means of freeing ourselves from their possessive grasp. In other words, through letting go of some unhelpful core beliefs, we can come that much closer to experiencing our authentic Self, allowing it to express itself and flourish in all of our interactions. This concept of being restored to our True Self is a common theme in many spiritual practices, and as you will experience firsthand through the nourishing of your Authentic Spirit dimension, it is key to unleashing that authenticity.

So how does our belief tree function? Take a look at the following diagram. We begin with *core material*, the events of our life that have shaped our understanding of ourselves and the world. Some of this is consciously remembered, but most of it has already been incorporated into the ways we think, feel and act, and the original events may have vanished from active memory altogether. What has occurred over time, however, is a series of processing steps that imbeds a specific conclusion in our unconscious, a *chained association*, about what has happened to us. These can be pretty straightforward associations, or profoundly complex ones. As one straightforward example, I might conclude somewhere along the way that I am clumsy, awkward or uncoordinated, perhaps because I had a lot of injuries and accidents as a child, or because I was told I lacked coordination by a frustrated parent, or because other children teased me about being clumsy or awkward – or all three. That conclusion can then be reinforced by a series of related memories and outcomes of choices I have made or continue to make. For instance: "If I try out for the track team, I'm going to make a fool of myself just like I did all those other times on the playground." As a result, I then begin to make all of my decisions on a set of operating assumptions about my own clumsiness. This naturally leads to behaviors that unconsciously reinforce those assumptions. If I am afraid to exercise because I am embarrassed about my body's lack of coordination, and instead choose sedentary activities, my muscles will weaken and I will gain weight. And, when I get up from my computer game to grab a snack in the kitchen, won't it be a bit more likely that I will trip over the clothes hamper, slam into the wall and crush the airplane model I so carefully mounted there? And of course the thought that arises immediately from the depths of my psyche is that, well, of course this happened, *because I'm clumsy!*

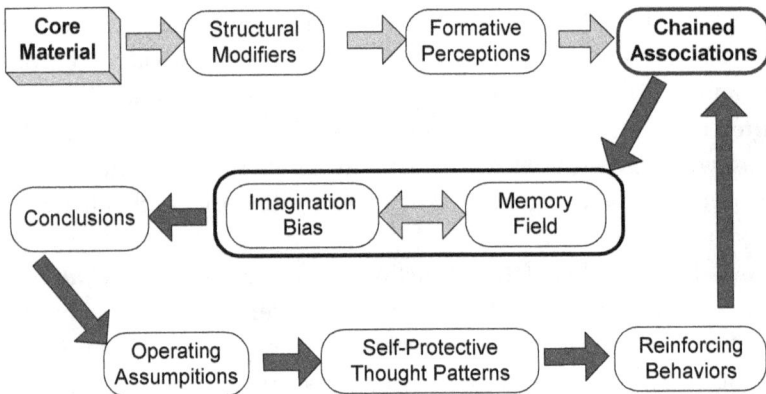

```
  Core                Structural           Formative            Chained
 Material   ──▶        Modifiers   ──▶     Perceptions  ──▶    Associations
                                                                   │
                                                                   ▼
 Conclusions  ◀──   Imagination   ◀──▶    Memory                   │
                       Bias                Field                   │
     │                                                             │
     ▼                                                             │
  Operating    ──▶   Self-Protective  ──▶   Reinforcing  ─────────▶
 Assumpitions        Thought Patterns       Behaviors
```

In order to break a chained association, we need to challenge it. We must dig down into our beliefs and ask a simple question: Why? Why do I believe that about myself? What makes me think or feel this way? Why do I react the way I do in this or that situation? Are my assumptions valid? Is this belief based in fact? Where did it come from? What does it mean? And so on. The following dialogue illustrates the beginning of this process and is taken from one of my client interactions. The client, whom we will call Jeff, is trying to manage some anxiety about a newly initiated romantic relationship, and has come to me to talk it through.

Jeff: Every time I think of getting together with Adrianna, I panic. I break out into a sweat and can barely speak. When she calls I'm even afraid to answer the phone. I'm terrified.

Todd: So these feelings are pretty intense.

Jeff: Yes!

Todd: Why do you think this is happening?

Jeff: I don't have a clue!

Todd: Can you describe another situation where you experienced feelings like these?

Jeff: No...uh, not in a romantic relationship anyway. I mean, I've been a little nervous before, but nothing like this.

Todd: What was that like, when you were nervous before?

Jeff: Well...you know, just getting to know someone. Isn't everybody nervous? About putting my foot in my mouth – that sort of thing.

Todd: Okay. So what about other situations? Have you ever felt as anxious as you do now?

Jeff: Hmmm. Yeah, I guess I felt this way at my last job interview, two months ago. It surprised me then, too. It was like I'd never had a job in my life...or ever accomplished anything before. I felt so stupid!

Todd: Why stupid?

Jeff: Maybe that's the wrong word. Incompetent is more like it. Or...inexperienced. Huh.

Todd: (after a moment) You seem thoughtful.

Jeff: I guess when I think of getting together with Adrianna, it's sort of the same feeling. Like I'm too inexperienced.

Todd: More inexperienced than you have felt in other relationships?

Jeff: I guess so, yeah. She's older than most of the women I've dated. And she really seems to have her act together. I just don't feel like I do. I guess that's what's making me freak out.

Todd: Why do you feel like your act isn't together?

Jeff: It's like at the job interview. I mean...I'm nearly forty! Why hasn't my career taken off yet? Why haven't I gotten married? Why don't I own a house? It's like I missed the boat or something. When I think someone's going to start asking about my life, I freak out. I clam up.

Todd: So you feel like you haven't accomplished enough?

Jeff: Are you kidding? I haven't accomplished anything!

Todd: I'd like to take a look at that statement, if that's okay.

Jeff: Sure.

Todd: You've shared with me before that you graduated college near the top of your class, that you've traveled extensively around the world, that you have a number of good friends, and that your work was appreciated and rewarded at your last job. Do you feel these are accomplishments?

Jeff: Yeah...I guess they are. But...

Todd: (waiting expectantly)

Jeff: But they aren't top shelf. They aren't the big ones.

Todd: Such as?

Jeff: You know, like I said: getting married, buying a house, having kids.

Todd: Why are those more important?

Jeff: I don't know...because they just are. I mean, every time I call my mom she asks when she's going to get some grandkids, you know? And all of my friends are slaving away to pay their mortgages. I never wanted kids, but most of my friends are married and have started a family. Heck, some have already gotten divorced.

Todd: You mentioned slaving away at a mortgage. Is that what you want to do?

Jeff: (laughs) Of course not. I mean, I like the idea of having a house, just not a huge mortgage payment hanging around my neck. Actually, I kind of like having the extra cash around.

Todd: So you can travel, things like that.

Jeff: Exactly!

Todd: Of those things you think you are supposed to have accomplished, which ones do you really want?

Jeff: (after a pause) I guess I want to get married. I want a committed relationship. I just haven't found the right woman yet. Plus, you know, I like to travel, so it's been hard to settle down.

Todd: So if we diagram this out, it sounds like you're nervous about going on a date with Adrianna because you aren't married or aren't in a committed relationship. Is that about right?

Jeff: (laughs) That doesn't make any sense, does it?

Todd: Sometimes emotions don't have to make sense. But I'd like to try something....

Jeff: Okay.

Todd: Could you take out your cell phone? (Jeff takes out his phone.) Let's pretend for a moment you are about to call Adrianna. How do you feel about that?

Jeff: I feel a little silly. Otherwise, I'm okay.

Todd: No anxiety?

Jeff: (pauses) No, just nervous. Actually a little giddy.

Todd: Excited giddy?

Jeff: (smiles) Yeah. In a positive way.

In this dialogue we haven't yet burrowed down to the core material that underlies Jeff's fears, but that wasn't the goal we set for the session. Our goal was to try to help him manage his anxiety better. By the end of this short exercise he had encountered and resolved at least one belief – that he should *already be married* – that had contributed to his fear. Simply by digging down into a few of his assumptions, we quickly dissolved a conclusion he had made about himself and the situation he was facing. And that's all it took for the intense emotions he felt to dissipate, and he could then relax a perceived impedance to his own nourishment. In real world therapy sessions, resolution can actually occur this quickly. Or it may take a longer dialogue to uncover other chained associations that contribute to a core belief – for example, observations of adult relationships from childhood or the result of a series of failed romances experienced as an adult. But once any association is challenged effectively for a specific context, it is no longer part of the chain and loses its power – for that specific situation and often for others as well.

> **Resources:**   This exemplifies a cognitive approach to unveiling
> assumptions and beliefs that interfere with our well-being. If
> this approach is appealing to you, I encourage you to check out
> *Mind Over Mood* by Dennis Greenberger and Christine Padesky.
> It's a workbook for cognitive-behavioral methods to managing
> emotions, and provides a well-organized path down the road to
> discovering the full extent of your belief tree.

What do chained associations usually look like, and where do they come from? Chained associations are the learned relationship between certain influences in our environment, and the consequences of our earliest responses to those influences. Depending on our sensitivity to the influence, the intensity of the influence, and our stage of development at the time we were subjected to that influence, any number of cognitive and behavioral patterns may be synthesized from those experiences. Usually, they are created when we are very young as the result of intense or traumatic events. And, usually, the resulting association creates a response of caution, anxiety or fear. Fear, being one of love's greatest antagonists, is a potent impedance to holistic self-nourishment. Even if we know in our minds and feel with our hearts that something is good, wholesome and nurturing for our being, irrational fear can shut down our receptivity and prevent energy exchanges from occurring. The following chart, borrowed from *The Vital Mystic*, organizes some of the more common of fear responses, and many of the beliefs and assumptions that underlie them.

FEAR CYCLES

Driving Assumptions & Beliefs	Fear Category	Avoidance/Fulfillment Behaviors
Beliefs: I'm not lovable. I am weak and vulnerable. **Assumptions:** I won't be attacked or punished if no one notices me; I'll be able to keep coasting along and never feel threatened.	Social Conformance	• Never outshine anyone. • Always do what I'm told. • Never rock the boat. • Don't say what I really think or feel. • Laugh at jokes I don't think are funny.

Beliefs: The world is a dangerous and unpredictable place. I am ashamed (or unsure) of who I am. People aren't trustworthy. **Assumptions:** The social masks (personas) I maintain are all that keep me safe from abandonment or humiliation.	**Challenges to Identity**	• Be defensive when criticized. • Be quick to accuse others. • Remain the center of everyone's attention. • Constantly seek assurance or approval. • Use or abuse people to get wants met. • Goals and accomplishments become more important than process.
Beliefs: I must control myself. Nothing I do is acceptable. The world is unpredictable. **Assumptions:** If I control things around me, I can control the chaos of insecurities within me.	**Changes in Environment**	• Keep the same routine. • Don't take risks or try anything new. • Make everything perfect. • Over-plan to avoid the unexpected. • Obsess about financial security. • Always stick to the rules.
Beliefs: I can't handle it anyway. I'm helpless. **Assumptions:** Ignorance is bliss...because what I don't know, can't hurt me.	**Confronting the Unknown**	• Deny what I deeply feel. • Tune out when I encounter something difficult or frightening. • Run away from authentic relationships. • Use drugs and/or alcohol to stay numb.
Beliefs: I'm worthless and unlikable. **Assumptions:** No matter what I do, I will probably fail.	**Value and Purpose**	• Be very self-critical and pessimistic. • Sabotage success and disappoint people who trust me. • Become emotionally addicted to sex, relationships, work, food, etc.
Beliefs: It's all too complicated, confusing, and difficult. Besides, I'm incompetent, and I end up hurting people or getting hurt. **Assumptions:** It's better not to try than to succeed and have responsibilities.	**Responsibility and Accountability**	• Act like nothing matters. • Don't follow through on commitments to myself or others. • Turn everything into a joke. • Be suspicious of people who seem motivated and directed. • Be reactively nonconformist.

Beliefs: Either nothing is my problem to solve, nor is anything my fault; or everything is my problem to solve, and/or my fault. **Assumptions:** I must either punish or exonerate myself for the shame I feel by reliving, perpetuating, or compensating for the trauma and abuse I experienced as a child.	**Pathological**	• Be impulsive and self-destructive (eating disorders, self-injury, substance abuse, overspending, seeking abusive partners). • Become phobic, paranoid, irrationally jealous, or have other uncontrollable fears. • Be perpetually narcissistic, controlling and abusive. • Have little to no understanding or management of emotions. • Never have a satisfying intimate relationship, or be antisocial in general. • Be chronically ill. • Think dichotomously: i.e. only in terms of black/white, right/wrong, good/bad.

You may notice that every one of the driving assumptions and beliefs listed here can be challenged. They are stories, elaborate rationalizations that we invent to cope with a challenging world. As tightly as we may want to hold on to them, they are illusions. Yet once we start acting out the correlating avoidance or fulfillment behaviors, we begin to make our mistaken beliefs and assumptions come true. Such is the power of the human will that we can create damaging reality out of fearful fantasy. This validates and perpetuates our fear cycle, creating permanent substitution behaviors that deplete our nourishment centers even further, causing the underlying beliefs to be much harder to challenge or give up. But once we have paused for a moment to reflect on what we have invented, we realize why we are resisting positive change. Using a cognitive-behavioral approach or other technique best suited to our current mode of being, we can then begin to let go of what we recognize as outmoded and destructive ideas, and replace them with something better. We can cast out irrational and destructive fear, and replace it with authentic and supportive love.

Substitutions

When our natural appetites are satisfied with alternative nourishment, we can sometimes feel as though we are meeting our own needs when we are actually depleting or injuring ourselves. In response, if we can't identify authentic nourishment, we will accelerate our efforts more and more, until we find ourselves entangled in a spiral of cravings, compulsions and desperation. Eventually, we become so dependent on our substitutions that even if we are presented with healthy nourishment, we no longer recognize its value. When we have moments of clarity about this spiral we can see some our behaviors as those around us have probably come to see them: as addictions. Most of the time, however, our increasingly insistent need is such an obvious, integrated part of our thoughts, emotions and self-maintenance that we don't realize how unhealthy we have become. Until, of course, we become really sick, or begin to lose our friends and community, or lose our job and so forth. Even then, because the depths of our depletion are so great, we may turn to more extreme substitutions and along the same trajectory of our previous spiral. Left uncorrected, the outcomes for ourselves and the impact on those who love us can be dire.

You might assume at this point that we are discussing substance abuse or alcoholism, and these are certainly part of the spectrum of substitutions and distortions. But in *Integral Lifework*, anything can become an addiction; that is, we can unwittingly condition ourselves to rely on ineffective, non-nourishing or even destructive appetites as substitutions for real self-nurturing. Any imbalance, no matter how small, can generate barriers to wholeness, and when that imbalance is severe enough that it disrupts one or more nourishment streams entirely, we can call that an addiction. You could even say that someone who has an "addictive personality" is someone who simply hasn't learned how to nourish themselves in a balanced and holistic way. The journey of relearning healthy self-care can be long, painful and frightening, but it is nevertheless possible – as with so much in *Integral Lifework*, the key is realizing and accepting that certain energy exchanges have been interrupted. What follow are some of the more common substitutions that occur under this category.

Addiction to Adversity

When I began trying to understand how best to heal myself and help others, I noticed a pattern emerging in different behaviors I observed. In counseling couples, in mediating disputes in the workplace, in working with families ravaged by abuse, in reaching out to alcoholics living on the street, in helping people manage their chronic illnesses, and in the psychotherapy I myself received, I witnessed the same occurrences over and over again. At some point in the healing process, either during the maintenance period after much of the hard work had been accomplished, or right at the moment of discovering how a difficult conflict could be ameliorated, a new crisis would develop. A new area of disagreement, new symptoms of illness, the discovery of new stressors and so on would take over. Then, once the new crisis was put in perspective, anxieties were calmed and new areas of healing begun, another crisis would abruptly surface. It reminded me of the root fires we sometimes experienced in the woods of Massachusetts when I was a child. Fire would burn its way into the dry root network under the soil, so that even when the immediate fire was extinguished, a new blaze might burst up from the ground a while later, sometimes quite a distance away from the original blaze. And so the firefighting would continue for hours or even days.

People often choose to perpetuate their emotional root fires. Sometimes these cycles are short and severe, sometimes longer and subtler, but often they persist over months and years. So I began to wonder: What was going on here? I think there are many factors in play in these situations – the examples of our early home environment, our level of self-awareness, our willingness to let go of victim identities, etc. – but one element that threads through all recurring crisis patterning is a fundamental craving for adversity. Perhaps this stems from one of our primary drives, the drive to adapt to our environment. Or perhaps it is a craving for new, exciting experiences – another fundamental drive. And creating crisis does have potential for generating many different kinds of nourishment. It can nourish our body with adrenaline and endorphins; our intellect with problem-solving opportunities; our heart and sense of community with the bonding that occurs during shared challenges; a temporary sense of purpose; and so forth. And when challenge is completely absent from our lives, our being atrophies. So even when the crisis could be averted, or the outcome has little real importance or our relationships could be strengthened more constructively, we often choose drama over more sensible paths. By picking a side in a conflict – sometimes almost at random – we quickly over-invest ourselves in a particular outcome and throw our whole being into advocating a narrowly defined result, usually at any cost.

This sort of crisis invention can be seen everywhere, from a spontaneous, heated argument over politics or sports, to the enduring tensions of family disagreements, to impulsive, reckless and self-sabotaging behaviors at home or in the workplace. The dynamic is pervasive. When it runs amok, without the balancing forces of other primary drives (to successfully affect our environment, to survive and thrive, etc.), it can destroy our quality of life. But even if it doesn't dominate our existence in this imbalanced way, is there perhaps a means of satisfying the same needs without a rollercoaster ride of abusive anger, aggressiveness, hateful speech, risky behaviors, heartbreak or violence? I think there is. By consciously and caringly nourishing the twelve essential dimensions of our being, we can achieve the same satisfaction with much less divisive and destructive consequences. And because dialectic tension is also an important aspect of all nourishment, we can deliberately engineer a sense of anticipation, excitement and unpredictability as part of the exchange in each nourishment center. In these ways we can attenuate the more destructive impulses that might otherwise manifest.

Consider what often happens when a natural disaster threatens a community. Old animosities may be subordinated in a cooperative effort to survive. In the same way, when we consciously bend our will toward multidimensional nourishment, the will to destroy, compete, acquire or dominate is attenuated. These fulfillment impulses are still within us, but they are channeled into a larger stream of effort. Through practice, we come to trust that all of our needs will be met; that our drives to exist, adapt, experience and affect will ultimately be satisfied.

So we can shape an adversity that energizes us within the context of conscious nourishment. How much of a challenge is healthy for us will depend on who we are individually, and where we are in our journey. We must each discover what narrow band of deliberate adversity best stimulates our growth, and balance it with our desire for comfort and stability. I once counseled a couple who lacked Playful Heart or Healthy Body nourishment of any kind in their relationship. With greater and great frequency, they found themselves vehemently disagreeing over something with an intensity of anger that surprised them both. So they sought my help. When they began engineering Playful Heart and Healthy Body energy exchanges, the pattern of conflict attenuated. They would still disagree, but the anger and frustration behind those disagreements evaporated more rapidly, and the energies in the debate were more constructive. There were still arguments and accusations, but they stung less and ended in laughter more. Since more important, direct nourishment was now taking place, the desire to seek a muddled, lower quality nourishment through an emotional tug-of-war took a distant back seat. They thereby effectively replaced an adversity substitution with holistic self-care, satisfying the same primary drives – to adapt and experience – in healthy and positive ways.

Many times over, I have witnessed the extreme discord in people's lives alleviated through introduction of healthy, balanced multidimensional nourishment. Someone addicted to their own anger begins to laugh at what used to upset them. A couple in constant conflict begins to relax and enjoy each others' company. People addicted to caffeine, violent sports, confrontational debate, risky sexual behaviors and any number of other adversity-inducing substitutions discover they are no longer in the thrall of those addictions. Even cognitive spirals like negative self-talk, depression, anxiety and fear begin to loosen when multidimensional nourishment kicks in. And sometimes, if the area of depletion can be rapidly identified, all that is needed to interrupt the addictive pattern is targeted nourishment that addresses the specific deficit.

How is it that we come to rely on such substitutions and nourishment distortions, instead of naturally caring for ourselves in healthy ways? Sometimes we simply never learned how to nurture ourselves in some dimension – it was never discussed in our presence or exemplified for us. Sometimes we were discouraged at an early age from nourishing ourselves in some way. Sometimes the pervasive sentiment of surrounding culture undervalues certain kinds of energy exchange and encourages us to dismiss them. Sometimes one generation passes on certain substitution behaviors to the next. Sometimes we have structural disadvantages in particular nourishment centers that exacerbate these challenges. And so on. There may be any number of reasons why we haven't been able to support our whole being in a balanced way. So we simply need an introduction to dimensions we have overlooked; we need integral practice to open doors to our neglected aspects of self.

Addiction to Comfort

Just as we can become addicted to adverse experiences, we can also become overly attached to a sense of comfort and stability. When this happens we become dependent on familiar environments and routines, a familiar diet of order and structure that provides the illusion of safety. Always eating the same foods at the same time, for example, or never missing our favorite TV show, or trying to keep our home environment looking and feeling the same way at all times. And of course we can become quite upset when the safe and familiar are abruptly changed or rearranged in some way. The unexpected guest who sits in our favorite chair and starts handling our knick-knacks; a café that no longer offers our favorite pastry; the cancellation of a routine event we have always looked forward to; the day we counted on being sunny turning to rain. In the most extreme cases, our very ability to function can be crippled when too many of the comforts and routines we rely upon are taken away. From an outsider's perspective, our paralysis may seem inexplicable, but from the inside it can feel like the Universe itself is coming unglued.

Like our craving for adversity, I think this addiction can also be traced back to primary drives, but in this case it is existing and affecting – rather than experiencing and adapting – which are being emphasized. To exist and affect, we believe we must effectively control and maintain order to achieve reliability and predictability. Of course we all need to feel relatively secure and maintain a modicum of continuity in our lives, but when our self-nourishment becomes too imbalanced or multiple dimensions of our being are neglected completely, a growing desire to control external variables can be an attempt to compensate for that chaos and depletion. Whether this manifests as a mildly controlling personality or a full blown obsessive compulsive disorder depends on the individual, but the root causes are often the same. An extreme deficiency of almost any type of essential nourishment can lead us down this road.

And just as comfort addiction shares similar causes with adversity addiction, the remedy is also the same: we can soften excessive compulsions to create comfort and stability through balanced, multidimensional nourishment. Are we missing something in our diet?

Do we lack emotional support from our community? Are we overcommitted to a career or set of choices that contradict the legacy we desire to leave behind? Have we been resisting actuation of what we know to be our life's purpose? Any of these can lead to severe deficiencies in essential nourishment. By identifying what is missing in our integral practice, we can quickly adjust our routines to include some nutritious food for our most depleted areas. It is a life-changing shift.

What becomes almost inevitable when nourishment is disrupted for long periods of time is the exaggeration of either comfort or adversity addiction patterns – and sometimes even both. The addictive thoughts, emotions and behaviors keep superficially satisfying one or more fulfillment impulses and primary drives and mask underlying depletions. The resulting lack of essential nourishment just amplifies the addictive craving and perpetuates the spiral. What is the ultimate result? Sickness and pain, suffering and grief, despair and self-destruction. Once the cycle has begun, it is often very difficult to see our way out of it; and it can happen at any point in our journey, regardless of how skillful we have nurtured ourselves in the past. That is why regularly assessing our own self-nourishment is such a critical step in sustaining a healing and effective long-term integral practice.

So these, then, are the two extremes of substitution nourishment: seeking comfort in a compulsive or fixated way, or seeking adversity in a compulsive or fixated way. And sometimes we may even perpetuate both, generating a crazed rollercoaster ride for ourselves and everyone around us.

Examples of Substitutions

In order to better understand what substitution behaviors look like, let's consider some real-world examples.

- Bruce is socially unskilled and isolated, and has trouble managing the stress of interacting with others. In the past, he has turned to alcohol and inappropriate sexual behavior to cope with that stress and the frustration of his loneliness. After nearly dying from his alcoholism, Bruce decided to cut back on his drinking. He also avoided situations where he might be tempted into previous sexual patterns, and eliminated the stressors from his life that seemed to be spurring him on to compensate in self-destructive ways. This was very liberating at first, but he soon found the old anxiety creeping back into his life despite his self-enforced isolation. So he turned to computer games and spent a majority of his time in this alternative reality. One way of describing this is to say Bruce was trading one addiction for another. In these situations, it is common to replace one form of inappropriate nourishment with another without understanding what is really lacking. In Bruce's case, what was most lacking was essential nourishment in nearly all of his dimensions. That is, in twelve out of twelve nourishment dimensions, Bruce was not able to successfully care for himself – he had simply never learned to do so effectively.

- Juan was not happy with his life. He had been sabotaging his survival by instigating conflicts at work and, as a result, getting fired from a series of jobs. In the frequent periods of depression that followed losing each job, Juan would binge on junk food and gambling as ways of feeling better about his predicament. When we examined each area of self-nourishment in more depth, it became clear that Juan had not addressed four of the twelve dimensions: Playful Heart, Empowered Self-Concept, Authentic Spirit and Fulfilling Purpose. As we delved into those areas, it became clear that Juan had confused one area of nourishment, Pleasurable Legacy, with these other four. In devoting himself to his family and children in the past, he had assumed that he was being nourished spiritually, creatively and with a sense of personal purpose. But he wasn't, he was just nourishing his sense of legacy. And so, after his children left home and he divorced his wife of many years, there was nothing left but gambling, bad food and risky behavior at work to fill the void left by his first substitution.

- Christina depended on marijuana and sex to feel okay about herself. Without them, she felt panic and chaos would quickly take over her life. In her case, Supportive Community turned out to be the most depleted dimension of her nourishment. In order to feel accepted and connected with others, Christina relied on sexual intercourse. When this substitution failed her, she turned to marijuana to escape the pain and self-examination that would facilitate her healing. This substitution then began to interfere with other areas of nourishment as well, and so her overall well-being began to suffer. But at the root of the problem was that very first substitution: believing that sexual connections with others could effectively create a Supportive Community.

- Patricia was addicted to cathartic *ahas*. She would attend evening classes and weekend retreats to learn spiritually-oriented techniques of self-discovery and connection with the ground of being. After each of these experiences, she would coast along for a time on an exulted high of insight and resolve. When she felt that high slipping a little, she would quickly sign up for another event that promised to immerse her in a new approach to spiritual growth or accomplishment. And although Patricia was able to nourish herself in many other areas, one dimension that was entirely absent from her life was Playful Heart. In all her seriousness to ensure she was on a healthy, self-nourishing track in all her other dimensions, she lacked any real sense of freedom, excitement or contentment about day-to-day life. So her cathartic *ahas* had become a substitution for the joyful, carefree playfulness that was missing in her life.

As you read through those examples, one thing you may notice is that it could have been any combination of undernourished areas that resulted in the same behavior. In the past I have attempted to map correlations between specific depletions and common substitution behaviors, but I have as yet uncovered no consistent relationships. Any depletion in one or more dimensions can lead to any number of substitution patterns. And the more extreme the depletion, the more extreme the attempts to substitute with ineffective or destructive appetites. However, one of the most striking correlations I have tracked over the years is how reversing such substitutions can eliminate unhealthy behaviors, thought patterns and even illnesses almost instantaneously. That is, once we discover what is lacking and address it head on, we are rapidly set free from the seemingly unrelated maladies we have struggled with over time. In order to make the time and space in our lives to target an undernourished area, we must let go of the substitution – as our addiction ramps down, our authentic nourishment can ramp up.

And finally, one of the more potent examples of substitution recovery was Dan, who suffered years of severe, debilitating depression and even an attempted suicide before rediscovering how to fully nourish himself. Traditional talk therapy hadn't helped. Antidepressants fogged his mind and took away his sex drive. But when he started singing and playing guitar again each day, his depression all but vanished. For years he had set his music aside for what he felt were more important career choices and personal relationships, sublimating his creative ideas and self-expression into his work, romances and friendships. Simply returning to what he had loved as a young man effectively cured him. And this exemplifies a persistent irony: that many people already know on some level what is lacking in their lives, they have just rationalized their way around it in order to achieve specific goals or nourish themselves in other areas. The new mother who gives up writing poetry because she feels she should devote all her energy to her child; the husband who shrugs off doing any more camping trips because his partner has no interest in joining him; the professor who stops expanding her intellectual horizons because she reaches tenure. In these situations, an ongoing journey of integral practice peels away the illusion of comfort and complacency invented through longstanding habits, and reveals the potency of dreams we left behind.

Alienation from Our True Self

Life is a maze of mirrors, reflecting our own state of being and consciousness back to us. What we perceive around us is not reality – it is an illusion constructed of our own perceptions, assumptions and imagination. Realizing this fact does not make finding our way through the illusion any easier. The walls we perceive still seem solid and our reflection still stares back at us, waiting for our next move. What awaits us at the end of that maze? Perhaps there is no end. Rather the process of finding our way through its corridors is our destination; the process of discovering wholeness. Wholeness is many things, some easy comprehend from afar, and others that can only be experienced and understood personally and close-up. Wholeness is a mode of being that relaxes all the impulses within us that cause our own suffering. It offers us a joyful, contented and fearless emotional state. It integrates everything we are – all that we perceive as good, bad or ugly – into a powerful, directed force in the Universe. Wholeness infuses us with ineffable mystery while grounding us in concrete realities of action and responsibility. Wholeness extends our consciousness, our will, and our entire being into a much broader realm of interconnectedness than we could ever have imagined. Wholeness transcends on countless levels the sum of our parts.

So how do we engage the maze on this journey of discovery? How can we find our way? How will we understand the countless reflections moving ceaselessly around us? And how do we separate what is real from what is pure imagination? For much of our lives we will tend to deal with these questions reflexively or unconsciously. We follow our parental examples, or allow our peers to pressure us into one mode of being or other, we absorb the cultural memes that have evolved over centuries to cope with human survival, we follow the habits we have unknowingly created over time, or we submit to our biological imperatives. Sometimes we meet people who challenge us to awake from our unconscious momentum, or encounter ideas that erode our habitual foundation of assumptions, and these external agitators are blessings if we incorporate them into an increasingly conscious journey. But the more potent proponent of freedom will always be our own soul as it struggles to comprehend itself. If we listen to its call, if we attend to its promptings, the mirrored maze without will be shaped and clarified by a mirrored maze within. As we encounter our soul – that spiritual intelligence that has, according to some belief systems, journeyed eons to bring us to this moment – the purpose of the maze becomes clear: it is a sacred opportunity to manifest boundless creativity in every choice; it is an imperative to heal, grow, change and transform in resplendent harmony with the Universe itself. It is a miracle waiting for us to happen.

How can I be so confident that this is the case? And why should you believe me? Well, I'm not...and you shouldn't. I have begged, borrowed and invented language to wrap around some personal and inexpressible experiences and observations, but I still have rigorous doubts about both that language and my understanding of what has happened. Writing in this way isn't always an easy choice. It might be more expedient to claim I am channeling ancient wisdom or the mind of some angelic being, or to quote other more authoritative persons to support my conclusions. In moments of weakness I may fall back on some conventional crutches – all of these things do, after all, contribute to my understanding of the Universe and my place in it. But if I truly believe in the power of every human soul to find its way through all the muck and glory of life, then I must trust my own soul as well. And that is where my primary evidence resides. As we have already discussed, anointing external resources with more power and authority than our internal resources is a dangerous habit. And our soul is perhaps the most powerful resource of all. So as I write, I will find no comfort or constancy in something or someone outside myself. Getting to know my own soul is lonely vigil, but a necessary one.

So what is the substance of these mirrors all around us? Well, we build them as we go along. We fabricate them from each of our relationships, from the consequences of each choice we make, and from the ways in which we nourish each dimension of self. Relationships, consequences and dimensions of nourishment – those frame our path. If we pay close attention to these mirrors as we make our way, while intimately getting to know our own soul at the same time, we can compare the images projected back to us with what our innermost Self knows to be true. Wherever we cannot see the essence of our being reflected, we know there are barriers to wholeness. Wherever we encounter an absence of love, a diminishing of our felt experience of compassionate affection, there is something for us to work through. Wherever we cannot sense the spiritual essence of what is, we are dealing with an illusion.

If we pay close attention to the mirrors of life's maze both within and without, we will always be able to synthesize the truth. And if we have not yet fully learned to nourish ourselves in all dimensions, the distortions in those reflections will rapidly become evident – as suffering, dissatisfaction, purposelessness and cognitive dissonance. Really, every nourishment dimension is an opportunity for barriers, and every barrier is an opportunity for nourishment. But at the center of it all, as the cornerstone of *Integral Lifework*, is mystic activation. It is through mystic activation that we encounter the essence of our being directly. And the deeper we delve into that connection with our True Self, the clearer our prioritization of energy exchanges will become. Now we see in the mirror dimly, but then we shall see face to face.

Unfortunately, many aspects of the human experience tend to alienate us from our True Self. When we rely on external influences to motivate or guide ourselves, of course. Or when we enter into codependent relationships. When we become addicted to ineffectual nourishment. When we forget the primacy of love in our hearts. When we invest all our energies in egoistic satisfaction. The list is endless. But no matter how completely we lose ourselves in such distractions, our soul still waits patiently for us at the core of our being. It is never too late to begin that inward exploration, and once begun, it will generate its own momentum and reward. When we encounter the ground of being through spiritual practice, we recognize the underlying essence from which our soul is formed, and strengthen the intimate bond with our spiritual self through this intimate understanding. And the stronger and more rounded our spiritual nourishment becomes, the more easily we can evoke our authentic essence from moment to moment. This is the unguarded secret of all spiritual traditions: that the Beloved, the Brahman-Atman, the Buddha nature, the Kingdom of Heaven – all ultimate and perfect spiritual realities – wait patiently within.

Karmic Barriers

There is another factor that weaves itself into all nourishment, and that is karma. Most faith traditions hint at specific consequences for all our actions, and some even include thoughts and emotions as players in this causality. For instance, if I do not honor my parents in this life, I will be lonely in my old age; because I was a pedantic tyrant in a previous life, I must learn compassion and tolerance in this one; whenever I engineer calamity to be visited upon others, calamity will manifest in my life three times over. Although historic discussions of karma are found mainly in Hindu, Jainist and Buddhist writings, religious literature of all types is riddled with such warnings. Regardless of our own spiritual beliefs, it is helpful to consider that we may in fact have some karmic work to do. Not necessarily because of a universal spiritual law, or because a spiritual agent is watching over us, or because we have agreed to the terms of a karmic contract before we entered this life, but because our unconscious carries the burdens and joys of our past deeds with us wherever we go. In a purely psychological sense, we cannot escape our past. The patterns of pain, suffering and loss unique to our experience will repeat over and over again until they are interrupted with love. So it is important that we acknowledge that karma exists, even if we can only accept it as a psychological phenomenon. Personally, I believe karma is a spiritual law, and that karma is accumulated and expressed over multiple lifetimes. This belief has some practical applications as an *Integral Lifework Practitioner*, because it can shed light on things like chained associations and core beliefs that developed in a past life. But sharing this belief is not necessary to appreciate the immediacy and power of karmic barriers.

What does karma mean for our self-nourishment? It means that nourishment in every dimension is moderated by karmic debts and assets, and until we recognize this, we will be unable to fully nurture ourselves, and will likely expend much effort in unproductive ways. The common experience of "beating our head against a wall" illustrates one consequence of intentions and actions that have not accounted for karma. When we find ourselves frustrated over and over again, keep failing in our efforts, and sense a general resistance either within ourselves our from our surrounding environment, there is often a karmic component to the lessons we have yet to learn. Either that, or we have not yet come to know our True Self, are struggling with willfulness and egoism, etc. In the case of karma, the remedy is fairly straightforward. First, we must set aside whatever intentions or efforts are encountering resistance. Just let them go. Then, we must discover what attitude, orientation or effort is required to generate positive karma and liberate us from our karmic debt.

Exercise: Generating Positive Karma Depending on your spiritual orientation and beliefs, there are a number of ways to practice this process. At its center is the formation of a specific question in our heart of hearts, and our longing for its resolution must be felt. That question is this: "How may I heal, and what may I heal, so that I am best able to love?" Whether you ask this of Deity, the Universe, your Spirit Guide or your innermost Self is less important than feeling this question deeply and genuinely within. Sometimes just sitting quietly and holding this question in your heart while directing your attention inward towards the center of your chest will evoke startling responses. What we are looking for here is some insight and discernment into how to shape our thoughts, felt desires and actions in ways that will work through whatever negative karma we have accumulated in this life or previous ones, and then generate an ever-increasing store of positive karma moving forward. If we remain relaxed, open and expectant, we will gain clarity about the road ahead. If we then align our intention, attention and follow-through with what we discover about ourselves, we can support holistic self-nourishment as we move forward and ameliorate any lingering karmic barriers to well-being.

As with any of the other influences we have discussed, karma weaves itself into all twelve dimensions. If we are struggling with self-nurturing in a particular nourishment center, then investigating the breadth and depth of our karmic bank account in that dimension is an essential pursuit.

> **Resources:**   For a better understanding of karma, try a web search on the topic. For a scientific approach to evidences of past life influence on the living, the work of Ian Stevenson is fairly compelling. His *Twenty Cases Suggestive of Reincarnation* is both skeptical and persuasive. For a less rigorous or detailed but more entertaining read, Tom Shroder's accounts of Ian Stevenson's work in *Old Souls* might also be worth a try.

Egoism & Willfulness

The human will is a powerful thing. As we have touched upon already, it is the mechanism through which we translate our whims and wishes into action. Our will also participates in forming cogent ideation from our physiological impulses, emotional reactions and the promptings of spirit – thought is, after all, a potent precursor to most action. But there are different qualities of will and different ways our will can be directed. Although there are many subtle gradations of will, let's concentrate for now on the extremes of willingness and willfulness. What makes these two opposites? Consider a time in your life that you were willing to do something, but you really didn't want to do it. For instance, when I am asked to pose in a photograph with friends, I am willing to participate, but I really don't enjoy having my photograph taken; like many photographers, I prefer being behind the camera instead of in front of it. Still, I am willing, and seldom even express my resistance. But the resistance is there. Okay, now consider a time in your life when you wanted to do something more than anything else, but things kept getting in your way. I remember once, when I was eight years old, I wanted to go to a friend's birthday party...and wanted it very badly. The problem was, I had a fever. I begged and pleaded with my stepmother to go, but she insisted that I had to stay home. I threw a tantrum. She spanked me with a wooden spoon. I kept crying and hollering and carrying on, and she spanked me again, this time breaking the spoon across my bottom. At the peak of my inconsolable grief, I barely made it into the bathroom in time to throw up into the toilet. I guess that must have convinced me that I really was too sick to go to the party, because afterwards I sought out my beleaguered step mom and apologized.

As an adult, frustration still happens when we can't get something we want, and although the flavor and volume of our tantrums have hopefully gentled a bit since we were young, we can still get pretty upset when our will is thwarted. A flat tire on the way to an important meeting. We can't find the clothes we want for our weekend trip. Trying to get in touch with a friend or loved one and failing over and over. Discovering the food in the oven is burnt a few minutes before our dinner party begins. All the standard interruptions to our desired outcomes. And when we keep pushing despite these interruptions and despite any negative impact our efforts are having on ourselves and others, this is willfulness. In willfulness, we are hell-bent on a particular outcome, and so we create a bit of hell for ourselves.

In contrast, if I dial down the intensity of my will, let go of trying to forcefully control outcomes, and apply just the right amount of effort so that I don't exasperate myself, I demonstrate my willingness without willfulness. And what are some positive results? For one, I can maintain equanimity in the face of failure. For another, instead of being locked up in anger or despair, my mind is free to think creatively and flexibly about the situation. In my previous books I have talked about *wishing without wanting*, and really this is a form of being willing without being willful.

There are many ways to describe willingness without willfulness. Some of these descriptions have positives connotations in Western culture, and some don't. But the ideas of detachment, trusting the Divine, not sweating the small stuff, generosity of spirit, acquiescence and so forth are woven throughout our greatest wisdom traditions. These same traditions warn against willfulness, calling it acquisitiveness, avarice, covetousness, attachment and so on. Willfulness also has many names in Western psychology, tendencies which are frequently described as unhealthy cognitive and behavioral patterns. Obsession, compulsion and autocratic or controlling behavior are a few of those. Yet all of these definitions are variations on the theme of willingness vs. willfulness.

Can I have passion, devotion and commitment to something without being willful? Of course, because passion, devotion and commitment are felt convictions that indicate a necessity for action; the question simply becomes what is the most appropriate action to take. If we can't accept variable outcomes or even consider new ways to approach a challenge, we are being willful. If we can be flexible in our expectations and how we approach each situation, we demonstrate willingness without willfulness.

So why is this important in integral practice? Because willfulness interferes with nourishment, and willingness facilitates nourishment. Willfulness perpetuated illness, but willingness heals us. Willfulness confines our will to emotions, thoughts and deeds that prevent growth and transformation, while willingness expands and frees our will to facilitate growth and transformation. And what about love? Can we love deeply or authentically if we are preoccupied with willfulness? No, for love demands openness, flexibility, forgiveness and letting go – all qualities of willingness without willfulness. In addition, love is the single most powerful force to overcome resistance when we are willing and able, but still a little ambivalent. So love and willingness are cofactors in any transformational process, and whenever love is absent, willfulness naturally tends to take root.

What is egoism, then? Egoism is a moral orientation in which all things relate to self, and all perceptions, ideations and efforts are constrained by what has the greatest perceived benefit to self. Willfulness is therefore the natural consequence of egoism, in that our whole being stubbornly and aggressively insists that everyone and everything around us attend to our fulfillment and our will. When we are young, our first efforts at individuating from our parents and establishing our own distinct identity involve a lot of egoism and willfulness. Echoes of my own childhood tantrum are easily observed in the willfulness and egoism of most young children. At this age, we have discovered that we are separate from our parents, have an independent will, and can exercise that will to serve our ego. We also believe that everything that happens around must of necessity have something to do with us. All of this is a natural process in the progression of our self-identification. As we grow, however, if we do not learn how to relax these early perspectives and impulses we will impede our own nurturing; what may once have been helpful internal resources will now disrupt our well-being. A thirty or forty year old becoming utterly despondent because they don't get what they want is an unsavory event to experience or observe. Thankfully, there is a proven avenue of transforming willfulness and egoism into more productive responses.

The concept is simple, the practice is difficult. To replace willfulness, we must learn acceptance, openness and willingness. To replace egoism, we must learn humility, compassion and letting go. These qualities are of course evidences of an expanding love-consciousness, so refining compassionate affection in all dimensions of self will go a long way in reforming willfulness and egoism. But we can focus on these barriers individually as well. For instance, we can learn to detect willful impulses in ourselves from moment to moment, and soften them by learning to accept what is; by letting go of expectations and outcomes and rejoicing in the miracles that unfold around us. And egoism can be addressed in the same fashion, through increased self-awareness and gentle adjustment of egoistic responses by broadening our arenas of affection; that is, by integrating the well-being of others – according to their individual needs and sovereignty – into our own motivations. Over time, this is a natural consequence of the personal transformation brought about by integral practice.

In my experience and observation, there are certain cultural and psychological conditions that preclude relaxation of egoistic willfulness to a fairly extreme degree. Among those are borderline personality disorder, bipolar disorder and narcissistic personality disorder. These are particularly challenging because people suffering these barriers lack consistent or accurate self-awareness. Targeting nourishment in the Authentic Spirit, Restorative History and Flexible Processing Space dimensions can help improve self-awareness and, over time, enable compassionate inclusion of the well-being of others in these situations, but the structural barriers such conditions present often demand extraordinary effort. In many ways, Western culture also perpetuates egoism and willfulness by promoting a sense of entitlement, permissive self-gratification, and an "I/me/mine" orientation to the world. This serves commercialistic interests well in the short run, but it is crippling to both personal and cultural evolution in the long run. In Part V, Love's Expansion, we will examine ways to challenge this cyclone of self-absorption and propagate a more mature response to wants and needs.

In conclusion, the following is a tale taken from Norse mythology. Just for fun, see if you can discern whether Odin is willful and egoistic in his quest for knowledge, or if instead he exemplifies willingness and letting go.

> Once there was a god named Odin whose thirst for knowledge was unquenchable. Over the long years that a god lives, he acquired many valuable insights into the workings of the world, sacrificing much along the way to gain them. For instance, in order to acquire the knowledge of Norse runes and their power, Odin hung for nine days and nights on the tree that spans all realms of existence, the Yggdrasil. He was even wounded with his own spear while hanging there. At last, he received the runes he saught. He also had more comfortable ways of obtaining knowledge. When he sat on this high throne, Hlidskjalf, in his great silver hall, Odin could see all that occurred across the nine worlds. And even when he wasn't on that throne, each night his two ravens, Hugin and Munin, would bring him reports of all the happenings in the realms they flew.

But Odin did not know everything, and on one occasion this became uncomfortably clear. Odin consulted a seeress – a Volva, a Priestess of the Wand – as he sometimes did, and learned that a great calamity was coming, one in which a horrible battle, earthquakes and flooding of the Earth would wreak a destruction so great that the Earth itself would be reborn. She called this cataclysm Ragnarok, and foretold that Odin himself would perish in it as he and the other gods battled with giants. This caused Odin some concern, and he decided to seek out even greater resources for wisdom and knowledge than he already possessed in order to deal with it. Perhaps he could forestall this prophecy, or at least prepare himself.

Now there was a fountain deep in the earth, guarded by an ancient giant named Mimir, and it was called the Well of Ages. The water from this fountain was magical, and brought wisdom to anyone who drank it – even prescience about future events, so the rumors claimed. Each day the giant Mimir dipped his ornate drinking horn, the Gjallarhorn, into the spring and drank, so that he became very wise over the years – almost as wise as he was old. Occasionally, brave seekers would find this hidden place and ask for a drink, but the price of wisdom Mimir exacted was so exceedingly high that few were willing to pay. One day a new seeker arrived at the fountain, and that seeker was Odin. He was clad in a cloak striped with fur and carried his magical spear Gungnir, which never missed its mark. Odin and Mimir, both knowing as they did of the great battle that was foretold, eyed one another as the enemies they would one day become. At last Odin said, "Mimir, I would drink of this fountain to gain all knowledge and wisdom." With barely a hesitation, Mimir shook his shaggy head and replied, "No." "But I will pay whatever price you ask," Odin insisted. Mimir, being infinitely wise and knowing all that was inevitable, sighed and considered. "If you pluck out your eye and cast it in the well, I will let you drink."

For Odin this was a bit unexpected. He considered the price, which seemed excessive. Odin shrugged. "All right then, my eye for one long drink," he said. So he set down his spear, flung his cape back over his shoulder, and quickly stooped to drink – Mimir had not, after all, indicated a definite order in their trade. The effect was instantaneous. Odin knew the breadth of the heavens and the depths of the sea and all that was to come...all at once in a furious rush. At last, Odin's thirst for knowledge and wisdom was fully quenched. It was not, however, as satisfying as he had thought it would be. For among all else he now saw Ragnarok and everything that would be lost. His beautiful Valkyrie, the lives of countless gods and men – even the sacred Yggdrasil itself would be shaken. He saw it all. And there was more that surprised him, for he also saw with infinite wisdom that the Earth's violent rebirth was not only inevitable, but necessary...yes, and even good. When he saw his own death during that rebirth, it brought a pained grin to his face.

Mimir grinned back at him knowingly. "You have what you came for. Now give me your eye," said the giant. Odin hesitated. He had gone back on his word many times before when he thought his cause worthy, but for some reason what he now knew prevented him from following that familiar course. He frowned, looking down at his spear and remembering the pain in his side as he'd hung from Yggdrasil those nine long days. What was a quick plucking out of an eye compared with all his past suffering? "Hmf," he grunted as he gouged his eye from its socket. Then he threw it in the fountain. "There it is," he said, studying Mimir with his one remaining orb. "Yes," said the giant, "there it is." And Odin left.

Now all that Odin learned at the Well of Ages cannot be told, but what would happen later at the battle of Ragnarok shades this tale with questions. After all, can a god fight as well with only one eye? Could it be that the wolf giant Fenrir took advantage of Odin's half-blindness, and was thereby able to swallow him whole? Could losing an eye for wisdom – even the wisdom to avoid his own demise – have actually led Odin to his end? It seems this is one snake that devours its own tale.

Mimir, in the meantime, discovered an interesting consequence to having the fiery eye of a god in his precious well. Odin's orb, it seemed, had transformed the spring water into mead. Still, Mimir drank it daily. Did his wisdom grow as it had before? We will never know, because he soon stopped drinking water from the Well of Ages altogether, losing his head over another matter that involved warring between the gods. But in his wisdom Mimir would have known that, wouldn't he? So perhaps he drank Odin's mead for comfort, knowing how things would eventually work out. It seems that great wisdom and foreknowledge did not really help either of them in the end.

Stress

Long-term stress kills people. How it kills is not entirely understood, but there are plentiful theories. Concomitant, sustained increases in hormone levels such as cortisol in people under stress have been tied to everything from shrinking brain tissue to immune system impairment to hyperglycemia and lower bone density. Other stress-related hormones such as norepinephrine may increase Interleukin-6 protein levels in cancer tumors, leading to accelerating tumor growth.[4] Ongoing research at Ohio State University has shown numerous correlations between stress and diseases – they have even found that allergies worsen during stress and anxiety. For years a general correlation between various stress factors and heart disease or heart attacks has been routinely observed, though the connection may be indirect – such as stress first leading to increases in blood pressure and cholesterol, which are risk factors for heart-related illness. Regardless of the specific mechanism, stress interferes with just about every dimension of nourishment. So what can we do about it?

The good news is that if we attentively nourish ourselves in every dimension, stress will be greatly reduced. In fact, in *Integral Lifework* all types of stress – physical, emotional, mental, spiritual – are the result of interrupted nourishment. And yet despite our best efforts, stressors can still insert themselves into our lives. Life events like relocating, having a child, starting a new job or retiring from one, experiencing a death in the family, going though a marriage or a divorce, buying a house, experiencing financial difficulties or becoming physically ill can all produce a heightened stress response. And since many of these events may be out of our control, or even an important and necessary process in our own growth or survival, eliminating stressors may not always be an option. Change is our lifelong companion, and depending on the extent and abruptness of the change at any given time, it will induce different levels of stress in us. So one way we can respond to increased stress is with increased multidimensional nourishment. In times when sudden or severe changes occur in our lives, we can learn to reflexively expand energy exchanges in all twelve dimensions to help compensate. This requires extra time and effort, but just as we must adjust the rest of our lives to the limitations sudden changes, we must adjust our lifestyle and integral practice to provide maximum nourishment in our time of greatest need.

The effect of improved self-care on stress is already well established. Additional physical exercise, meditation, supportive social interactions and satisfying sex all have proven benefits for stress reduction. From my experience and observation, immediate benefits can be experienced from increased nourishment in every other dimension as well. For instance, when we discover and actuate our life's purpose, we relieve stress at many different levels at once. For one, arrival at a personal vision for our life puts things in perspective, and thorns and hurdles that once inspired anxiety or frustration quickly recede into background noise. For another, the intense satisfaction of living out our purpose further insulates us from life's stressors. And the same is true of every other nourishment center, because each one anchors us a little more firmly amid the storms of existence and infuses us with additional energy to manage whatever comes. Balanced, holistic energy exchanges increase our overall resilience and pliancy, allowing us to respond more fluidly to change. However, keep in mind that any abrupt new investment in expanded nourishment routines can actually add to stress in the short run. It is, after all, yet another major change. So it is helpful to ramp up slowly and add new components to our integral practice one-at-a-time, rather than biting off more than we can effectively chew.

What happens when we increase routine integral practice to manage stress is that we transform stress itself into nourishment. Rather than medicating away our stress or distracting ourselves from it, we are allowing stressful situations to stimulate our being in healthy ways. We are balancing out antagonistic situations with compassionate self-care, and this allows us the energy and breathing room to integrate the changes we can't control so they become part of our whole and steady state, or to modify the tensions we can control so they can become part of our dialectic energy exchanges. Further, we enhance our ability to translate the golden intention – our desire to augment the good of All – into meaningful action, regardless of circumstance. We deepen our capacity to love by exercising compassionate affection in times of adversity. We strengthen our internally dependent fulfillment orientation and exorcise any lingering codependency. We enhance the harmony and stability of our most important relationships, while allowing the rush of adventurously being to draw us forward. As with so many other barriers to nourishment, stress provides us exciting opportunities to alchemically transmute impedances into facilitators; to change lemons into lemonade, and lead into gold.

Counterproductive Desires & Impulses

There is, I think, an unfortunate misunderstanding in modern thinking about appropriate ways to manage our desires and impulses. In the context of *Integral Lifework*, all desires and impulses originate in some way from our primary drives, and are either effective or ineffective in their facilitation of nourishment. Some are filtered through our personas as old survival responses. Some become dominant fulfillment impulses that, usually as a result of chained associations, translate into our core values. Others are created through recently developed habits and disciplines. And some are externally encouraged – I shy away from the term externally generated, though sometimes it may seem that way. For instance, after a particularly inspiring musical performance, I may want to sing out loud, or play an instrument, or incite others to join a jam session in my home. But the impulses and desires to musicize are already inside me as part of my self-nourishment matrix. In the same way, advertisements on TV or radio might key into some latent longings, and my unconscious processing of their suggestions could soon have me purchasing the advertised brand of goodies. All of these responses, though, lead at some point to a conscious choice to fulfill that desire or impulse, and this is where management comes in.

How many approaches we have to this subject! Some schools of thought insist we deny, renounce, suppress or reject certain morally questionable proclivities, while encouraging others that are perceived as honorable and proper to flourish. Another tradition might advise we prioritize virtuous impulses over egocentric ones, and sublimate those that do not serve a greater good. Another option is to relax such reflexive desires altogether, quieting the mind and heart so that our responses are conscious and thoughtful. And yet another way of thinking extols the virtue of indulging any and all desires and impulses without sorting through them at all. The list of choices isn't endless, but it sure is extensive, and the variation in consequences can be extreme. After all, how I manage my impulses and desires will determine my acceptance in society, my ability to maintain relationships, my overall mental, emotional and physical health, and perhaps, if some belief systems have it right, what happens to me after I die. So how do we decide what approach is right for us?

Allow me to propose a different way of looking at things. What if desires and impulses, no matter how destructive, narcissistic or antagonistic, aren't really the issue at all? What if something else entirely is the determining factor in how these proclivities impact our lives? Earlier in this book and in pervious writings I have suggested that a foundation for the most positive and effective outcomes is a pronounced transformation of intention, in essence shifting from a self-absorbed focus to what is of greatest benefit to everyone and everything: a golden intention, the good of All, which is inclusive of self. It is further proposed that what, exactly, the "good of All" looks like for each of us is less important than simply holding that benevolent intention in the forefront of our consciousness and allowing it to dominate our decision-making process. And if this golden intention possesses us entirely, how could any choice be faulty or ineffective, even if it produces unexpected outcomes? After all, we have dedicated ourselves to a greater cause. But...we humans are especially adept at fooling ourselves. We can excuse the most self-indulgent acts with a sleight-of-conscience, rationalizing this or that extravagance as benefiting the good of All, when really, in our heart of hearts, we know we just want it for ourselves. In effect, it isn't the desire or impulse that is problematic, it is our own willfulness, along with the nefarious creativity with which we can circumvent what is healthy for us, for those we love, and for everyone and everything around us.

So how can we set ourselves free from an apparent enslavement to this self-destructive rationalization? When love-consciousness indwells us, when it takes us over completely, all of our desires become its eager subjects and humbly submit to its will. Nothing is inappropriate or ineffective, because love is guiding and filtering every urge. Whenever we are truly in love, that love saturates all thoughts and intentions and chases all our worrisome shadows out into the Light. We discussed the road to that state of being in Part III, and as one approach to managing our most willful proclivities we can return to parenting styles. If authentic love can be demonstrated when managing a willful child, why not a willful urge?

Here is an example. A client of mine, Jonathan, has been struggling with what he considers inappropriate sexual urges for many years. He is painfully aware of how he has unconsciously manipulated situations to facilitate his desires, despite many attempts to train himself away from those habits. Now, it is important that Jon not feel judged by me in our therapeutic relationship, but I can agree with his own observation that his impulses are interfering with his well-being, especially in his ability to create and sustain intimate relationships. Remember that, in *Integral Lifework*, addictions to certain behaviors are almost always substitutions for nourishment in dimensions that have become depleted. For instance, Jon has never had a meaningful long-term intimate connection with anyone, and has a great well of fear surrounding the concepts of intimacy and vulnerability in any relationship. But he is also bravely willing to confront those fears, and that is of course the long-term solution to his struggle. But what can he do in the meantime?

Well, in Jon's case it doesn't take him long to figure it out on his own. Instead of struggling against his desires, he tearfully accepts them as part of himself, without judgment, guilt or shame. That is a hugely cathartic event. "I won't have to struggle anymore," he says, and it's a great relief to him. By *integrating the ugly or unbelievable* (a channel within the Empowered Self-Concept nourishment dimension), Jon is able to forgive himself for his sexual impulses, and begins parenting them with love. That is, he sets clear boundaries for them, enacts proportionate consequences when they behave disruptively or unlovingly, and otherwise creates an authoritative and egalitarian style of interaction with them. And it works. His impulses become not only an acceptable part of his life, but a loved and cared-for part of his life. As a result, they are much less disruptive to his well-being and overall nourishment. They become better behaved children. Soon, Jon finds himself dating again, and although his sexual desires and impulses are intensified by these interactions, he now has the tools and strength to manage them effectively. He is no longer a slave to his hungers, fears, anxieties or self-loathing.

The application of authentic love to almost any impulse-management scenario will have similar results. The impulses don't disappear, but they do mellow. If I say to my sugar craving, "You can have some sweets later, after lunch, but not before," the craving not only subsides in the moment, but is of course much less pronounced once I' have eaten a meal that includes complex carbohydrates. So here again the mitigation of any potential barrier occurs through introducing balance. Balance, patience, forbearance, self-discipline, love – however we want to describe the moderating effort, the result transforms impulses and desires that could undermine our well-being into patterns of thought, felt desire and action that support our well-being and the well-being of others. In Jon's case, the Empowered Self-Concept was his chief focus, but for someone else it could be another nourishment center altogether. As with other barriers, discovering what dimensions are depleted and targeting nourishment in those dimensions often has rapid and dramatic results.

PART V

LOVE'S EXPANSION

ARENAS OF AFFECTION, ARENAS OF ACTION

At the center of all loving interactions is empathy. To be able to empathize with the conditions of others, to be able to place ourselves in their position and appreciate their experience is the heart of intimacy. As differentiated from sympathy, which simply amplifies and perpetuates emotional pain, empathy engenders a readiness to respond in the most loving ways possible. And the empathic connection in turn adds invaluable input to our discernment about how best to care for ourselves and others in each situation. Over time, as we expand that empathy into new arenas of affection – new horizons of compassionate action – we come to identify with realms beyond our immediate, self-referential experience. We differentiate less and less between "self" and "other" in terms of priorities of action. Our moral valuation begins to shift, so that we seek the benefit of others because we recognize the rightness of such action and the inclusion of those others in our sense of self. This is a natural byproduct of multidimensional nourishment over time. So one way we can begin to define arenas of affection is by revisiting the levels of moral development described in Part I, and seeing how they might impact our developing sense of identity as love-consciousness matures within us.

SELF-IDENTIFICATION	STRATA OF MORAL VALUATION
Formless Infinite Self Equates both Being and Non-Being (or Non-Identification) and Compassionate Integration of All Other Self-Identifications	**Applied Nonduality** Translation of mystical, nondual consciousness into unfettered being where loving kindness harmonizes with spiritual understanding; a persistent, all-inclusive love-consciousness that integrates previous value orientations and current intentions into a balanced, purposeful flow
All-Being Identification with Progressively Broader Inclusion of Consciousness & Being Together with All Supportive Systems	**Spiritual Universality** Through intimate connection with an absolute, universal inclusiveness of being, moral function is defined by a guiding intentionality of "the good of All" as revealed by a successive unfolding of spiritual awareness, intuition and dialectic processing
Shared Spirit Identification with All Beings as Defined by Shared Spiritual Understanding	**Transpersonal Holism** Appreciation and acceptance of pluralistic value system and the necessity of moral ambiguity – as guided by discernment of intentional, strategic outcomes that benefit the largest majority possible
Earth Life Identification with Every Living System on Earth – All Its Individual Components & Supportive Environments	**World-Centric** Appreciation and acceptance of interdependent, globally inclusive systems and the need for individual and communal responsibility with compassionate effort in support of those systems
Human Society Identification with All People Everywhere	**Principled Rationalism** Commitment to a clearly defined set of reasoned moral principles that intend to benefit all of humanity, with a corresponding individuation of identity from affinitive and beneficial communities
Affinitive Community Identification with All People Who Share the Same Values or Experience	**Cooperative Communalism** Acceptance of communal role and necessity of collaborative contribution to human welfare without a need for competition or positional authority, with facilitative conformance to a community's shared values
Beneficial Community Identification with All People Who Benefit Each Other	**Competitive Communalism** Acceptance of communal role to participate in mutually beneficial community, usually in competition with others for personal positional power and influence, and without necessarily conforming to that community's shared values
Committed Greater Self Acceptance of the Identify of "self" as Larger Than Associations with Group(s) or Ideas	**Contributive Individualism** Fully individuated from tribe and committed to own well-being and wholeness, and interested in efforts that appear "good" or helpful to others as framed by (morally relativistic) individual experience and interaction

Tentative Greater Self Identification with a Possible "Self" Larger Than Associations with Group(s) or Ideas	Opportunistic Individualism In the process of individuating from tribe, morally adrift except for a sense of obligation to own well-being and wholeness, with minimal concern for the impact of that process on others
Secure Tribal Position Identification with "My People"	Defensive Tribalism Championing correctness of primary social group(s) and propagating the distinct definitions of rigid rules (law & order, right & wrong, black & white) of the group(s) defines most moral function
Insecure Tribal Position Identification with "The People I Want to be My People"	Tribal Acceptance Conformance with and approval or acceptance from primary social group(s) governs moral function; what is "right" or "wrong" is defined by what gains or loses social standing within the group(s)
Ego Identity Identification with Ego	Self-Protective Egoism Acquisitive, consumptive, hedonistic patterns to protect and sustain ego in a self-absorbed and self-centered moral orientation with indifference to the needs of others, as moderated by fear of personal gains being lost
Formative Identity Developing Ego and Ego-Identity	Self-Assertive Egoism Aggressive promotion of own wants and whims above those of others as a moral imperative in most situations, as moderated by fear of personal pain or punishment
Unformed Identity	Egoless "Raw Need" Naïve state: volition is centered around unrestrained basic needs fulfillment in every moment

Have you ever observed the identity shift that is described here in yourself or others? Even if the experience is fleeting, this actually can happen quite frequently. It occurs something like this: As we strengthen each dimension of self, we can feel safe, confident and grounded enough to be vulnerable and intimate with others within that dimension. And as we moderate our barriers across all dimensions, we can confidently express our authentic being from moment to moment in more of our relationships and interactions. At some point we then integrate progressive nourishment in all of its dimensions into an entirely new mode of being. As a result, often without realizing it, we progress from a narrowly confined identity to an ever more expansive and inclusive identity. It is precisely this process of identity shift that is reflected in each stratum of moral valuation. First we catch glimpses of each new stratum as we mature, sometimes resisting our progression, sometimes leaping forward, sometimes slipping backward. But somehow we keep growing until we can comfortably inhabit each new stratum completely. Ultimately, if we can entirely let go of our previous conceptions of self, there is a sense of being that embraces non-being or non-identity along with everything else.

How does this sense of self impact our arenas of affection? Paralleling these transformations of identity are the concrete realms of action within which we consciously focus our efforts. The flow of compassion we initiate in ourselves for ourselves never ceases or fragments, but our perception of that self – the felt sense of our boundaries of being – expands to include more and more interdependent phenomena. We become more, we love more. And since love-consciousness is prerequisite to this evolution, love-consciousness grows continually in harmony and resonance with All that Is (according to our current understanding of what that means) until there is nothing left to encompass. We become everything, love becomes everything, and everything becomes love.

As a felt experience all of this much more easy to comprehend as it unfolds experientially in our lives. But consider what love's expansion means in the context of integral practice. How will we nurture the twelve dimensions as our identity expands? What will that nourishment look like for us? Remember that this is really just a continuation of caring for self, and that just as with individual self-nourishment, how our love-consciousness propagates will be unique to our own attributes and circumstances. It is up to each of us individually to determine what our personal impact will be and how we will choose to love. Nevertheless, it will be helpful to examine some examples of how love actuates within those broadening ranges of identity. So just as with our initial examination of the twelve dimensions of nourishment, what follow are some suggested departure points for your own evaluation and synthesis. In many ways the recommendations for each scope of engagement simply offer up a question: *what would you choose to do here?* Each new horizon presents exciting opportunities to throw open the shutters of our being. When we are ready and willing to do so, we thereby invite necessary illumination into our innermost self, and allow compassionate affection to flow unhindered from our center out into the world.

Our Closest Relationships

Our closet relationships are certainly the primary testing ground for our nourishment, growth and transformation. Whatever heights of spiritual insight we may attain, whatever bliss we encounter through holistic self-care, whatever realm of perfected Love and Light we have nurtured within ourselves, our most intimate relationships will become the reality check of our accomplishments. This is because exchanges in these relationships demand the most from us. We are at our most vulnerable. Our expectations of trust and safety are at their highest. And the pressure we put on ourselves – to be authentic, to show love and kindness, to invest in the relationship, to be supportive, to succeed – can often be extreme. The closer we are to someone, the deeper our empathy will be for their pain, and the more our suffering will affect them. On many levels, allowing an intimate connection to develop with anyone is a tremendous risk. Which is why all of our insecurities, ego struggles, self-worth issues, doubts, inconsistencies, hypocrisies, mismanaged emotions, self-deceptions, weaknesses and other delightful foibles rush into plain sight whenever those we love the most are near. Once we recognize this, we can allow our closest relationships to help us remain honest about both who we really are, and where we are in our journey. If we are brave enough to face the mirrors of our dearest friends, they will offer us our greatest opportunities for self-awareness and integrity.

Authentic Intimacy & Family

The beginning of authentically loving others is authentically loving self. If the qualities of love-consciousness permeate our being, love will flow naturally out from us to envelop everyone we meet. And when that love is reciprocated, authentic intimacy occurs. Purely on the surface of things, if we demonstrate genuine interest in the well-being of others and attend to their words and actions actively and with a thoughtful presence, people tend to open up and share themselves much more readily. But beyond that, if what flows through us in those moments of interaction are equanimity, empathy, receptivity, loving kindness and confidence, then the initial spark of an open and caring heart will quickly build into an all-consuming flame of connection. For these qualities are the foundation of love-consciousness, and open the door to every truly

intimate moment we will ever experience. Yet each quality has little to
do with an exterior, conscious effort in the moment; rather, they are an
aftermath, a consequence of a thousand previous conscious decisions to
love the self. Equanimity, empathy, receptivity, loving kindness and
confidence – these form an elixir compounded of past and present
personal disciplines, and are the concrete evidence of our lengthy
journey through the Land of Light.

There is ample discussion of romantic relationships, family interactions
and friendships throughout other chapters, so it seems redundant to say
more at this juncture. But clearly the nature of every interaction can be
assessed with tools like the Relationship Matrix, and governed by the
characteristics of authentic love. The influence of our family on our well-
being is of course tremendous.   The expectations of our parents,
grandparents, siblings – anyone we identify as part of our family of
origin – serve as our conscience and guide for much of our life; we can
never be completely free of their influence. And yet, at some point in
our process of becoming an adult, we must learn to differentiate what is
the voice of our family and what is our own, distinct vision of our life.
Whether that vision can be understood or supported by our family
should not interfere with our self-actualization. And, if members of our
family of origin antagonize our well-being in some way, we must find a
way to forgive and honor them while still maintaining a clear boundary
around our sense of self.

Turning that same principle around, we must also recognize the
significance of the influence we wield when forming a family of our
own, and wield it carefully. For most people, there is usually a moment
of weakness at some point in their most intimate relationships when they
realize they are, in that moment, parroting the very unhelpful words
they heard from their parents and swore they would never utter
themselves. And such is the power we have over those we love as well.
Whatever we offer to our loved ones – whether anger and disapproval or
joy and support – will linger in their unconsciousness long after we have
had our say.   Such is the vulnerability and responsibility of true
intimacy, and, for all of the reasons just elucidated, this is why we must
model true love through how we love ourselves. The more secure we
are in the compassionate affection we hold for our own being, the more

effortlessly we will translate the affection we feel for others into constructive and nurturing actions.

Community & Society

Earlier, in our discussion of Supportive Community, many of the specifics of constructive communal relationships and interactions were enumerated. Now we will build on that foundation and examine how targeted nourishment for a malnourished society might begin.

The Evolution of Memes

Like any complex organism, societies evolve and change over time. Because human social evolution involves human consciousness, the cycles of that evolution appear quite different than elsewhere in Nature. In much the same way that humans have used selective breeding to emphasize desired traits in domesticated animals, we have also created social institutions that selectively emphasize one particular avenue of social contract, aesthetic or worldview over another, allowing those selective memes to dominate our culture for a time. This process of memetic propagation often begins with just a few individuals, and expands outward across many arenas until social institutions have formalized its cultural acceptance. In fact, *Integral Lifework* is modeled on this very principle, and the success of concepts and practices like authentic love are dependent on memetic propagation. So carefully considering the evolution of memes can inform how we go about effectively caring for our community and society as a whole.

Once we become conscious of how memes evolve and expand, there is real opportunity to enhance positive and lasting change. Keep in mind as you review the stages below that memes come in many different forms, with just as many potentially destructive outcomes as constructive ones for the affected culture. Memes, like viruses or bacteria, can sometimes seem more concerned with their own survival than the survival of their host. In addition, a meme can present itself as nourishment, when really it is the most depleting kind of substitution.

How does this self-perpetuating process occur? Here are some proposed
stages of memetic evolution:

- **Inception.** A host – a group or individual – at ground zero uncovers
  a new approach, idea, insight or pattern that reprioritizes thought
  and action, and either a new meme takes form, or an old meme is
  reborn. Sometimes this occurs as a result of a latent or suppressed
  appetite in a culture or subculture, and sometimes the meme itself
  invents an appetite within one or more nourishment dimensions.
  Once the meme gains a host through which to replicate itself, it can
  begin to interact with other memes in the host's belief-space,
  encourage attempts to reinforce itself in the host's supportive
  behaviors, and then probe the broader ideosphere of the
  surrounding culture.

- **Success.** By demonstrating how the new meme enhances one or
  more forms of nourishment, the ground zero inception takes deeper
  root in the host and the meme gains breadth, depth and substance.
  The impact and strength of the meme relates to how depleted any
  nourishment dimensions it addresses may have been, as well as how
  full-spectrum the meme is; that is, how many nourishment
  dimensions are addressed simultaneously. In particular, memes that
  can only operate in one processing space (mental spacetime, etc.) are
  inherently weaker than memes that thrive in two or more. Another
  way to look at this is to ask the question "How may fulfillment
  impulses does this meme satisfy?" If it satisfies several in a new
  way, it will tend to be more enduring than memes that satisfy fewer
  fulfillment impulses.

- **The Island Effect.** Observing its positive impact, others begin to
  adopt the meme and it gains momentum as a cultural phenomenon;
  its host expands. These early adopters may be conscious or
  unconscious of the meme's influence, and they may be either an
  arbitrary cross section across many cultural strata, or a select,
  isolated group. Initially, the new meme will tend to either encounter
  resistance in the surrounding culture, or quickly fade away. No
  matter how successful the meme is for individuals, or how quickly it
  initially spreads, memes usually require resistance to become strong
  enough to survive. Just as with the principle of dialectic tension in

nourishment, without resistance a new meme is more of a "flash in the pan," fading quickly into the background noise of life. This resistance may come in the form of conflict with competing memes, or cultural ostracism, or persecution, or reflexive dismissal and criticism. Thus the successful meme creates a cultural island and slowly becomes evermore concretely established.

- **Winnowing.** At this stage the meme either breaks out, propagating across multiple socioeconomic strata in its parent culture, or it fails and dies. If memetic competition is too strong or the environment too resistant, the meme may encapsulate itself like bacteria in an unfriendly environment, and become dormant until factors change in its favor. If there is no resistance or competition, the meme tends to weaken and denature itself, perhaps lending its conceptual DNA to other memes. If there is just the right balance of propagation and resistance – a narrow band of memetic facilitation – the meme thrives and becomes more established.

- **Emergence.** This is the meme's individuation process. Because the meme has passed and initial threshold of fragility and possible extermination, it now begins to assert itself more aggressively. This might occur in the form of challenging other widely accepted memes for dominance, or rebelling against its former oppressors, critics and persecutors, or adapting itself to other dimensions of nourishment. A successful emergence finds the new meme permeating wider and wider arenas of affection, and gathering supportive structures (i.e. interdependencies with other memes, or a *memeplex*) that strengthen it.

- **Stabilization.** Here the meme calms down a bit, like a rebellious young person finally settling into a more adult identity and donning a mantle of responsibility. There is often broad cultural acceptance of a meme at this point, as well as the first stages of the meme's institutionalization. That is, just as social morays can progress to accepted moral valuations and eventually become codified as law, a stabilized meme concretizes into social institutions across all strata of society. Instead of a fad, movement or revolution, the meme is now a de facto standard, fully formalized into the status quo.

- **Prime of Influence.** Whatever impact the meme will have on its parent culture, it has now reached its peak, cascading across all of society and spawning its own child memes and fortifying its supportive memeplex. As with any of these stages, this one may last for years, decades or even millennia, spontaneously absorbing other memes in whirlwind of memetic syncretism, spreading virally across several different cultural and subcultures, and either deliberately or inadvertently suppressing any competing memes as a consequence of its dominance and momentum.

- **Distortion.** Like any other organic thing, memes eventually grow old and die. As part of that process, memes at this stage become inflexible, bloated and heavy. They can no longer adapt to or integrate new memes or other changes in the surrounding culture. And although institutions that embraced the meme may still have positional authority in the culture, their real influence is waning. At this stage we often see cultural proponents of this meme acting towards other, newer memes in much the same way that their oppressors, critics and persecutors behaved when their own meme was new. As a result, the meme becomes increasingly distorted as it tries to hold on to some vestige of power. The further the meme declines in this way, the less it resembles its initial vitality or energized differentiation from other memes.

- **Dormancy or Death.** After a meme has been sufficiently weakened by distortion and declining influence, it passes away. That passing away can take many forms. For instance, the old meme could be dramatically usurped by a fresh new meme and disappear entirely. Or it might be absorbed into other extent memes, subordinating itself as part of their memeplex. Or it might encapsulate itself within another meme, waiting for an appropriate moment to resurface. Memetic death can be sudden or prolonged, but in the end the true substance and import of the original meme is usually forgotten. Whatever its revolutionary differences at one time, its relevance is lost in modern context. Unless, of course, it is somehow revitalized and reborn.

- **Rebirth.** Given the right circumstances, timing and receptivity in a willing host individual or group, any meme may be rediscovered or retooled in a new way. Once this happens, the evolutionary process begins again with Inception, but this time with the added energy of a previous history. In other words, an old meme that is revived will have more authority and appeal than a completely new meme, and will tend to become established much more quickly.

As a metaphor for observable patterns in human culture and history, the meme is a convenient concept. Whether religious movements or health fads, pervasive cultural attitudes or rarefied workplace etiquette, a popular product touted in mass media or a new method accepted only by a cadre of influential specialists, memes can be huge or tiny in both their scope and significance. But is a meme more than a metaphor? At this time, I believe that memes exist as artifacts of will, agents created by thought and volition that act independently inside and outside of our consciousness, traveling through many different systems of communication and utilizing many different media – including media we haven't yet recognized or identified – in order to proliferate through a collective host. Regardless of what memes actually are, however, the concept provides a useful placeholder for processes we can readily observe but not yet fully explain.

With this in mind, imagine a world where authentic love is the dominant memeplex. What if every person on Earth could nurture themselves so completely and unconditionally that they felt unlimited compassion for everyone and everything at all times? This is the vision I cherish in my heart as I write, teach classes and collaborate with clients in *Integral Lifework* sessions. I believe it is possible. But how will this memeplex take root? Will the idea that there is an effective way to holistically nourish ourselves and others – and that this process flows from and results in authentic love – succeed against the memes of greed, prejudice, aggression, chaos, egoism or the plethora of other destructive impulses derived from ignorance and fear? So far, I have observed true love prevail time and time again in my own life and the lives of others. It seems to me that love is the solid ground, the steady state, to which all things must eventually return. We need only create the spaciousness in our lives with which true love can make a home.

> **Resources:**   For a broad and inclusive introduction to memetic theory, try Susan Blackmore's *The Meme Machine*. As of this writing many excellent resources are also available through a simple web search of "memetics." Interestingly, memetics itself seems to have recently passed from the Island stage to the Winnowing stage of its evolution; so…time will tell.

The Marketplace

Because I was raised in Western culture, I tend to view society in the context of capitalism. Like most Americans, I was enculturated into the Randian ideal that society consists mainly of interdependent market forces whose sole purpose is to enable my individual satisfaction and empowerment. The answer to the question of John Galt's identity was hammered home over and over again throughout my childhood: everyone who wants to participate in commercialistic opportunism *is* John Galt, and it was my privilege and responsibility to embrace the John Galt brand of self-actualization.   And yet, as I observed the consequences of this philosophical orientation, I began to question the viability of that brand. In particular, I began to realize that although business ownership in a competitive marketplace is one of the most exciting and stimulating adventures society can offer – and thus one of the most potentially nourishing enterprises available to us – the ever-increasing concentration of power and influence in U.S. corporations seemed to be at odds with the nourishing aspects of capitalism.   In particular, as I experienced corporate America firsthand and educated myself about its workings in the world, it became increasingly clear that corporations were often deliberate in their oppression of individual liberties and disruptive to our personal and collective well-being. Patterns created by supposedly rational self-interest seemed at odds with holistic nourishment.

When we take the time to examine the record of corporate influence on society, it quickly becomes evident that any efforts we undertake to nourish our community and culture must address this influence first and foremost. Let's consider a potent example. The following excerpt is taken from the 2004 Executive Summary of the *United States Final*

Proposed Findings of Fact regarding federal litigation against tobacco companies:

> "In response to this growing body of evidence that smoking caused lung cancer, Defendants and their agents joined together and launched their coordinated scheme in the early 1950s. Defendants developed and implemented a unified strategy that sought to reassure the public that there was no evidence that smoking causes disease. At the end of 1953, the chief executives of the five major cigarette manufacturers in the United States at the time – Philip Morris, R.J. Reynolds, Brown & Williamson, Lorillard, and American – met at the Plaza Hotel in New York City with representatives of the public relations firm Hill & Knowlton and agreed to jointly conduct a long term public relations campaign to counter the growing evidence linking smoking as a cause of serious diseases. The meeting spawned an association-in-fact enterprise ("Enterprise") to execute a fraudulent scheme in furtherance of their overriding common objective – to preserve and enhance the tobacco industry's profits by maximizing the numbers of smokers and number of cigarettes smoked and to avoid adverse liability judgments and adverse publicity. The fraudulent scheme would continue for the next five decades."[5]

Reading the rest of this Executive Summary is chilling to the heart, mind and spirit. The tobacco industry's' fraudulent scheme just kept on expanding. Cigarette companies began engineering more deliberately addictive tobacco products – all the while publicly denying that nicotine was addictive at all – which they then aggressively marketed to children and teens in order to create lifelong consumers. They knew that, if their efforts were successful, this product would eventually kill millions of people, but they deliberately worked to conceal this fact from the public through deceptive advertising (i.e. offering "light" or "low-tar" cigarettes that supposedly mitigated health risks), lying to Congress, destroying and suppressing evidence, and spending millions on public relations campaigns. This addiction-creating, lethal subterfuge continued until lawsuits and the leaking of internal corporate documents exposed the ruse some fifty years later. Shockingly, even after tobacco corporations lost their case in court and were ordered to change marketing practices and pay millions in perpetual settlements, they continued targeting young people, minorities and women to expand a smoking consumer base.[6] And of course these corporations are still peddling their lethal product today. This classic example of corporate influence has resulted in the suffering of countless families and a massive burden on society regarding the long-term health care of smokers. In the meantime, the corporate executives responsible for this horror continue to retain their wealth, their personal freedoms and a powerful lobby in Washington D.C.

There are of course thousands of other cases that illustrate how corporate culture does not subscribe to nourishing objectives – or even the prevailing moral valuation of the society in which it operates – and I don't wish to overstate the obvious. However, a few more large-scale examples will, I think, drive the point home:

- Henri Nestlé invented infant formula in 1867. In following decades, the Nestlé Corporation began marketing infant formula all around the globe. In search of ever larger markets, Nestlé began targeting populations in the developing world, using tactics that promoted their product as a healthy, modern and sophisticated alternative to breast feeding. By flooding those markets with enough free samples to effectively interrupt breast milk production in mothers who used those samples, they deliberately induced dependency on their product. These efforts, along with similar strategies from Wyeth, Bristol-Myers and other corporations, exacerbated serious health problems and increased mortality in those infant populations.[7] An international boycott of the company begun in 1977 did raise awareness of this issue and establish standards for marketing of infant formula through the World Health Organization. However, as late as 1997, Nestlé was still using the same strong-arm marketing tactics to get mothers hooked on its product. [8] Even in the U.S., government programs and corporate ad campaigns have conspired to supplant breast feeding with formula feeding.[9] As of this writing, a survey of articles about the benefits of breast feeding conclusively indicate that it is far superior to infant formula and can significantly reduce risks of infant illness and death; those articles also indicate the dangers of substituting or even augmenting nutrition with infant formula.[10] Today, three decades after the boycott was begun, Nestlé is still producing its infant formula, still aggressively marketing the product around the world, and, although their corporate website now offers a caveat about the importance of breastfeeding, Nestlé still promotes the nutritional efficacy of its infant formula product despite all evidence to the contrary.

- In December of 1984, the Union Carbide pesticide plant leak in Bhopal, India, released enough methyl isocyanate (MIC) into the surrounding population to kill over 7,000 people within the first three days, and eventually lead to the deaths of an additional 15,000 people by 2005.[11] This happened despite repeated warnings to Union Carbide about dangers at the plant, and specifically the type of "runaway reaction" that would eventually cause the leak. To avoid accountability, local Union Carbide officials first denied the toxic cloud released was just an irritant like tear gas. The corporation then argued in U.S. and Indian courts that neither had appropriate jurisdiction over its operations in Bhopal. Five years later, Union Carbide settled with the Indian government for $470 million, and was thereafter ordered to subsidize care for disaster survivors for eight more years. For the first six months of 1989, Union Carbide's total sales were about $4.5 Billion, and their net profits were about $387 Million, so this settlement would have eaten up just a tad more than a half-year's profits at the time – except that it was covered almost entirely by Union Carbide's insurance policies, so it had hardly any impact at all. The Bhopal chemical plant site was never adequately cleaned up, and heavy metals and caustic chemicals from the plant continue to disrupt the health and well-being of tens of thousands of people.[12] To date, Union Carbide has also not released the full chemical composition of the gas cloud, which has greatly hampered efforts to treat victims. In 2001, Dow Chemical Corporation acquired Union Carbide for $7.3 Billion, creating the second largest chemicals manufacturer in the world after DuPont. Bhopal's sister plant, located just West of Charleston, West Virginia, has continued to experience a number of OSHA violations, accidents and life-threatening leaks, the most recent of which was in August of 2008.[13]

- DuPont Corporation has been manufacturing Teflon products for several decades now. Over the years, it has become obvious despite

DuPont's efforts to conceal and deny the fact that one of the chemicals in Teflon, a PFC called PFOA, presents a substantial risk to human health and the environment, and has been leaching out of their products and production facilities for years.[14]   In particular, high concentrations of PFOA have been measured in the blood of DuPont's plant workers and in the drinking water of populations surrounding their plants.   Yet despite documented cancer, reproductive issues and liver toxicity in animals from DuPont's own research on PFOA, despite a disproportionate increase in birth defects among DuPont's factory workers, despite 3M discontinuing the production of all PFCs in 2000 in response to growing concerns about PFC toxicity,[15] despite the EPA declaring PFOA a "likely human carcinogen" in 2005, despite the off-gassing from the normal use of Teflon cookware killing pets and producing flu-like symptoms in humans, and despite the fact the PFOA persists in a nearly indestructible state wherever it ends up (human blood, the environment, etc.), DuPont still manufactures Teflon. We can still purchase Teflon products in nearly any retail store. And DuPont is still the largest chemicals corporation in the world.

These are all well-documented instances, and because of these and other large-scale events the public is, at least on a surface level, aware of the intrusive dangers of corporate America. There is even periodic outrage about corporate misconduct. A shoe manufacturer is using sweat shops or child labor to produce a popular sneaker. Diamond mining and oil drilling companies tacitly endorse terrible working conditions at their facilities and the violent repression of local populations. Pharmaceutical companies are exposed as concealing lethal side effects of their most profitable drugs. High finance brings the global economy to its knees with risky subprime lending and other reckless schemes. Companies formerly headed by highly placed government officials are revealed to be immersed in war profiteering and bribery of foreign officials. Buildings and bridges collapse on people because developers used faulty materials to increase their profit margins. All of these things and more have roused consumer indignation in recent years. However, a majority of Americans still unwittingly support such heinous corporate proclivities with their daily purchases – because corporate misconduct is simply that prolific.

Consider also that the language of business has permeated U.S. culture as well, slowly gnawing away at its moral underpinnings. "It's just business" has entered the popular vernacular as an acceptable excuse for callous behavior that promotes personal gain over the welfare of others. "The bottom line" has become a ubiquitous justification for decisions that effectively treat people like property. And "making good business sense" seems increasingly to be the only kind of sense that matters in American culture. Except for a thin veneer of corporate philanthropy, concepts like compassionate affection are routinely excised from business environments, processes and an ever-broadening business lingo.

In my own life, I witnessed firsthand events that undermined any trust I might have had in corporate culture. When I worked for the U.S. military at a vehicle repair facility, I inventoried sheet metal parts that cost the U.S. government – and thus every taxpayer – thousands more than they should have because of no-bid contracts. When I worked at a major U.S. retailer, I witnessed folks who had spent their entire adult lives committed to that company systematically forced out of their jobs just before they became fully vested and could draw a retirement pension. When I was a technical consultant, I was routinely asked by corporate executives to misrepresent the truth – to employees, to government agencies like the EPA and the SEC, to any customers I came in contact with, and so on – in order to protect corporate interests and insulate executives from personal accountability. In the patient advocacy I have provided, I have seen over and over again the grievous impact that profit-driven procedures and drugs can have on people's well-being. And, when I was myself a mid-level manager in a Fortune 100 company, I saw close-up the desperate, driving greed and ethical ambiguity that neatly explained everything I had observed to date in U.S. corporate culture.

After twenty-five years of trying to operate conscientiously and compassionately within various business environments, I concluded that capitalism in its Western implementation is for the most part a dehumanizing system of exchanges. Products that appeal to temporary, sensational gratification win out over those that nourish genuine need. Communication that inflates the importance of one dimension of nourishment vanquishes balanced, full-spectrum approaches. And the more any dimension of nourishment is commoditized and commercialized, the lower the quality of nourishment that is actually being delivered. Foods lose their nutritional value. Other products become so homogenous that only those of exactly average tastes and exactly average means can appreciate them. Necessary diversity and competition is crushed by consolidation, the faddish impulses of consumers and the profit incentives of shareholders. Great ideas are discarded or overridden by superior marketing campaigns or anti-competitive business practices, often resulting in the lowest quality outcomes for the majority of consumers with the highest profits for a minority of producers. Whole industries rise and fall according to these rhythms.

This kind of commercialism disparages self-nurturing. It limits or prevents integral nourishment, rewarding the shrewd, deceptive and divisive above the caring and compassionate. Ultimately, it results in scarcity rather than abundance. And because the fundamental metrics for success of almost all businesses involve profit margins, market share, share price and return on investment, the resulting competition is understandably cutthroat, calculated to benefit whoever wins regardless of the means used or consumer well-being. To raise an argument that business only responds to existing demand – and thus shouldn't be held accountable for outcomes antagonistic to individual or societal well-being – is specious. The demand for gas guzzling SUVs, cigarettes, diet pills, sugary/caffeinated/alcoholic drinks, gruesome entertainment, anabolic steroids, fatty fast food, toxic children's toys, non-stick frying pans and a host of other harmful products is a result of deliberate, extensive, relentless and well-targeted marketing. Yes, the reflexive whims of uneducated consumers have answered those profit-driven invitations, but corporations initiated the cycle by synthesizing artificial needs out of thin air. By inventing sales concepts that exploit half-formed fears, impulsive desires, latent longings and low self-worth, they create demand where none exists.

Consider these advertising hooks: "modern convenience," "more for less," "you deserve it," "cheaper is smarter," "have it your way," "because you're worth it," "we're someone you can trust," "look sharp, feel sharp," "newer is better," "people who don't buy this are stupid...." Are any of these really true in the long run? Of course not, but we can be persuaded to feel they are true just long enough to make a purchase. And since there is no opposing persuasion to moderate pointless consumption, and because we do feel fractionally more powerful, excited or elated for a short time after spending our money, the cycle reinforces itself endlessly. There are consumer protection agencies and advocates, but just as the stern warnings of parents can't compete with the influence of teenage peers, so the muted advisements of such organizations can't compete with the sexy, groupthink appeal of ubiquitous, well-funded ad campaigns.

In this way the current American commercialistic model depends on the minimization of self-reliance and authentic self-worth, and on the continual devaluation of the True Self in order to shift our fulfillment focus toward externals. If I am a fundamentally unattractive, unsophisticated, incompetent, unwell person who feels entitled to immediate alleviation of my resulting unhappiness, then clearly I must consume my way out of these conditions, relying solely on the superior wisdom of others. That is the real message behind all modern advertising: that we must voraciously consume our way to happiness and wholeness, because those conditions cannot be found within ourselves; we are empty vessels waiting to be filled. The result is a deliberate amplification and perpetuation of abject dependency, which in turn sustains an endless cycle of human suffering. In a profound irony, even popular spirituality trends in the U.S. distract people from the authentic Love and Light within themselves, emphasizing instead the saccharin substitutes of cathartic experience, egoistic empowerment, moral rectitude or cultish tribalism. This really isn't spirituality at all, it's just another externalizing falsehood that justifies conspicuous consumption.

And of course our individual capacity to love and the arenas of our affection are limited by consumerism as well. If we are forever preoccupied with the pseudo-nourishment offered by alluring externals, and if we are kept from understanding the breadth and power of our own being through perpetual busyness, how will we ever be strong enough to explore love beyond our own self-absorption? How could we even perceive the limitless horizons of love-consciousness? Instead of expanding our compassion outward into the world around us, we will be competing with everyone else for what little love can be found close at hand – at the mall, in the movie theater, over the Internet, in our cell phones…anywhere but in the uneasy quiet of confusing solitude or the demanding reciprocations of empathic companionship. We could be producing energy exchanges that heal, grow and transform whatever and wherever we engage, but instead we have become fixated on consuming within smaller and smaller circles of nourishment, until all that remains is an artificial representation of self – a hollow, shriveled shell that has forgotten its own soul.

Through countless examples of insatiable avarice and wanton turpitude, it is impossible not to conclude that the corporate memeplex is aggressively opposed to true love in the individual and the collective. On a national and international scale, it pointedly antagonizes the ideals of democracy, free speech, civil liberties, and those self-evident truths in the U.S. Declaration of Independence that represent the fruits of affectionate compassion. In fact, corporations consistently constrict life, liberty and the pursuit of happiness by every definition but one: material gain. And despite the pro-corporate rhetoric of well-funded PR campaigns, material gain does not in itself equate well-being. In an integral memeplex, material gain may be a natural consequence of acts of kindness toward and from others, or an intermediate goal that is framed within the qualities of love. But material security is not an end in itself, because this would mean once again transferring the innate power of our being into externals. Nearly all spiritual traditions in the world try to convey the principle that such acquisitiveness distracts from, rather than supports, wholeness and wellness. And with very few exceptions, corporations have not acted in favor of authentic love or any of its chief characteristics, they are not soulful or compassionate – or human in any way – but instead reinforce externalization of all types of nourishment and the destruction of social cohesion. And of course this makes perfect *business sense*, because patterns of depletion, aggression and dependency serve corporate profits much more handily than patterns of nurturing, cooperation and self-reliance.

How did it come to this? And how do corporations continue to get away with these sorts of atrocities and remain immune to proportionate accountability? In part what makes corporations so powerful is their enormous concentration of wealth, which allows them tremendous influence over individuals, communities and governments. How many reports do we hear each month about corporations paying off dictators, or cutting deals with armed rebels, or supplying weapons to criminals, or bribing public officials, or funding political campaigns, or drafting self-serving legislation, or settling lawsuits with people in quiet nondisclosure outside of court? And so the wheels of international commerce are lubricated with the blood, sweat and tears of innocents, the greed of corrupt government officials, and the wealth of the affluent. But this is only part of the equation. Another part, which is not widely recognized or understood, is that corporations in the U.S. have been granted the legal protections and privileges of individuals without an equivalent level of social responsibility. They have been granted *corporate personhood*.

To fully explore the topic of corporate personhood is beyond the scope of this writing. However, suffice it to say that successive rulings of the U.S. court system have, over time, increasingly granted corporations the same rights every citizen is accorded by the U.S. Constitution. But rights such as freedom of speech, freedom of conscience, the right to lobby Congress, the right to due process and jury trials, the right to contribute to political campaigns, protection from unreasonable search and seizure and so forth were never meant to apply to corporations; that is clear to anyone who has examined U.S. history with any rigor. The purpose of the Bill of Rights was to ensure that the authority of governance rested with the people, for the people and by the people. The misinterpretation of "person" as used in the Constitution to represent anything but human beings is a gross violation of the spirit of that document. However, as a result of concerted efforts by corporations to empower themselves, they have effectively sabotaged the democratic institutions of the United States, and greatly weakened the relative power of governments and individuals to thwart corporate agendas.

And finally, the incestuous marriage of corporations and political institutions has solidified the dehumanizing influence of corporate culture in the U.S. and around the globe. Whether it is the World Bank forcing economic globalization down the throats of developing countries, or the IMF backing the disruptive and sometimes violent resource grabs of expanding corporations, or the WTO methodically enlarging a type of "free trade" that benefits corporations but not workers or consumers, all of these institutions are the creations of world leaders fulfilling the self-serving vision of large corporations. And the more intimate corporations become with political institutions, the more predictable the outcomes. The wealthy become wealthier, the poor become poorer, global cultures are homogenized, human rights are decimated and the Earth is despoiled.

Most fiscal conservatives recognize that the rule of law is necessary to facilitate commerce – without stable governments and reliable economic systems, risk assessment and profit projections become unpredictable. But unless governments are large, somewhat intrusive and very well-funded, the rule of law is really a sham, becoming little more than an orchestration of corporate agendas at its best, and at its worst a bureaucratic façade that mires real justice in overcomplicated legalism. For if government isn't endowed with more power than corporations and made transparently accountable to its people, how can it protect society from corporate misconduct? How can it discipline public officials corrupted with corporate payola? How can it champion any cultural values that might interfere with the routine abuse and exploitation that occur in pursuit of profit? How can it protect us from the self-serving agendas of other special interests? It can't. As we have seen repeatedly around the globe and throughout human history, a weaker government means a weaker rule of law.

Despite the inspirational speechifying of Margaret Thatcher, Ronald Reagan and other influential figures who have subscribed to a Friedmanesque, neoliberal economic philosophy, the "market revolution" they touted has failed dismally. Smaller government and deregulated capitalism succeeded in liberating greed but little else, instead driving the capitalist wedge ever deeper between the wealthy and the rest of society. No invisible hand has righted the wrongs of overreaching corporations, and the rising economic tide has only elevated a callous minority of masters above a drowning majority of servants. When we add to this landscape a perpetual "war on terror" that defends this economic system – a system dependent on endless expansion and growth – U.S. capitalism increasingly resembles the feudalism of medieval Europe. In this scenario, corporations assume the role of powerful lords, governments take the part of vassals loyal to those lords, terrorists fulfill the function of uncivilized invaders, politicians are the knights sworn to defend corporations, and the rest of us become indebted peasants constantly afraid for our lives.

Clearly, in order to propagate the meme of true love in the world, corporate barriers to nourishment must be eliminated. There are several ways we can approach this challenge, beginning with an awareness of our own responsibility as caring citizens to advocate change. For example, we could attempt any or all of the following:

1) Reign in corporate power by revoking corporate personhood as a legal concept and restoring the intended authority of the electorate.

2) Hold corporations, their managers and their owners to a higher level of accountability to the rule of law through more rigorous application of regulation, penalization and incarceration.

3) Provide more tools for consumers to make ethically informed choices about their product, service and stock investment purchases, effectively managing corporate behavior through consumer behavior.

4) Empower democratic governments at all levels to restrict the size of corporations, the concentration of wealth in any one corporate entity, the availability of resources (labor, natural resources, etc.) to corporations, and the access to specific markets allowed any company.

5) Change the relationship between consumers and producers so that respectful and empathic interdependence is acknowledged and reinforced, and shared values are clarified.

6) Give populations direct, democratic control over corporate charters; for example, allowing corporations to be dissolved and their assets auctioned off as the result of a simple majority vote in a ballot initiative.

7) Constitutionally mandate a separation of corporations and state in much the same way we have separated church and state in the U.S.

8) Restructure the IMF, WTO and World Bank to support a different economic model than globalization a la Western-style capitalism; a model in which human well-being and human rights are valued more highly than corporate privileges and profits, where funding is not tied to Western-style free market reforms or sociopolitical conditionalities, and small, local business is considered more favorably than transnational megaconglomerates.

9) Create incentives for corporate profit-sharing and fixed ratios by industry for the highest and lowest employee compensation.

10) Educate corporate executives, board members and shareholders about the cultural value of empathy and kindness, hoping that this will inspire more compassionate business practices.

11) Institute new standards for worker, consumer and environmental safety that are based on something similar to the EC's *precautionary principle* (i.e. *Vorsorgeprinzip*) rather than a traditional risk-benefit analysis.

12) Free the news media from its dependence on corporate sponsorship.

13) Insulate or segregate financial markets from all speculative derivatives trading – just as any other form of gambling is regulated.

14) Reengineer the U.S. monetary system so that all credit is publicly controlled rather than issued by profit-driven banks. That is, abolishing the fractional reserve banking system, wrestling monetary control from private banking institutions and returning it to the U.S. government.

There will, of course, continue to be powerful resistance to such remedies; those who consistently gain from the prevailing system of commercialized exchanges are threatened by changes and alternatives. As if in response to such possible threats, corporations have assiduously built a system whereby consumers must submit to unethical, greed-centric business practices in order to nourish themselves in any dimension. If current trends continue, the implications are ominous. There will be no publicly funded alternatives to challenge the bias of corporately controlled media. There will be no new art but only repetition of formulas that have sold well in the past. There will be no spirituality that involves interior discipline, only empty rituals and cathartic distractions. There will be no philosophical debate, no profound ideas, no encouragement to grow or evolve on any level except for the innovation of new consumables and new ways to market them. Education will consist only of preparing workers for specialized tasks and inculcating an unquestioning devotion to the cycle of production and consumption. All products will be manufactured by people without basic human rights. The destruction or disruption of natural environments will weaken the Earth's self-sustaining cycles and everything living within them. False nourishment that addicts, sickens and ultimately terminates human beings will become the sole foundation of a declining global economy. All wealth and power will be concentrated in those merciless few who perpetuate this status quo for their own gain. Authentic love, because it interrupts the style and essence of this mode of commerce, will be dismissed, repressed and greatly feared.

Hints of this potential outcome have been evident for some time, and with each passing year our options for substantive nourishment decreases while our fanciful choices increase. That grilled salad at the local fast food chain isn't really any more nutritious than the old grilled chicken sandwich, but we are repeatedly sold on the idea that it is, and that repetition wears us down. In the meantime, the locally owned ethnic restaurant has gone out of business because they couldn't compete with the volume-based pricing, misleading advertising and underhanded resource acquisitions of the fast food chains. Which is why the idea of competition resulting in the best outcome for the consumer is such a ridiculous falsehood. The only metrics that consistently win out are lower prices for commodities and higher profits for bigger businesses. Nearly everything else – quality, diversity, dimensions of nourishment, ethics, consumer health and safety, environmental health and safety, you name it – are woefully diminished as a result.

If the current marketplace rewarded practices, products and services that were deemed beneficial via metrics more sophisticated than commoditization and profitability, the landscape would evolve differently. What would the world look like if all commerce was grounded in trust, cooperation, friendly competition and compassion for the well-being of humanity and the Earth? What if business values and language emulated loving interpersonal values and language? Among other things, we would likely already have cheap alternative energy, healthy foods would be ubiquitous, healthcare would be free and effective, teachers would receive much higher salaries, our air and water would be clean and human activity would no longer contribute to global warming. If love guided the marketplace instead of greed, self-destructive attitudes of entitlement would be replaced with self-expansive opportunities for real happiness.

An Integral Solution:
Fulfillment Orientation, Relationship, Information & Identity

At the root of all of these challenges is imbalanced nourishment on an individual level, easily and quickly correctable through widespread adoption of integral practice. In *Integral Lifework*, the focus of individual effort is active, creative and productive. To generate interior energies and offer them in loving exchange is the heart of its alchemy. Here the answers to our most difficult questions, the conditions for our greatest joys, and the vision and power for our unique contribution to the whole are all within us, just waiting to be tapped. *Integral Lifework* opposes Western commercialism's assertion that all answers, joys and life vision are available outside ourselves, at discount prices, if we will only act quickly – and without reflection – on our most shallow consumptive impulses. It counters these impulses with introspection, empathy, patience, discernment and love. What if, instead of acquisitive self-indulgence, the source of our confidence, joy, strength and purpose were love, forgiveness, generosity and kindness? In 2009, as the global economy experiences a major reset, the world is once again reminded that externalizing our well-being only guarantees one thing: that we will end up live beyond our means if we keep relying on the external satisfaction of our needs. Will we heed this admonition?

If we apply the same principles of authentic love to the marketplace as we have to other arenas, it can help evolve a model of integral commerce. The first step is really an individual choice to exit the flow of consumerist culture and tend to the wealth of our inner life, and that begins by simply switching out mollifying substitution activities for holistic nourishment in each of the twelve dimensions. Once that is accomplished, we can begin to reshape the local and global marketplace into a more friendly, nurturing and supportive setting.

For instance, we could inspire a new relationship between consumers and providers of products and services; a caring, compassionate relationship based on mutual appreciation, affection and trust. We could reinitiate a sense of interdependence and connection, establishing lasting exchanges on other levels besides monetary so an authentic relationship can exist. For example, when I speak to someone at a company, I should be able to view their picture, know a little about their life, understand what position they have in the company and why they are working there. In essence, I should be able to meet them as a whole human being. Likewise, they should have some idea who I am, what I have purchased from their company, how I have interfaced with their company in the past, and the quality of those previous interactions. It should be the meeting of two human selves, not a selfishly insistent need interacting with a strict set of company policies, or a credit card number interacting with an automated point-of-sale system. Some companies have implemented publicly accessible employee blogs and online consumer forums, and perhaps this is a start down the right path. But it is not enough. There should be more points of interaction and understanding for genuine intimacy to exist, and all of the principles of high quality relationship (compassion, sovereignty, boundaries, etc.) must be present in some form for an integral marketplace to take root.

On the consumer end of things, clearly the more consciously we consume, with as broad an awareness as possible about how our consumption affects other arenas of affection, the more loving and responsible that consumption will be. There are two fronts to this approach. The first addresses effective self-nourishment: Does this act of consumption truly nourish me, or am I substituting for something else? This will become increasingly clear to us as we deepen our commitment to integral practice and experience its benefits firsthand. The other front concerns values. Does this consumption further my personal values or does it contradict them? Many different organizations, movements and fads have attempted to address this concern. Vegetarianism, organic food production, Voluntary Simplicity, targeted boycotts of disreputable companies or harmful products, class action lawsuits, consumer protection agencies, investigative reporting, the "going green" movement, Chambers of Commerce, regulatory agencies and so forth have all made their contribution to values alignment between producers and consumers. And of course the Internet provides access to much of the information both consumers and producers require to navigate a values-based relationship, but not in a way that is objectively organized or easy to search. For instance, if I web search "earth-friendly teddy bears made in the U.S.A.," I have no way of quickly or easily fact-checking the sites that come up.

To remedy this I would propose that a clearinghouse be established for both consumers and producers, so that every layer of production, distribution and sales can be scrutinized through existing avenues of data mining and reporting. Anyone should be able to search that clearinghouse based on customized criteria, with an easy-to-understand rating system for each set of values. The goal would be to quickly and easily answer questions like these:

- How much labor does this company outsource, and where is it outsourced to?

- Does this service provider support fair labor practices? What is there record in this regard? Am I paying for sweat shops, prison labor, illegal immigrants, workers from oppressed populations if I spend my money here?

- Does this manufacturer participate in environmentally responsible methods?

- What was the outcome of lawsuits against this company, and how many lawsuits or settlements have there been for the last three years?

- Is it a public or private company? Who owns a majority of shares, who are the members of its board of directors, and what are the personal values, goals and ethical profiles of those owners and board members?

- Are executives and managers held accountable for implementing values-driven business plans? Is exploration of personal values part of the hiring and managing process?

- Were animals used in product testing? Are products harmful to animals?

- Has this corporation ever participated in bribing public officials? In drafting legislation? In lobbying efforts?

- What is this manufacturer's overall record of reliability and cost of ownership for all its products?

- What level of customer satisfaction has been independently verified, and can it be sorted by demographic?

- How well are female employees compensated at this company compared to men? What about minority employees? Do they hire older employees? Have they ever forced out aging workers?

And so on. Perhaps there would also need to be some additional, independent fact checking of the data, but in my own research I have almost always found the information I needed already available...it just took a while; probably longer than most folks would ever wish to allot for making simple purchasing decisions. This process can and should be made simpler for everyone, to facilitate conscientious consumption and build into our commercial relationships something that all other relationships demand: transparency, honesty and accountability. The goal here, of course, is not to encourage conformance to the letter of the law or appearances of propriety – under the greed-centric model, corporations are already very good at playing that game. What this is about is changing corporate culture, its values orientation and the nature of exchanges in a capitalistic system. It is about empowering people to be able to express caring and kindness in their choices, something that is currently extremely difficult to do.

Perhaps most critically, repairing this situation will also require a potent reorientation of individual and collective identity. If we strongly identify as needy consumers – of ideas, of values, of stuff – then we will never view ourselves as contributors to society, nor will we generate much compassion for ourselves or anyone else. If I view myself as a producer, as a creator of ideas, values and useful products, then I can appreciate my contribution to the whole. And if I do not identify as a compassionate producer who cares about the well-being of everyone, then at every step of the production and consumption exchange my contribution to the whole will always be less important than the benefits I reap – from persuading workers to sacrifice their quality of life to persuading consumers to buy something they don't need. The ultimate goal, then, is really for all of us to become compassionate producers. Consumption should only be a byproduct of our efforts to achieve collective good, starting with being kind to ourselves. And so we come full circle to multidimensional nourishment. For if I can nurture my own well-being, I will be much more able to offer products and services that help others nurture themselves. The first step in healing a "passive consumption identity disorder" is cultivating active, conscious, integral self-nourishment that holds the good of All as its governing intention. And thus compassionate affection can retain the highest value in all exchanges, and a truly integral marketplace is born.

On some levels, all of these suggested reforms are really half-measures. Any system whose inherent structure permits profit to take precedence over people naturally interferes with compassionate affection. Obsessive concern over profits will always result in products and services that conform too readily to superficial wants or manufactured needs rather than authentic nourishment. Wherever material exchanges are prioritized above sound nourishment principles, supportive relationships and compassionate affection, business transactions will aim to placate fears, enlarge egos, satisfy self-centered impulses and forsake skillful nurturing in favor of immediate gratification. But if we can elevate compassionate relationship to the top of business priorities and drive free enterprise with the golden intention rather than greed, the incompatibility between true love and Western capitalism can be moderated. In fact, profit can then become an instrument of accountability, an indication that business is contributive rather than destructive. I believe most responsible business owners already know this.

There are many additional approaches that can accelerate the healing of an unloving economic system, and these are discussed at length by other writers, including those listed among the resources below. Whatever the stages of transformation will be, it is clearer now than at perhaps any other point in recent history that the linkages of compassionate affection to business practices must be rapidly and radically restored. Let us begin to act before we begin to forget.

> **Resources:**   For a helpful discussion of some of the underlying problems of the global marketplace and possible solutions, you might try *Alternatives to Economic Globalization* by the International Forum on Globalization. I also recommend researching the web regarding "corporate personhood" to understand the debate over that topic, as well as exploring *Defying Corporations, Defining Democracy* from POCLAD, which defines both the personhood challenge and some possible solutions. To shed light on the destructive machinations of corporate power, consider reading Noam Chomsky's *Profit over People: Neoliberalism & Global Order*, Naomi Klein's *The Shock Doctrine: The Rise of Disaster Capitalism*, Andrew Bacevich's *The Limits of Power*, and Greg Palast's *The Best Democracy Money Can Buy*. The poet David Whyte's efforts to reintroduce soulful compassion in the workplace might also be of interest. You could also search the web on "microfinance" to appreciate a more inclusive and compassionate approach to economic development, with some detailed and helpful resources at www.grameenfoundation.org. And of course E.F. Schumacher's *Small is Beautiful: Economics as if People Mattered* is a good read for anyone interested in this arena.

State & Nation

As citizens of the largest and most influential democracy on Earth, Americans have a unique opportunity – and therefore a more pronounced responsibility – to contribute to the well-being of millions around the globe. Caring for ourselves and our closest relationships, reinventing our communities, propagating constructive memes and reforming our economic system are all excellent first steps along the road to lasting positive change. Now we arrive at politics. Perhaps as never before, the U.S. political system is beleaguered by paralyzing and self-destructive trends. For decades our political leaders at all levels of government have run rough-shod over the supporting principles of a sound democracy. After systematically weakening the legal framework of our government, special interests now are free to write their own, self-serving legislation, then fund the campaigns of politicians who will vote that legislation into law. These politicians routinely compound such political favors to the point of illegality, but are rarely held accountable for their corruption. Political ideologies have become so polarized that opposing parties are now more preoccupied with demonizing, sabotaging and obstructing each other than with effectively running government. And the most cherished traditions and institutions of U.S. democracy – the Judiciary, the Constitution, the Congress, the Executive Branch, the election process – have increasingly been sidestepped, dismantled, diluted or distorted beyond recognition to serve the short-sighted power grabs of a political elite.

Although I myself am among those who are filled with relief, joy and hope to see such an intelligent and articulate person as Barack Obama gain our highest office, this new and promising administration remains the product and purveyor of a crippled political system. And although I share the optimism that much constructive change is in the offing, it is unrealistic to expect any individual or administration to entirely reverse decades of political entropy. In fact, such expectations would be yet another reflection of the disempowering externalization that permeates American culture; no leader should be expected to solve all the ills we ourselves have created, and created by trusting past leaders to solve all our ills for us at that. It is tremendously beneficial to our democracy that so many young people have been energized by the political process in the 2008 election, but it would be a devastating loss of much-needed involvement if those young people do not take on a mantle of constructive effort beyond electing and supporting their candidate.

Could an integral approach to politics help in some way? I think it can, and with a fairly straightforward approach: by translating the twelve dimensions of nourishment into the framework of a more interdependent political process, a more engaged electorate, and a more compassionately effective agenda. I will make an initial, brief and somewhat insubstantial sketch of this here – one that is admittedly concentric to my own experiences, interests and prejudices. Rather than detailed remedies, what I am most interested in here is exploring what components of the U.S. political landscape could be reshaped into more nourishing and transformative forces for good. I would encourage others with interest and expertise in the political arena to explore these questions and develop more specific models of integral politics.

First a note on some concepts and terms I use in the following descriptions. "Communally funded" means some combination of governmental funding, private funding that is incentivized by public policy, and individual donations and volunteerism. "Communally commissioned" indicates a process where entities or individuals compete for communal funding. "Communal involvement" means that citizen stakeholders are invited to contribute to a local, state or federal process, much the same way people are summoned for jury duty today, via appointment to citizen commissions or other temporary decision-making positions. The objective with all of these communalities is to engage people in what is happening in their own governance, creating opportunity for people to become producers and active citizens, rather than remain passive consumers. This is also a deliberate redistribution of power. There is still a role for government agencies, elected officials and private businesses, but now randomly selected citizens mitigate those power concentrations and the traditional quid pro quos. Another desired effect of this approach is that the additional expense incurred by the new mechanism of communal involvement is offset by a reduction in the size of government institutions, as well as the ever-hoped-for savings possible through increased fiduciary oversight.

Healthy Body. From the examples of Europe and Asia, and some of the more progressive ideas here in the U.S., it seems as though public policy could greatly encourage a healthier population through any of the following:

- Communal involvement in urban and interurban development and planning that is centered around walking and mass transit, with integrated living, working, recreating and business communities, rather than geographically segregating these functions and relying on automobiles to ferry people from one enclave to another.

- Shifting agricultural subsidies away from large corporations to smaller, more diverse and more local food production, with an emphasis on and incentives for organic methods, and some level of communal involvement (i.e. consumers reconnecting with food production).

- Aggressively legislating and enforcing environmental and consumer protections against industrial contamination of soil, water, air and all consumer products, while at the same time incentivizing environmentally friendly technologies.

- Reinvigorating noncompetitive fitness programs and providing diverse physical recreation facilities in public schools.

- Establishing a national healthcare program as a non-profit public service, where health outcomes are prioritized and incentivized among providers as more important than billable procedures. In addition, a rigorously integrative model could be used to treat the whole person, with an emphasis on preventative medicine. Primary care providers would serve smaller patient populations and develop more well-rounded relationships with patients. And, finally, all supplement and pharmaceutical advertisements and marketing would be banned from the general media.

- A cultural shift that integrates regular exercise into workplace environments.

Playful Heart. The arts are the lifeblood of any culture, and more than advocating additional menu items for consumption, all levels of government should take part in revitalizing community involvement in the arts. And by "the arts," I mean any form of creative self-expression. For example:

- Increasing curricula, communal involvement and communal funding for the arts in public education.

- A substantial increase in communally commissioned art for public spaces, to be owned by the public in perpetuity.

- The establishment of communal performance spaces, with communally funded productions of theatre, music and other performing arts made available to the general public at a greatly reduced cost.

- Increased communal funding for arts festivals, no-fee arts competitions, adult education for the arts, and so on.

- An increase in communally funded broadcast media and web content that provides non-commercial arts and arts educations programming, including locally produced, communally commissioned media from and for all age levels.

Supportive Community. In addition to the individual efforts encouraged through *Integral Lifework* practice, vital communities could be encouraged in many ways. For instance:

- In addition to the performance spaces just mentioned, we could revitalize urban community centers, libraries, and community colleges, relying primarily on communal funding and involvement.

- Incentives such as tax benefits, employment benefits and community recognition for people who remain in any location for more than five years, or who offer an extraordinary amount of their time and resources to community involvement.

- Instituting regular community celebrations which do not encourage material expectations or exchanges, but instead reinforce communal sharing, creativity, ceremony and unity. For example, a holiday where only gifts which have been hand made are exchanged, or a festival where people join together in song and dance, or a half hour each month where people everywhere pause in meditation or prayer.

Expanding Mind.   A rich educational experience at all levels seems central to this dimension, as a does access to ongoing resources that promote both learning and the open exchange of ideas.

- Reinvigoration of K-12 education. Enumerating the ideas and debates about how this can be accomplished is a topic for another time. However, there are a few clear and critical areas that must be addressed for nourishment to occur. For instance, both students and their parents must experience increased accountability for their investment in and commitment to education. This accountability cannot occur just through grades, scholarships or the promise of college, but must also include increased societal valuation of the educational process and outcomes. Learning for learning's sake must become important to our culture again, something that parents and students are proud of and passionate about – something that intrinsically matters. No educational system can successfully convey knowledge of history or the arts, critical thinking skills, practical job skills, or the foundations of math, science, language, literature or anything else if the surrounding culture doesn't value that process or the people providing it.

- Elimination of all barriers to higher education; if the desire is there, the doors should be open.

- Communal involvement in forums, think tanks and political discussions held in communal performance spaces and broadcast over communal media.

- Communally funded basic access for every American to the Internet, including no-cost, no-ads hosting of a personal web page.

Fulfilling Purpose.   This is really about providing opportunity and resources for people to clarify their life focus early on, as well as shift that focus later in life if they encounter a need to do so.

- Establishing a comprehensive, integral approach to aptitude and interests assessment early in life, with repeated examination of developing skill sets prior to young people entering college or starting a career.

- Communal resources and support for adults to reassess their career choices and begin a new direction when necessary for their well-being or the well-being of their community.

Authentic Spirit. Somehow we must encourage space in our culture for each individual's communication with their innermost Self and an abiding connection with the ground of being. To facilitate this, we might:

- Include basic, non-denominational meditation practices and surveys of mystical literature in age-appropriate curriculum in public schools.

- Encourage designated periods for prayer, meditation and mystic activation in the workplace.

- Promulgate standardized approaches to non-denominational mystic activation for the general public (which is clearly one of the chief goals of *Integral Lifework*).

Restorative History. In the broader societal context, it seems that integration of historical realities into the present sociopolitical landscape should be the purview of educational institutions, commemorative works of art in public spaces, regular retrospection in communally funded media, and communal remembrance of people who have contributed to our individual and collective well-being. In particular, including equal time for both the less attractive aspects of U.S. history and the most heroic seems appropriate, as it creates opportunity for both collective celebration and collective healing.

Pleasurable Legacy. This is the reason for society's existence and the inherent purpose of this arena of affection. What clearer charter could we have than "life, liberty and the pursuit of happiness?" The question merely becomes how best to facilitate this vision.

Flexible Processing Space. In many ways, political orientations reflect the dominance of different processing spaces among values subcultures. For example, folks from one political affiliation might lean more toward mental spacetime, and folks from another toward emotional spacetime. At the city, county, state and national levels, therefore, this nourishment dimension could be translated into providing equal footing for all political perspectives, and increasing the opportunity for political groups to exchange ideas and synthesize solutions that integrate the full political spectrum.

- Establishing a communally funded non-governmental organization dedicated to triangulating common ground among different political affiliations, translating partisan rhetoric into constructive dialogue, clarifying party positions in values-neutral language, educating the public about the political process and party histories, fact-checking the data supporting various positions and popular initiatives, informing the pubic about how to engage in the political process, and so forth.

- Engineering representation of parties outside of the current two-party system in the Presidency and Congress, through reforms in primary systems, campaign funding, redistricting, etc. – for example, instituting a direct popular voting process for all elections, abolishing the electoral college, and creating redistricting process immune to party politics.

- Increase the accountability and transparency of the judiciary. I have only some vague ideas about how either might be accomplished, but it seems that term limits, limited communal campaign financing, full public disclosure and interpretation of past rulings, and independent oversight with disciplinary purview would be a good start.

- All political advertising (for initiatives, candidates, judges, whatever) could be strictly formatted to allow equal time for all viewpoints, with rigorous fact-checking of all claims on both side presented immediately following each ad.

Empowered Self-Concept. This is the fertile ground where cultural memes intersect with therapeutic relationships. A communalistic approach to self-governance will, I believe, help elevate self-worth through its liberation from consumerist complacency and externalized fulfillment. Such an approach intends to emphasize the quality of sovereignty and self-reliance intrinsic to authentic love. However, the creation of authentically caring citizens begins with individuals healing themselves. Which means the resources for such healing must be widely available and easily accessible. From my admittedly biased perspective, some form of integral therapy and education similar to *Integral Lifework* should become the gold standard around which all integrative counseling is constructed, as well as a model for primary triage and preventative care, which is then made available to everyone as part of the national healthcare system. Integral concepts and practices could also be introduced through communally funded wellness education programs, as well as through public K-12 education curricula. Imagine if young people understood how to holistically and compassionately nourish themselves at an early age? How many substitution and depletion behaviors (acting out, suicide, teen pregnancy, drug use, dietary issues, etc.) could be averted if our youth and their parents empowered themselves with multidimensional nourishment?

Satisfying Sexuality. Here we can advocate for social policies that promote understanding and education about human sexuality and sexual orientation. This education should aim to disentangle the confusion over sexual identity, romantic involvement and authentic intimacy. It should effectively free people to be who they naturally are without guilt, angst, shame or ignorance, while at the same time discouraging the use of sex as substitution nourishment.

Affirming Integrity. At a governmental level, this dimension could be about expanding the independence and influence of watchdog mechanisms within society.

- The press is not free if it is dependent on corporate sponsorship, so advocating independent news sources produced through communal funding and involvement seems prudent.

- Watchdog departments in all branches of government should be given more influence than purely advisory roles – they should, in fact, directly inform policy development.

- All political campaign financing could be limited to equal portions of communal funding for all registered candidates, as well as for each pro and con position on each ballot initiative.

- It seems reasonable that voters have the right to vote incumbents at any level of government out of office, even if there is no competing or preferred candidate. Over time, I believe this one measure alone could create a more vital and engaged democracy.

- Once government can establish its independence from corporate influence, careful torte reform could limit frivolous lawsuits and discipline attorneys who instigate them. As of this writing, however, the threat of hefty punitive damages are one of very few regulating mechanisms that have successfully reigned in irresponsible corporate business practices.

Most of these ideas are not new, but they do seem to fit neatly into the nourishing landscape of the political arena of affection. These proposals offer a taste of the efforts required to align a state or nation with the balanced nurturing of *Integral Lifework*. At its root, compassionate affection is most relevant at the individual level, and effective proliferation into wider arenas of affection is dependent on the integral practice of a critical mass of individuals. Public policy cannot supplant individual sentiments and behaviors, but it can nudge them in a more positive, self-nourishing direction. Regardless, though, I would welcome critiques, suggestions or insights into the broader development of these nourishment centers within a sociopolitical context, and I look forward to what others can contribute.

Resources: For information on education reform, check out www.edutopia.org. To explore the foundations of an effective community, check out Peter Block's *Community: The Structure of Belonging.* For interesting discussions of alternative voting systems, stop by www.fairvote.org. To explore healthcare reform, try a web search on "international healthcare models."

Planet Earth

Our planet has sustained life for millions of years and provided for the exponential expansion of our species and others with awe-inspiring results. How these results occurred is, I think, less important than recognizing and appreciating the miracle of life itself. The mere existence of complex, interdependent flora and fauna should be enough to inspire profound and undying affection for the Earth. Is there a benevolent guiding force behind it? Is Nature truly an interconnected, self-regulating, counterpoised system? Or do islands of life represent arbitrary successes amid equally arbitrary cataclysmic extremes? Although such questions are intriguing in a scientific sense, they can distract from the fundamental debt of gratitude we owe this planet for our being. Because the Earth is, we are. That alone is enough reason for us to respect, admire and cherish our oasis amid unfriendly space. I will offer some additional justification for our affection, but as with all other arenas the question remains as to how best to express it. Is it enough just to conserve natural resources? Do a little recycling now and again? Give money to organizations that promote environmental protection? Lobby Congress to list a few more endangered species? Buy some organic produce? What does it really mean for our heart of hearts to love the Earth, and how does that translate into action?

The cycles of the natural world have supported humanity for millennia, but they also interfere with our priorities. As much as we often thanklessly rely on those cycles, we are quick to resent instances when Nature thwarts our desires. The sudden storm that delays our trip. The unwelcome weeds that flourish in our gardens and lawns. The wild predators who steal our livestock and sometimes dare to attack humans. The poisonous creatures who threaten the safety of our children. The mice and rats who invade our homes to capitalize on crumbs fallen from the table. The insects that likewise won't respect the boundaries of our domicile. The birds and bees that inconsiderately anoint our freshly washed vehicles with hard-to-clean spatter. In a part of San Diego close to where I live, a battle is being waged over a small crescent of beach where seals like to sun themselves and birth their young. Some of the residents here feel their children should be allowed safe access to that stretch of sand, while others wish to protect the safety of the seals. The Navy has likewise been defending its right to conduct ultra-low frequency communications tests, despite the fact that these have consistently disoriented and injured marine life off the San Diego coast. In all of these instances, the natural world just gets in the way of human habitation, and consequently must either be subdued or destroyed.

So for many people, Nature isn't something that inspires or nourishes, it is instead an irritation, something unpleasant to be managed or, if it becomes too threatening and cumbersome, annihilated altogether. And with an increasing amount of the human population concentrated in urban areas, where rivers have been paved over, trees grow in rows and all food comes in sterile, neatly packaged containers, the opportunity to develop affection for Nature is almost nonexistent. I feel quite lucky to have spent my childhood freely exploring the woods of New England and the unpopulated beaches of Oregon. There was always evidence of humanity to be found – a rusting pitchfork, the collapsing foundations of an ancient farmhouse, huge driftwood logs from a timber harvest, a crumpled beer can, an abandoned shoe – but it was subordinated to a backdrop thriving wilderness. Since both of my parents loved the outdoors, I also experienced the most rugged and inaccessible of natural landscapes when I was young. My father took me canoeing over rugged rapids (and even the occasional waterfall). My mom liked to walk old logging roads and explore abandoned houses deep off the beaten path. I was encouraged to ski, camp and even attend an Outward Bound style summer program where twelve kids spent two weeks hiking the White and Green mountains without any contact with civilization. So I had an advantage over many city dwellers in this respect, and this early exposure to the wonders of Nature helped shape my worldview.

But even if we didn't experience this wonder growing up, it is never too late to fall in love with planet Earth. Spending a few weeks camping in America's National Parks and Monuments will soften even the most hardened heart. To see the sun set over endless snowy peaks in the North Cascades. To watch wolves playfully cavort in the sprawling meadows of Yellowstone. To breathe in the vastness of the Grand Canyon or the towering beauty of Zion. To awaken in the silent intensity of Yosemite's alpine lakes. To lose all sense of time and space in the rolling stillness of White Sands. There is no end to the wonder awaiting those who explore our national treasures, and thanks to the insightful effort of previous generations, that path is available to anyone almost anywhere in the U.S. It's really just a choice to take a risk and immerse ourselves in the wild. Even though I live in a huge city, I am less than an hour from relatively untouched wilderness, and regularly make my pilgrimage to that sacred alter. When I don't make the time to hike in the wild, I will at least spend some time watching the waves come in at the beach or breathe in the trees and grass of a nearby park. And if I am too exhausted to even make those short treks, I will play half hour of the BBC's *Planet Earth* series or peruse a National Geographic magazine, or send gratitude out my bedroom window to the glowing moon, or listen to the birds call to each other as they fly over my home. In some regular way, I choose to remind myself of the bigger picture, of the natural forces that sustain me, of the gifts of beauty, exhilaration and awe that the Earth continually offers. Through this choice I gain both the perspective and the renewal my being craves, and any lingering resistance to the potential inconveniences of Nature sloughs away.

In terms of integral practice, the opportunities for integration with Nature are plentiful. I can meditate in Nature, I can exercise my body there, I can rejuvenate my heart by witnessing her wonders, I can worship without expectations, constraints or self-consciousness within her embrace. Along these lines, I think it is paramount that we honor the cycles of Nature in some way. That we recognize, appreciate and offer gratitude for day's waning into night, for Spring's arrival and Summer's departure, for the lovely and awe-inspiring phases of the moon, for the ebb and flow of tides and a cool, dense fog acquiescing to bright, warm skies of deepest blue. And if I want to share this beauty in a social exchange, or volunteer to give back to my community, or support my conviction that at least some wilderness should remain untamed by human habitation, there are all kinds of levels of community integration available to me through government and nonprofit organizations. And so expressing the love I feel for the wild becomes an easy consequence of immersing myself in exchanges with Nature. Of course I will work to protect endangered species and what remains of their pristine habitats, just as I promote the well-being of any loved ones in my life. To love is to act in beneficial ways for the object of that love; from this foundational intention, all we require is appropriate attention to what is occurring within and around us, and a modicum of self-discipline to follow through on what we know is good and right.

Now...what happens when the objects of our affection force us to choose between them – when they seem to compete for the same resources? For instance, if my affection for my country demands I support a strong military, should I side with the Navy, or with the whales and dolphins? What if I am likewise concerned about the safety of my family or my own livelihood when wolves and cougars are reintroduced into the mountains near my home? What if drilling for oil in a national wildlife refuge could relieve some of the financial burden on millions of Americans struggling to make ends meet? Are national security, job security or personal safety more important than protecting the Earth from humanity's destructive influence?

For me, the answer is obvious. The technological progress of humanity over the centuries has devastated natural environments to the point where the exploitation, depletion and pollution of the planet has endangered humanity itself. We are by any measure a weaker, poorer and less healthy species because we have, on the whole, disrespected Nature and abandoned harmony with natural systems. Historically, there have been very few examples of positive results from human reengineering of Nature. Whenever we harness, subdue or interfere with the Earth's natural cycles and bounty on a large scale, we tend to inadvertently harm ourselves, mainly because the unforeseen consequences of these efforts are disproportionately severe. For example, how could we have anticipated that fertilizing crops far inland with nitrogen would lead to huge die-offs of marine life in the Gulf of Mexico? Or that farming cattle, burning fossil fuels and cutting down forest would contribute to global warming? Or that trying to manage our bodies with chemistry (birth control, diet pills, sleeping aids, pseudofoods, energy boosters, anti-depressants, etc.) would lead to more serious health problems than those we were initially trying to address? And so on in a plethora of instances where we have sought to live outside of Nature's laws rather than within them. So if I truly love humanity – my family, my country, myself – I will not let humanity continue along the path of decimating Nature unchallenged. With every choice to race forward along a course that destroys what cannot be replaced or reengineer what Nature already provides, I am compelled to ask one simple question: is there another way?

Inevitably, there are always other ways to reconcile what we perceive to be competing needs. But it requires a commitment to effort, patience and discernment. Just as in any relationship, we cannot always demand everything we want along the timeline that we want it. High quality outcomes that benefit the good of All tend to demand greater time, energy and resources than we might initially anticipate. Despite what some pundits and politicians would have us believe, there are no free, quick or easy fixes. We cannot consume or produce our way out of global warming, health problems, caustic pollution or vanishing natural resources. There is always a cost, and so there must also be a willingness to transparently enumerate that cost and distribute it in reasonable and equitable ways. If we choose not to accept the impact of humanity's burgeoning population on the planet, and make the difficult choices those consequences demand of us, we will suffer. Yet if we can shift our governing intentionality from self-centered acquisitiveness to compassionate and inclusive love-consciousness, we will more easily be able accept the sacrifice necessary for mutually beneficial outcomes, even if that sacrifice is high.

As always, our alternative to love is to harden our hearts still further. Some people think nothing of cutting down a tree that blocks their satellite dish, or poisoning their own drinking water with pesticides, or dumping excessive amounts of that increasingly precious water on ornamental lawns, or shooting animals for sport instead of for food, or any number of other wasteful behaviors that generate a short term advantage for themselves while disrespecting Nature. But they learned this behavior from others who assured them they were morally acceptable activities, parents and friends and communities who insisted there would be no negative consequences. They learned how to silence their love for Earth, this sacred home that has shepherded life since its beginning, this miracle from whom we have derived nearly all of our most valued comforts, pleasures and treasures. And although to me this seems the harshest form of blasphemy against the heart of life itself, those sentiments and behaviors can be unlearned. Just as a child from an abusive home can heal, thrive and grow to become a compassionate and caring person, those who have been taught to abuse the Earth can learn to fall in love with her once more.

Shepherdess of Souls

Sun-warmed rock to sweat my thirst
  moonlit stream to quench it
    womb of every life we know
    Shepherdess of souls
      where do you lead us?
I follow with contented warmth
  safe within your gifts
  eager for lush promises
    unaware of who I am
What would you
  of this miraculous dust?
What hopes weigh your heart
  when we claim your summits
    or furrow your sweet valleys?
The scent of fall brings memories
  close to darkness
    kindling brighter fires
      intimate with nothingness
      summoning our passions
Warm rock, cold stream
  cradled, perfect balance
Light and dark
  thirst and satiation
  endings and beginnings
You will always be the center
  of everything we are
    and everything that we become

The consequences of renewing our passionate affection are self-evident. When we learn of attitudes or behaviors that have negative impacts on the Earth, we work tirelessly to change them – first in ourselves, and then in our community, our nation and so on. In my own journey, I have come to a conclusion that until humanity learns how to live nondestructively and in harmony with the Earth's natural systems, human population must of necessity decrease rather than increase. Although consumerist attitudes and capitalist enterprise are the main mechanisms of reckless annihilation, the critical mass amplifying those mechanisms to truly unsustainable proportions is a human population that grows exponentially. In 2008, our global population approached 6.78 billion. In 1964, the year I was born, global population was less than half that figure. In the centuries before year 1800, not even one billion people had ever lived on the planet at any one time. And yet, with the exception of compulsory and authoritarian attempts at population control in parts of Asia, we just keep reproducing and devouring natural resources without a second thought.

In all likelihood, the results of our overzealous misuse of the Earth will eventually begin to regulate population whether we choose to do so willingly or not. Increased desertification, proliferation of tropical diseases, depletion of easily accessible potable water and other basic resources, mass migrations in response to rising sea levels, and the inevitable social unrest that accompanies all such events will naturally attenuate humanity's global presence. And yet, if enough people fall in love with this planet both deeply and quickly, we can soften the impact of our past missteps. For a little while longer, the decision to live in a conscious and loving relationship with the Earth will create a gracious blessing for future generations. Within the next few decades, however, that freedom to decide our own future as a species may be taken away from us, if we do not act with wisdom and love.

| Resources: | An inspiring vision for an Earth-friendly humanity can be found in Thomas Friedman's *Hot, Flat and Crowded*. You might also try web searches on "low impact living" or "sustainable lifestyles." A search on "zero population growth" will also provide ample information and resources about the ZPG movement.

Beyond the Earth

There are of course other realms beyond the Earth, and I believe that as our identity expands to include those realms we will understand the most appropriate and loving actions to take within them. For example, as mentioned previously, affection for the Moon, her gracious impact on Earth's thriving ecosystems, and the echoes of that influence in human biorhythms seems an understandable extension of a celebratory joy in life itself. The Sun, the other planets of our solar system, the Milky Way, the dark matter of space…all of these ultimately have a place in our sense of being. As we come to know our innermost Self through spiritual practice, we will come in contact with the essence of the Universe. Our own soul and the ground of being are, after all, mirrors of each other; one essence is the seed, and the other is the tree. Our inner Light is a fragment of the Absolute, and our consciousness is part of a vast continuum of Mind. This is evokes the mystical aspects of integral practice, to be sure, but is nonetheless a natural unfolding of holistic self-care. Beyond such basic observations, however, this is an expansive subject for another time.

Assessing Outcomes

The metrics for success across all arenas of affection are essentially the same. Is there thriving? Is there wholeness? Is there health and well-being? Is there healing and equanimity? Is there a sense of unified purpose? Is there liberation from fear? Is there happiness? Are barriers transformed into nourishment? Is there a deep, abiding affection grounded in effectual compassion? Is there empowerment of the soul? Is there a felt connection with the ground of being? Is there illumination of the mind and perpetual gratitude in the heart? Is there acceptance and integration? Is there joy? Is there love? If all of these qualities are present, then that seems like a good beginning. If any of these qualities are absent, then we must discover what nourishment dimensions are underserved, gently engage whatever barriers we encounter, and lavishly nurture those dimensions in a targeted and loving way.

FALLING OUT OF LOVE

Crumbled and scattered
  my shattered spirit
    smolders fragrant in the dark

Grief blocks the sun
  burning my lungs with smoke
    stinging eyes and throat and hope

How can my heart fly again
  weighed down with this?

How can I lift my hands
  or take a step
    adrift in a pointless void
      where love is lost?

I stare without seeing
No sound consoles me
Something pulses through my veins
  a residue of wonder
    echoes of a vital essence
      spilled too greedily
      into fleeting vessels

No one understands
  not even my own flesh
    which breathes and sweats and heals
      chagrining my will to abandon it

I am afraid of what this means
I am afraid
  of Light's return

revealing what I have become:
a clod of scorched earth
a remnant of fertile ground
where bittersweet fruits
unwelcomely take root

If love is the greatest power known to us, binding the Universe itself together, how can it fail? It can't. The felt experience of love may vary from moment to moment, but love as a free-flowing, all-pervasive force remains a reliable constant; it is we who sometimes fall out of that flow. We are the ones who fail, and the grief that we feel when loving relationships end is the grief over a real and palpable death. Not the death of love, but the death of our own relevance in the Universe. For to falter in our most cherished relationships is to falter in our most fundamental purpose: to receive and transmit authentic and compassionate affection; to become an empathic antenna that participates actively in the unifying frequency of all matter. There may be other factors that contribute to our devastation and despair – perhaps we were too closely enmeshed with someone for either party's good, perhaps we were overly dependent on them for our own sense of well-being, and so on – but deep down our spirit knows that love really is the only reason for existence.

At the same time, however, in our grief and pain we may lose sight of a crucial truth: that the choice to reenter the flow of love is always available to us, no matter how far we have fallen. Yes, we will require time to heal. Yes, we may have newly formed barriers to nourishment we need to overcome. Yes, it will require commitment and effort to gather all those shattered fragments of self back together and step bravely forward into a new receptivity and vulnerability. But no matter what scars and shrapnel we carry in the worldly temple of our heart, mind and body, our soul remains intact and unperturbed, eager to engage in the dance of life if only we will allow it. What prevents us from healing? What arrests us in our grief so that we can't recover? What inhibits us from seeking help to find our way? In Part IV we explored the many barriers to self-nourishment, and any of those could be the culprit. But in the years I have accompanied individuals and couples through the healing process, one impulse stands out as the most prevalent in preventing our reemergence into love, and that is willfulness.

The road to our failure to reenter love is paved with stubborn resistance. Instead of forgiving ourselves and others, we stoke the fires of our anger and resentment. Instead of letting go of the past, we hold onto it, desperate to justify our identity as a victim of fate, or of human weakness, or of the callousness of people who have hurt us. In other words, we passionately refuse to take responsibility for our own well-being, and reject compassion for our own brokenness with equal fervor. And of course there is no guarantee, should we refresh our heart and seek to rejoin the flow of love, that we will not fail again or even many times over. There is no doubt that the spirit of love awaits us with open arms, but our circumstances, our patterns of thought and volition, and perhaps even deeper, more karmic barriers may continue to test our resolve. The will to love is akin to the will to live; it demands all courage and persistence with joys, hopes and victories that are both fierce and fleeting. For it seems that the very moment we grasp at love, the instant we remand its gifts to the prison of our rigid expectations, is the moment we lose everything. So the process of regaining love is much the same as the privilege of its keeping – in both we are forever letting go, until true love remains love's all-encompassing object.

Aside from an acute and devastating loss of love, there are others conditions where love seems absent, where the felt experience of compassionate affection distinctly ebbs. What is happening here? Once we gain the will to live and love, why would it seem to dissipate or attenuate? Our being is an organic thing, and like all organic things it requires care and feeding to survive. Supporting the conditions for love to thrive include nourishing ourselves holistically and overcoming barriers to wholeness, and often this is all we need to create the space and energy for love to fill each moment. You could even say that practicing *Integral Lifework* is intended as a guaranteed recipe for creating the perfect conditions for authentic love to fill us up. And once we acknowledge love's presence and power, it begins to sustain itself, organizing our existence to fulfill all of the necessary prerequisites like a gardener cultivating a plot of land. For anyone who has experienced this critical mass effect, it may seem incongruent to imagine how love could then drift out of our consciousness. But no matter how diligent or willing we are – and no matter how carefully we avoid the traps of willfulness or expectations set in stone – a discontinuation of the felt experience of love can still happen, and most likely *will* happen at some point. Why? It is my belief that each apparent absence or failure has an important lesson in store for us, if we open ourselves to the teaching. So that is what we will cover next.

Cloudy Days and Long, Dark Nights

Throughout our journey, there will be both occasional cloudy days, and lengthy occlusions of the sun of life. Sometimes we will merely be puzzled at the absence, and sometimes our confidence may erode entirely until cloying darkness and doubt challenge us to the core of our being. Some of these we might recognize as simply feeling blue – a melancholia that we know from experience will pass relatively swiftly. Perhaps these are caused by the weather, by shifts in our biology or by something we consumed, but as sad as we might feel, we trust that the clouds will eventually clear. These little hiccups in our well-being really remind us of how wonderful life can be. Like the first unfettered breath after a bad head cold, when we emerge from the shadow of a minor depression we appreciate our health and well-being anew. They are, in fact, helpful reminders to slow down, rest a bit, take stock of things and provide ourselves some added patience, forbearance and support.

For me, these cloudy days manifest as a steady increase in irritability and pessimistic thoughts. As soon as I sense myself "going negative" about things, I know my inner world has become overcast. And, once I recognize what is happening, if I don't take the opportunity to disengage from my busy schedule and give more attention to that inner world, I will get worse. I might sabotage some project I am working on, or add some turbulence to my relationships, or otherwise kick the anthill until those little critters are swarming all over the place and biting at my feet. If I keep putting off that necessary introspection and self-care, I may even become physically ill. In one way or another, I must slow down or take a break from highly energized productivity. And of course I have witnessed this same pattern in others; perhaps you have seen it in your own life. So what do you think is going on here?

As organic beings, we have organic cycles. Like the changing tides, or the phases of the moon, or advancing seasons, or the rising and setting of the sun, we have internal rhythms that govern our existence – perhaps much more powerfully than we would like to admit. This is true for women and men, children and elders, the sick and the healthy, those who are well-nourished and those who are not. It is an inescapable part of who we are. And as such, we need to honor the rhythms within. A great example of this is sleep. Our bodies might crave a nap in the middle of the day, and instead we push ourselves through the drowsiness. Instead of going to bed when we are tired, we might force our eyes open to watch TV, read or interact with friends. And we might fortify ourselves against the tide of our natural sleep cycles with caffeine, exciting entertainment or force of will. Like our need for sleep, our need for rest, introspection and variation in routine are just as often sidelined for the main attraction: that-all-important-super-urgent to-do-list, that obsession with mental spacetime. So when the signs that we need a break arrive – those dark clouds of sadness, negative feelings, crankiness, physical illness and so on – we must heed them in order to remain whole.

The Long Dark Night

There are other types of darkness that are considerably more severe than occasional cloudy days. Not only do they persist for longer periods, but they are much more disruptive and acutely felt. Among these are the long dark night of the soul. Although this can occur more than once in a lifetime, the long dark night is less cyclical in nature because it is induced by the arrival at specific spiritual horizons. Its characteristics may change slightly from person to person, but there seem to be more common experiences than not. Here are some of those:

- A seemingly uncorrectable interruption to one or more self-nourishment routines that have served us well in the past.

- A recurring experience of isolation, disconnection and even alienation from other people and our own sense of self.

- Unexpected feelings of loss, abandonment and grief.

- Moods that range from angst to anger to deep sadness, with joy and contentment somehow less accessible than they've been in the past.

- Confusion about priorities and goals, combined with a vague listlessness that saps our energy and motivation.

- Self-doubt, undermined self-confidence and an increasingly keen questioning of our own purpose, identity or habitual modes of operation.

- A sense that we have misplaced something, are missing some vital clue to our well-being, or are otherwise out-of-step with the flow of life around us.

- A loss of contact or connection with what we have associated with the bedrock of our spiritual nourishment – a separation from the ground of being, the Divine, the Absolute, the True Essence of things, and so on.

- A resurgence of desires to indulge in substitution nourishment or otherwise overemphasize one aspect of our being over another, mainly in order to fill the void that has abruptly intruded on our lives.

The first time this happens we might assume we are severely depressed, have contracted some sort of illness that is dampening our normal function, or perhaps are working through some kind of karmic disruption to our well-being. And although all of these may also be true, they are not the root cause of this particular condition. Instead, what we are experiencing is a new phase of personal growth, a phase that begins with separation and individuation from modes of being upon which we have previously relied. A metamorphosis that requires we be nudged out of our nest of comfortable habits and identity.

What initiates this process? I think if varies. Perhaps we have become too dependent on external structures we have created to support our wellness, and some part of us knows it is time to rock the boat or mix things up a bit. Perhaps our nourishment centers become inured to the type of exchanges we have cultivated over time, the same way our body can suddenly reject (through allergy, illness, severe immune responses, etc.) some food we have eaten all our lives. Perhaps the long dark night is a natural process of spiritual individuation that occurs for all conscious beings, encouraging a new level self-sufficiency in our spiritual connections. Perhaps we begin resonating with a different frequency in love's continuum, or nestle into some new pattern of consciousness, or cross the threshold to a new stratum of moral development and a concurrent expansion of our arena of affection. Whatever the impetus, all of our habits must be reformed to integrate with the change in resonance, and the resultant disorientation forces us to find new avenues of energy exchange – often in multiple dimensions at once. No matter how advance and balanced our integral practice, we must begin again, assembling new combinations of self-nourishment that are tuned to a new mode of being.

Of course we always have a choice. We can continue to suffer through our long dark night without attempting to change our dependencies or advance our compassion. We might even initiate some creative substitutions to regain our equilibrium. But, as a result, that darkness is likely to become more and more debilitating as our nourishment centers continue to stagnate. And no matter how stubbornly we try to reinvigorate what has worked for us in the past, we simply can't go back. Transformative practices have the tendency to do that. We may plateau at some phase of our journey for a time – perhaps even years – but new challenges and new awakenings are inevitable. So, just as those blue feelings on cloudy days signal an opportunity for rest and reflection, a long dark night is a signal become more vigorously awake, to step up to the plate and keep our eye on the ball. We are starting a new game and it's time to bone up on a few new skills and strategies; to boldly go where we haven't gone before.

Differentiating Healthy Darkness from Dangerous Depression

As with any condition, if the darkness we are experiencing is so debilitating that it is threatening our very existence, it's time to seek help. There is no point in rationalizing grave depressive cycles as crucibles for spiritual rebirth if they are destroying the vessel of our spirit. There was a time in my life when suicide seemed like a logical exit strategy away from pain and despair, but that was before I had written any books on mysticism, taught any classes about Integral Lifework, or grown much as a human being. The fact that I had not accomplished much of value (at least in my own depressive estimation) did little to counterbalance my personal woes, but a small voice within me pointed out that if I terminated this grand experiment prematurely, I would never know what my true potential was. So I decided to delay my own demise and immediately seek the support of a good therapist.

Depression is a crippling malady. It not only robs us of joy and passion, but impedes us from finding our way out of a downward spiral. But this unhealthy darkness is different from cloudy days and long dark nights of the soul, mainly because it has a different cause. Rather than a temporary interruption in self-nourishment, a full-blown depressive episode is the result of intense and acute nourishment depletion and seemingly impassible barriers to self-care. It is the consequence of one or more dimensions of self throwing in the towel – giving up on their contribution to our well-being and any hope of renewed nourishment. Essential parts of us are so injured and starving that death may really seem like a reasonable alternative.

So a helpful measurement of our depression's severity is its impact on all of our dimensions of well-being. If we are having difficulty with self-care in most of the twelve nourishment centers, we are experiencing something different than a gentle reminder to replenish our energy or a spiritual prodding to become more self-sufficient. These conditions may also be present, but they have been subordinated by a threat to our basic survival. Some part of us has become so broken that we cannot face it alone. And despite how we might feel about life and our own worthiness to become well, there is nothing to lose – and everything to gain – by seeking professional support in our time of crisis.

Enemies of Love

Perhaps the greatest enemy to love is indifference. Not caring seems to be more destructive that hate, fear, resentment or a whole host of other negative emotions, because at least these other reactions acknowledge some inherent value in their object and invoke energy around it. Even if someone harbors a murderous impulse against someone else, they still care about the conditions of that person's existence; they may desire to make those conditions worse, but a mechanism of valuation is still present. Indifference, on the other hand, erases value altogether, and eliminates the potential for any and all energy exchange. The condition of someone's existence becomes irrelevant. So if I pass a homeless person who is begging for money and feel resentment at their intrusion on my day, at least I recognize the potential for some sort of relationship between us; they can still have an impact on my life. But if I don't perceive that homeless person, if I walk by without recognizing their humanity on any level, then I deny all potential for connection. So, in a way, things like resentment, fear and even hate are distant echoes of love's possibility. An energy exchange is still taking place. But when indifference takes root, there is no longer any possibility for love.

Most other enemies of love are the children of indifference. Callous disregard for our own well being or the well being of others, for example. Or treating our body like a material object or mechanical device. Or conditioning our lives into a series of empty and meaningless habits. Or tuning out all emotional content in communication with others. Or indulging every whim without considering our responsibilities or the consequences of our actions. Or disconnecting entirely from our own emotional awareness. Or trivializing some dimension of self-care because we don't believe it is important. Or avoiding situations that require courage, effort, discipline or growth. All of these are indications of an underlying disability in the heart's empathic and compassionate function, and without that function a wide array of self-sustaining nourishment will be impeded. This is one reason why, when a person's heart becomes dead to the world around them, any strong emotion can be a welcome awakening.

Compared to indifference, other enemies of love are just junior demons trying to cut their teeth on our spirit. Doubt and disbelief, a crisis of self-confidence, deceptive manipulation, legalistic inflexibility, belittling dismissiveness, brutal abuse...all of these interfere with love, but they do not negate it. Energy is still being exchanged, even though it isn't positive or supportive. It is when we stop feeling and caring altogether that we can completely lose our bearings and forget how to rekindle love. This is one reason I believe antidepressants and anti-anxiety drugs should only be used for extreme interventions and for relatively short periods – just long enough to establish a few healthier coping mechanisms. I have seen firsthand the long term impact of such drugs, and it is heartbreaking. Slowly but surely, indifference about more and more of life's blessings and trials seeps into a person's bones when they rely on pharmaceuticals – or any external coping mechanism – to medicate away their deeply felt experience. And with that indifference comes disconnection, disaffection and, ultimately, a subtle alienation from their innermost Self and everyone around them. Feeling deeply, even if those feelings aren't always pleasant, is a critical companion to true love's journey.

Certainly there are exceptions to this approach. Someone suffering from bipolar disorder, severe chronic depression, suicidal impulses or paranoid delusions requires medication as part of their treatment. But it is impossible to imagine that the huge number of people currently prescribed mood enhancing drugs all have severe or debilitating psychological disorders. This trend is, I think, another symptom of a society conditioned to rely on externals for its well-being. And that orientation, as we have already explored at length, acts like a tall, thick wall that distances us from the bountiful love within.

PART VI

AN INTEGRAL LIFE

INTEGRAL LIFEWORK PLANS

What is the goal of integral practice? To nourish us in every dimension we have already identified, surely, but even more than that, to combine different nurturing disciplines into streamlined, self-reinforcing habits. These habits, in turn, introduce new kinds of energy exchange. That is, they create intentional nourishment efficiencies while strengthening our being in ways we could never have anticipated. Because of natural interactions between different parts of self, this principle has likely been demonstrated in our lives already. Perhaps physical exercise has made us feel better emotionally, or meditation has freed us of unhealthy habits, or regular laughter has sped our physical healing. The connection between mind and body has been appreciated for some time. *Integral Lifework* simply expands the definition of known interdependencies to include every aspect of our being – mind, body, heart, spirit and soul – and then adds interactions with our surrounding environment as a mechanism of exchange for all dimensions. That is, everything is interconnected within and without, and every relationship reflects every other. Because of this amazing design, nourishment can happen on many levels at once.

Now add to this the power of consciousness, which can either enhance natural energy exchanges or interfere with them. Our consciousness can lead us into a pit of despair and depletion, or up to soaring heights of self-transformation. So an *Integral Lifework Plan* is about consciously initiating harmony, transcending barriers to full-spectrum nourishment, and evolving ourselves into new stages of being. And all of this – the whole package of healing and transformative practice – is governed by a love-consciousness that inspires even as it sustains. In this way, integral disciplines honor and cultivate that single, most profoundly holistic force in the Universe; actuating an *Integral Lifework Plan* invites a perpetual commitment to true love.

How then do we effectively create integral practice that nourishes us according to our individual needs? Everyone brings different strengths, skills and insights to the table, so developing an *Integral Lifework Plan* is a unique process for each person. However, the goals of each and every plan are universal, and can be pared down to a straightforward outline:

1) **Envisioning Outcomes & Intermediate Goals**
    a) What are the end results we imagine for ourselves in various areas?
    b) What are the benefits of those outcomes?
    c) What are some milestones we can use to mark our progress?
    d) How do any of these accomplishments relate to our core values?
    e) In what priority or order do we wish to approach each goal?

2) **Assessing Nourishment**
    a) Developing awareness about current nourishment levels in twelve essential dimensions.
    b) Identifying depletions, substitutions and distortions of nourishment.
    c) Exploring the nature of persistent barriers to nourishment.

3) **Learning New Nourishment Skills for Depleted Dimensions**
    a) Applying targeted integral practice to address depleted dimensions and specific barriers.
    b) Emphasizing practices well-suited to our innate talents, current skills and interests.
    c) Harnessing well-nourished dimensions to replenish undernourished ones.
    d) Expanding our wholeness through cross-pollination of nourishment dimensions.

4) **Cultivating Loving Intentions**
    a) Evoking an authentic, felt experience of love for self, others and All that is.
    b) Translating that felt experience of love into concrete and effective action.

c) Relying on this felt experience as a primary motivation for healing, growth and transformation.

d) Expanding our arenas of affection consequent to evolving our strata of moral valuation.

5) **Practical Alchemy: Perfecting Integral Lifework with Combined Nourishment Practices**
   a) Building momentum and confidence to nourish many dimensions at once.
   b) Designing nourishment routines with the integral checklist.
   c) Allowing additive synthesis to occur.

6) **Fruits of an Integral Life: Assessing and Maintaining Progress**
   a) Identifying useful metrics.
   b) Spontaneous development of a *blessing presence*.
   c) Making necessary adjustments.

Envisioning Outcomes & Intermediate Goals

Think of intermediate goals as milestones along your journey, and outcomes as the consequences or benefits of having achieved those milestones. Milestones are very specific and measurable. For instance, let's say I want to be able to sleep through the night without being awoken repeatedly by back pain, and be able to do this without the help of medication. The outcome will be satisfying sleep, less fatigue and irritability throughout the day, less overall physical discomfort, and no more of that brain fog the medication seems to create. This outcome is an imagined result – an attractive vision I can hold in my heart and mind to draw me forward. A milestone I might choose for myself is sleeping through the night pain-free, without the use of any medication, for at least three days in a row. And in order to achieve the goal I set for myself, I need to first clarify to myself why these is important to me. That's where my values come in. Returning to the Values Alignment exercise in Part I, spend a few days defining your goals, outcomes and underlying values. When you have done this, begin to prioritize your list using the same technique; that is, ask yourself, "Why is this goal or outcome more important to me than that goal or outcome?" and so on.

Once you have your priorities clarified, you are ready to begin assessing your nourishment in-depth.

Assessing Nourishment

When I first began my formal *Integral Lifework* practice, I spent a year or so developing on-line nourishment assessments for my clients. I had developed other such instruments before, and was both excited and confident about how helpful they would be. To my chagrin, I discovered that, although the assessments promised to be accurate and useful in some ways, they had one unfortunate and unintended consequence: they were disempowering in a way that ran counter to the ethical framework and best practices of *Integral Lifework*. Such instruments invite people to rely on external assessments of their well-being, rather than encouraging the introspection, self-confidence and "felt sense" of each dimension necessary to sustain ongoing self-nourishment. As objective tools, they provided interesting data, but in the therapeutic context, they undermine the collaborative, client-centered model. If an objective of *Integral Lifework* is to encourage healthy self-sufficiency, then any nourishment assessment process should reflect that goal. So instead of any externalized instrument that aims for objectivity, I have decided to stick with an intersubjective approach that involves dialoguing with the client about different areas of nourishment and encouraging them to discover their needs, strengths and barriers in that context. Sometimes I rely on my intuition to shape my side of that dialogue, but mainly I offer the groundwork – philosophical questions, probing techniques borrowed from Hakomi, the downward arrow technique used in cognitive behavioral therapy, guided meditations, and so forth – which not only prompts people to find the answers within themselves, but to feel confident about what they find.

So, you might ask, how does this translate into the written format of this book? Well, it doesn't – at least not easily. Back in Part I, we explored a simple but effective Nourishment Levels exercise, and that is a great start. You can expand this exercise by reading through The Twelve Dimensions in Depth in Part III, and asking the same basic questions of each nourishment channel. How do you nourish yourself in each of them? How often? What areas haven't been regularly addressed? Why do you think that is? Trust your intuitive abilities and discover your innermost landscape. Once you've uncovered a handful of nourishment components that haven't been consciously or consistently nurtured, try comparing those dimensions to the goals and outcomes you have already prioritized for yourself. Do you detect any interdependencies, connections or relationships? Even if they aren't readily apparent, there is almost always an interaction between undernourished dimensions and seemingly unrelated challenges we have identified in our lives. You may intuit those connections, but even if they remain obscure, allow yourself to believe that a relationship exists. For instance, that something languishing in Restorative History will facilitate your relationship goals, or something as yet unaddressed in Empowered Self-Concept will help resolve a block in creativity, and so forth. The logic of *Integral Lifework* is the logic of being, so the shortest distance between two points is hardly ever a straight or obvious line. However, whatever the path of our internal interdependencies, our being already knows how it looks, feels and senses. We just need to find ways of listening to our own interior intelligence – a goal the exercises among these pages aim to achieve. To assist with this effort, please consult the "Index of Exercises" at the end of the book.

Targeted Integral Practice

In and of themselves, the basic mechanisms of nourishment routines can sustain us, but they will not create the momentum necessary for lasting healing or enduring transformation. For integral practice to be truly healing and transformative, three factors must be present with some consistency. First, a love-centric governing intention must permeate all activity. Second, internal transformative exchanges must translate into exterior exchanges – that is, interactions in ever-widening arenas of affection. And third, we must always begin by providing special attention to undernourished dimensions; we must first create targeted integral practice and expand out from there.

How do we accomplish this? One approach that has been helpful to many of my clients is to capitalize on well-nourished dimensions to assist more depleted facets of self. For instance, if I am very grounded and in-touch with my own body, but a little out-of-touch with my spiritual life, I can practice mystic activators that emphasize a physiological component to help accelerate spiritual nourishment. If I'm great at feeding my intellect, but tend to neglect my body, I can create mental puzzles or challenges as part of my physical exercise routine to make it more interesting and engaging. If I have a strong sense of purpose, but struggle to allow myself richly felt experiences, I can trick myself into playfulness by structuring that play around my chosen purpose – as a game, a celebration, a creative project and so on. By weaving undernourished channels into well-nourished ones, the confidence that accompanies our strengths will energize our weaknesses. The miracle of consciousness is that virtually any activity can become nourishing with appropriate attention, intention and follow-through. We just need to choose a place to begin, set our intention, and keep going.

Ultimately, we must cross-pollinate all of our energy exchanges. In other words, we need to introduce each nourishment dimension to all others and eliminate segregation and boundarizing in self-nurturing. In order to be completely whole, all of our nourishment practices should be able to relate comfortably with all others. One interesting way to evaluate this integration is the interplay of our relationships and nourishment environments. Would friends we seek out to for unstructured play get along well with those whom we primarily engage in intellectual stimulation? Would our intimate romantic partner feel comfortable spending time where we work? Would the places where we feel anchored to Nature be appealing to those involved in our life's purpose? If I introduce my spiritual practices to one of my supportive communities – say, an affinity group for one of my hobbies – would they respond favorably? And what about my family of origin? How would they react to any of my nourishment practices? You get the idea. The more compartmentalized our lives, the less complete we will feel. But the more harmoniously all of these worlds interact, the more our own sense of well-being and wholeness is cemented with integrity.

Practical Alchemy

Having come this far we can at last depart from theory groundwork, and explore the source and endpoint for all multidimensional nourishment:

a process that integrates all of the diverse elements enumerated thus far. After all, the ideal integral routine should fully nourish every dimension – and the promise of *Integral Lifework* is a comprehensive, individualized map for any person to do just that. All of the practices provided so far have been biased toward specific dimensions, but they really nurture several other dimensions at the same time. Each has the potential of becoming much more than a targeted exercise. Now we will broaden our focus to include all dimensions, all processing spaces, the satisfaction of all fulfillment impulses and nourishment prerequisites, the facilitation of widening arenas of affection, the broadest transformation of identity and the highest circles of intimacy. In other words, we will create practices that energize every level of exchange at once, while remaining centered around depleted or underserved nourishment channels.

This sounds like a tall order, but in reality the resultant disciplines are surprisingly simple. When we combine our practices in a certain way, we accommodate limitless quantities of new awareness, insight and energy, adding layer upon layer without things becoming awkward, unwieldy or overly complicated. How is this accomplished? By letting go; by doing without doing; by giving up our ego and giving in to love. In fact, when we relinquish set expectations and let things evolve organically within love-consciousness, an additive synthesis will naturally occur. That is, the facets of our practice will interact on their own to create something larger than the sum of their parts. This is how baseline disciplines offer us everything we need to heal, grow and thrive. This is practical alchemy, and it can support any chosen life direction, any set of beliefs and any mode of being – as long as each of these is rooted in authentic love that constantly expresses itself. What makes this approach so powerful is that there is nothing artificial or contrived here – the structures native to our human design are reflected and amplified by it. We were born to operate this way, and we are only becoming true to ourselves as we sustain and deepen our practice.

Recombinant Integralism

So, where do we begin? Let's look at an example where an initial discipline targets dimensions of nourishment identified as undernourished, and then builds from there. Let's say I have discovered the following depletion patterns in my life:

- **Healthy Body**
    - o   My sleep is low-quality and frequently interrupted
    - o   My quality of nutrition is inconsistent
    - o   I don't exercise enough
- **Supportive Community**
    - o   I feel isolated and disconnected from a community of shared values

- **Authentic Spirit**
    - o   I resist pursuing a connection with the ground of being

- **Restorative History**
    - o   I don't have healthy communication or constructive relationship with my family

- **Flexible Processing Space**
    - o   My processing space is fairly inflexible, and is mainly limited to mental spacetime

- **Empowered Self-Concept**
    - o   I have little confidence in my own ability to be skilled or effective (low self-efficacy)
    - o   My feelings of self-worth are just middle-of-the-road

- **Affirming Integrity**
    - o   I struggle with integrity around translating what I believe and feel into what I say and do.

Taken as a whole, this combination of depleting patterns might seem overwhelming. But watch what happens when we initiate an *Integral Lifework Plan* that creates practical alchemy:

1) **Week One** – I research and identify an established group whose charter or explicit function aligns with one or more of my core values, and which offers regular group activities that involve exercise.

2) **Week Two** – In preparation for my first group activity, I walk brusquely every day for thirty minutes to gain some conditioning. While walking, I pick out an integrity affirmation that is particularly relevant to me (for instance: "Because I am devoted to my own well-being, I seek understanding in my soul."), and recite it as a mantra, relaxing my mind into its rhythm and allowing its meaning and importance to course through me. As I do this, I pay attention to the sensations in my body and any emotions I am feeling. Throughout my walk, I keep reciting the integrity affirmation as a mantra and paying attention to my emotions and physical sensations.

3) **Week Three** – I plan to attend my first group activity the following week. Throughout this week, I continue my exercise and walking meditation routine, and I add something. At the beginning and end of the routine, I excite gratitude in my heart for the opportunity to go for a walk, to appreciate my surroundings, to care for myself, and for the possibility of finding like-minded people in the activity I plan to attend. I sincerely and joyfully thank the Universe for this unfolding moment and the healing I am experiencing right now.

4) **Week Four** – I attend my first group activity and see how it goes, and I continue my walking meditation and gratitude practice. If the group activity feels okay, I plan to attend again in the next week or two. If I need to find another group, I do so.

5) **Week Five and Six** – I continue my walking meditation and gratitude practice each day, and attend one or two more group activities. If I encounter resistance, disappointment or confusion in anything I have tried thus far, I can check in with my *Integral Lifework Practitioner* or other wellness resource about possible barriers.

6) **Week Seven, Eight and Nine** – In addition to my ongoing walking meditation and group activities, I begin a mystic activation practice for at least fifteen minutes every other day. And let's say I have now identified relationships in my family of origin as a major barrier.

7) **Week Ten** – In addition to my ongoing walking meditation and group activities, I begin a mystic activation exercise for at least fifteen minutes each and every day. I also reflect upon and journal about what needs to heal in my family of origin relationships.

8) **Week Eleven** – Continuing everything I have been practicing up until now, I spend one hour during the week writing a letter to a close member of my family with whom I have a particularly painful history or unhealthy dynamic. Using lots of "I feel" statements, I describe first how I feel, then how I would like to resolve those feelings through healing dialogue.

9) **Week Twelve** – Continuing everything I have been practicing up until now, I begin to address my diet and sleep habits. I try to get up at the same time each morning regardless of when I went to bed. Without being too rigid or harsh on myself, I try to implement the rule of thirds in my diet each day.

10) **Week Thirteen, Fourteen and Fifteen** – I continue everything I have been doing up until now, expanding the time I spend on my walks and in mystic activation whenever possible. I revisit any areas where I encountered resistance or disappointment earlier, and see if I can move forward any easier now.

11) **Week Sixteen** – I continue everything I have been doing up until now, and revisit the letter I wrote my family member. I consider how I might have a conversation with them about this. I experiment with an empty chair exercise, where I read my letter aloud as if they were seated in the chair in front of me. I review my Integral Lifework Plan and assess how I am doing in each area, where I can improve on my own, and where I might need some assistance.

Gradually this process builds on itself, with each component supporting all the others. What happens – slowly at first and then with increasing intensity – is that my being is conditioned to expect high quality, full-spectrum nourishment. If I abruptly stopped nurturing any dimension after week sixteen, I would likely become aware of the deficit as a felt need very quickly. My body would miss those walks; my spirit ache for the attention I gave to its processing space; my heart sadden over the loss of my new social connections. This is how we tune into multidimensional nourishment as the benefits from additive energy exchanges become clearly evident. My sleep is more satisfying and sound. My hunger for unhealthy foods attenuated. I can enjoy and even rely upon different processing spaces. Confidence in my own abilities – especially in facilitating these nurturing habits – improves, along with a growing sense of self-worth. After all, I am successfully caring for myself now! What remains is to translate this momentum into healing the unhappy elements of family relationships. This may take several attempts, and might or might not involve challenging interactions with those family members, but the strength I have gained through consistent self-care will carry me over that hurdle. And, when I have fully articulated my desire for healing and attempted to communicate it, my newfound inner strength will help me maintain healthier boundaries, constructive communication styles and emotional honesty in those and all other relationships. I will overcome past barriers that inhibited self-care, and continue to affirm my own integrity.

What is really occurring in this example? Mainly the combining of a handful of previously discussed exercises into a routine that addresses specific nourishment deficits. And if you have experimented with those exercises, you may already intuit which ones you can combine into a practical alchemy suited to your unique situation. Built into this alchemy is the self-reinforcing power of compassionate affection: I initiate this journey because I care about my well-being and effectiveness in the world, and the journey itself strengthens those convictions because it connects me with myself, with others, with feelings of contentment and competence, and with the essence of love itself. The caring relationship I create with each part of my being is reflected in the caring relationships I create with others around me. And so, without being entirely conscious of what is happening, I transform a self-limiting scarcity of nourishment into a thriving banquet. All I did at first was preen my feathers and flex my wings a bit, and suddenly I have taken flight. By combining a few seemingly lesser elements in a certain way, I can create precious gold.

This is how we can heal hurts, treat illnesses, revitalize heart and mind, and awaken lasting contentment in our lives. In a matter of weeks or months – and over the course of ensuing years – this is how we can actualize true love in every moment. This is *Integral Lifework*.f

Integral Checklist

To appreciate how any practice can provide multidimensional nourishment, you might consider using the integral checklist that follows. We have already discussed most of the terms in the checklist, so all that remains is to ascribe an emphasis for each nourishment parameter that a particular practice provides. The following example uses the mystic activation exercise introduced at the end of Part I. Eventually, you will be able to use this checklist to evaluate any new nurturing activity, and thereby determine its potential value as part of your integral discipline. The idea here is to eventually depart from relying on routines suggested by any external source, and invent some on your own.

Integral Checklist for Mystic Activation	
NOURISHMENT PARAMETER	**EMPHASIS**
Nourishment Prerequisites	As set by intention, potentially any or all
Nourishment Dimensions	Depending on context of practice, any or all
Processing Space	Depending on type of mystic activator, any or all
Dialectic Tension	Yes – comfort routine & sacred space contrasts with challenges of interior discovery
Maturity Factors	As set by intention, any or all
Moral Valuation Strata	As set by intention, operates in contributive individualism or above
Elements of Motivation Diagram	Any or all
Mode-Change Methods	As set by intention and dependent on type of activator, all are available

Arenas of Affection	More expansive with persistent practice
Intimacy Potential (Circle of Intimacy)	Begins in convenience, ends in devotion with persistent practice
Overcoming Barriers	Useful in routing energy around structural barriers as well as dissolving chained associations and stress-inducing patterns
Desire/Impulse Management	As set by intention, very effective
Relationship Factors	With persistence and as set by intention, all high quality factors both facilitate the practice and are reinforced by the practice
Fulfillment Impulse Satisfaction	Discovery, Understanding, Maturation, Fulfillment, Sustenance, Autonomy, Union, Affirmation, Mastery, Imagination, Exchange

Note how intention and context can change the emphasis for each nourishment parameter. This is true for many self-care habits, but mystic activation is particularly potent in this regard. Ideally, any integral practice should populate as much of this checklist as possible – no nourishment stone should be left unturned. Over time, we can keep returning to this checklist to reexamine how a particular practice nurtures us. But this is not a formula set in stone. Remember that the intention, attention and follow through you apply to any combination of activities will shape their nourishing benefits. These are the three legs of the integral easel. When any one of them is missing, integral practice is diluted. When all of them are present and supported by a growing love-consciousness, integral practice has miraculous outcomes.

Resources: Systems of integral practice have existed in various forms for a long time. The mind-body-spirit integrations of Yoga, certain martial arts and the spiritual disciplines of mystically oriented religions, for instance, are excellent resources for informing a practice. As for books, *The Life We Are Given* by George Leonard & Michael Murphy is a helpful resource, as is *Integral Life Practice* by Wilber, Patten, Leonard & Morelli. If you want a real challenge, you could also explore Sri Aurobindo's *A Synthesis of Yoga* to appreciate his approach to integral practice.

Loving Intentions

As much time as we have already spent on this topic, we can always spend a little more. To be able to cultivate loving intentions and translate them into effective action is what all miracles are made of. To then expand those intentions and actions into wider and wider arenas of affection is proof positive that love-consciousness has taken root and blossomed into fullness. Wherever we are in our journey, the felt experiences of gratitude, affection, empathy, tenderness, charity and the myriad other expressions of true love should always be simmering within easy reach of our heart, mind, body and spirit. If we lose our way in unintended overemphasis of one dimension or other, we need only remember the fountain that springs eternal from the center of our being. When darkness and distraction overwhelm us, we must return to love. Amid all the astounding abilities and accomplishments that humanity has manifested, the quality of compassionate affection holds the greatest promise. If we can govern the immense power of our collective vision and will with the golden intention, the full depth, breadth and mystery of the Universe awaits our arrival. How could we ever turn away from such an incredible journey?

Fruits of an Integral Life

The justification for any approach to living and loving lies in the fruit it produces. And when we enliven all our dimensions of self-nourishment with affectionate compassion, that fruit is delicious. To taste such results is to believe in the value of integral practice. Yet "tasting is believing" is circular, self-referential reasoning. After all, is it a genuine experience that we are healing and growing, or merely an elaborate rationalization? Is it real fruit or just fruit-flavored Cool Aid? So it is always beneficial to set up some metrics for evaluating *Integral Lifework* as one would any other approach. Thankfully, that is fairly straightforward, because the resultant personal transformation and impact on our immediate relationships is both sweeping and relatively rapid. As a quick overview, here are some measurable objectives and benefits:

- Enhancing physical healing for acute and chronic illness

- Expanding creative energy and insight

- Increasing clarity in personal goals and life direction

- Overcoming obstacles in our spiritual journey

- Resolving immediate or longstanding emotional challenges

- Improving and enriching intimate relationships, friendships, family relationships and work relationships

- Creating healthy, nourishing patterns of interaction with others

- Promoting overall harmony, wholeness and wellness within and without

- Discovering effective, compassionate ways to create positive change in the world, and expanding our energy to enact that change

These outcomes revolve around the steady evolution of compassion and caring for each dimension of self. They then expand that love outward to embrace broader and broader arenas of affection. They also steadily nudge us into the narrow band of optimal function for each maturity factor. In fact, routinely returning to that chart and evaluating how well we are balancing each area can be an invaluable aid in our progress, so I encourage you to try that.

Integral Lifework accelerates a straightforward upward spiral: as we improve our energy exchanges, we increase vitality in that dimension; as our vitality increases, we feel more joy, hope and excitement; as we feel more joy, our natural response is appreciation and gratitude; as our gratitude becomes more constant, our compassionate affection blossoms spontaneously; and, coming full circle, our burgeoning affection in turn inspires and permeates our integral practice, making our energy exchanges that much more effective. So increased vitality ultimately inspires love, which energizes nourishment, which fortifies vitality. We will sense this upward lift the longer we practice – that is certain. But in order to construct a set of meaningful milestones for our ongoing efforts, let's also take a look at some real-world success stories.

Examples of Healing, Growth & Transformation

During the past few years of working with folks in San Diego and – via web consultations – in other parts of the country, every one of my clients has improved their overall well-being to some degree after initiating integral practice. All the credit for this improvement of course belongs to them, because it was their disciplined intention and effort that created such positive outcomes. Instead of substituting client names, I will briefly summarize the challenges they faced and the impact of their efforts over a short period of time – usually just a few weeks.

Body & Mind

- **Environmental allergies, after eight weeks of targeted integral practice and barrier resolution:** Improved tolerance to identified allergens. Elimination of all medication. Improved energy and abatement of depressive thoughts and feelings. Thorough identification of depletions, barriers and substitutions, with planned strategies for resolution.

- **Chronic insomnia, after two weeks of targeted integral practice and barrier resolution:** Regular, satisfying and contiguous sleep in ensuing months. Improved energy and mental clarity. Improved ability to manage mood swings and begin addressing causes of depressive thoughts and feelings. Partial identification of depletions, barriers and substitutions, with acknowledgement of resistance to resolution.

- **Candida, after six weeks of targeted integral practice and barrier resolution:** Rapid cycle flare-up frequency reduced and flare-up symptom intensity abated in ensuing months. Energy, physical appetites and physical self-confidence greatly improved. Depressive cycling of thoughts and emotions interrupted. Renewed interest in pleasurable activities, self-discovery and growth. Identification of depletions, barriers and substitutions with partial resolution and plan for ongoing resolution efforts.

- **Excess weight, after eight weeks of targeted integral practice and barrier resolution:** Steady weight reduction toward target weight and increased ability to maintain weight loss in ensuing months. Improved feelings about body-image and social confidence. Improved physical energy and sleep. Heightened enjoyment of, and renewed interest in, favorite activities. Identification of depletions, barriers and substitutions, and commitment to path of resolution.

- **Severe depression, after six weeks of targeted integral practice and barrier resolution:** Reduction in intensity of depressive and self-destructive thoughts and feelings, and improved ability to manage self-destructive thoughts and impulses when they arise. Improved enjoyment of life and ability to set positive goals, remain motivated and follow through. Elimination of behavioral patterns that contributed to depressive cycles, and improved ability to recognize and interrupt other negative patterns of thought and emotion. Identification of depletions, barriers and substitutions with partial resolution.

- **Obsessive-compulsive thoughts and behaviors, after ten weeks of targeted integral practice and barrier resolution:** Substantial reduction in obsessive-compulsive and self-destructive patterns of thought, emotion and action. Improved sleep and energy. Improved quality of interaction with others with more positive, self-supporting relational outcomes. Identification of depletions, barriers and substitutions, with suggested path to resolution and a tentative commitment to follow through.

- **Addictive behaviors, after two weeks of targeted integral practice and barrier resolution:** Abatement of addictive cravings and behaviors and improved ability to manage substitution impulses. Identification and partial resolution of depletions, barriers and substitutions.

- **Low of self-worth, after six weeks of targeted integral practice and barrier resolution:** Greatly improved compassion and affection for own being and willingness to continue appropriate self-care. Identification and resolution of depletions, barriers and substitutions.

- **Patterns of destructive anger and frustration, after three weeks of targeted integral practice and barrier resolution:** Elimination of anger as initial emotional response to frustrating situations. Abatement of frequency of frustration and improved management of emotions. Identification of depletions, barriers and substitutions, and commitment to a path of resolution.

- **Crohn's Disease, after three weeks of targeted integral practice and barrier resolution:** Gradually reduced medication and abatement of flare-ups and flare-up symptoms in ensuing months. Identification of depletions, barriers and substitutions with suggested path to resolution, with some resistance to follow-through.

- **PTSD, after four weeks of targeting integral practice and barrier resolution:** Abatement of anxiety and paranoia. Improved confidence and goal-setting. Improved management of depressive emotional cycling and anger responses. Identification of depletions, barriers and some substitutions, with suggested path to resolution.

- **Suicidal ideation, after three weeks of targeted integral practice and barrier resolution:** Elimination of suicidal thoughts, insomnia and self-medication with food and alcohol. Renewed interest in life and life goals. Identification of primary contributors and suggested remedies to underlying depression. Partially identified depletions, barriers and substations.

Relationships

About half of my *Integral Lifework* clients define healing in their most important relationships as a high priority outcome. Usually, these relationships are with family members and romantic partners, but sometimes it may be a close friendship or work relationship that they wish to heal or strengthen. Here are some of the relationship challenges they courageously took on:

- **Lack of intimacy and a perceived breakdown in communication in a long-term marriage, after four weeks of joint targeted integral practice and barrier resolution:** Rejuvenation in quality and frequency of intimate sharing and sex life. Increased openness, empathic listening and honesty in daily communication. The beginning of a shift from codependence to interdependence and self-sufficiency. Partially identified depletions, barriers and substations with suggestions for ongoing exploration and remedy.

- **Anger and resentment towards close friend and perceived loss of closeness, after three weeks of targeted integral practice and barrier resolution:** Reconnection and clearer boundary-setting in target friendship, clearer understanding of unhealthy relational dynamics and how to manage them, and more empathic communication with attenuation of rescue responses. Fully identified depletions, barriers and substitutions, with a detailed plan for ongoing resolution.

- **Antagonistic and sometimes destructive relationship with parent, after two weeks of targeted integral practice and barrier resolution:** Clarity about codependent dynamics and awareness of major triggers. Attenuation of frustration and hostility. Initial efforts at self-sufficiency. Identified depletions, barriers and substitutions, without a fully developed plan for ongoing resolution.

- **Increasing frustration and sense of failure and alienation in new romantic relationship, after six weeks of targeted integral practice and barrier resolution:** Identification of unhealthy relational dynamics and communication disconnects. Rejuvenation of sense of safety in the relationship and hope for its future. Identified depletions, barriers and substitutions, with one party committed to ongoing resolution efforts, and the other hesitant about doing the work.

Personal Vision and Life Direction

Either as a side road along the way to other desired outcomes, or as a specific goal, gaining clarity about the personal vision for their lives has been extremely important to many of my clients. Once this topic arises, it may only take one or two sessions to generate the clarity desired to energize this nourishment center. I often encounter clients who feel lost amid a swarm of conflicting demands and priorities, which they often perceive as coming from outside themselves. The expectations of parents, the presumed and real needs of a child, the expressed desires of a partner, a boss or coworker's demands, and so on. This swarm of external influences often becomes a constant distraction from appropriate self-care, and as a result we can quickly become so depleted there seems no escape from the constant pull of those externals. Although there can be other mitigating factors, what has consistently freed clients from this oppressive sense of outwardly focused effort is a rediscovery of personal purpose. Once we clearly frame our life's work, we can prioritize our responses to externals much more easily. Then, as we develop our conviction and compassion around our life's mission, we can decline requests or demands that don't align with that mission without feeling disappointment, agitation or guilt. This epiphany has liberated so many people from increasing depletion, frustration and despair I thought it deserved special mention here.

Examples of this unfold nearly identically from one person to the next. Once a genuine purpose has been identified, we can ask ourselves a simple question in the face of each new external expectation, request or demand: "Will my response in this situation fulfill or further my personal vision?" Abruptly, our priorities become crystal clear, and feelings of resentment, worry or stress over what others expect of us all but disappear. In order to completely believe in our individual purpose, of course, that purpose must align with our core values, talents and acquired skills, and that alignment is what many of the introspective practices outlined thus far can encourage. But the revelation that we have a purpose – and that this vision can channel our thinking, feeling and volitional energy into a blaze of productivity – is the most effective insulation available against the storm of conflicting expectations that constantly swirls around us. When returning clients express feelings of being adrift or struggling with choices, one of the first questions I ask is: "Have you checked in with your purpose lately?" Even when our personal vision shifts or evolves over time, if we can return our finger to its lively pulse we will always find our way back to clarity and directedness.

More Arenas of Healing

The list goes on. With many other similar examples to draw upon, the conclusion I have come to thus far is that *Integral Lifework* can be effective in addressing a broad range of physical, emotional, psychological, spiritual and relational challenges. In many ways, I believe this is mainly a result of the quality of compassionate, self-empowering effort *Integral Lifework* encourages people to embrace as they learn to heal themselves. Any and all of the failures I have witnessed in this work have been either the result of my own inability to empathically connect with a client, or a client's resistance to self-awareness in exploring a difficult, life-long barrier. When my own empathy has failed, it is usually the result of engaging too many clients in a week or some other imbalance in my own self-nourishment. In terms of client resistance, I well remember one client being quite emphatic about it: "I don't want to deal with my past!" she said. "It's unpleasant. I don't want to dwell on those uncomfortable memories." And yet, if we avoid processing our primary barriers to self-nourishment in even one dimension, our lack of empathy for self will prevent us from progressing toward wholeness. And if neither practitioner nor client can uncover a path to these empathic connections, avenues to addressing the causal factors of suffering will tend to remain closed. Without true love, there can be no true healing.

A Blessing Presence

Before I began my own integral practice, I was not a peaceful person. I was plagued with anxieties, fears, angers and grief. My every choice was either colored with confusion and doubt, with codependent responses, or with natural but unmanaged impulses that led to feelings of guilt or remorse. The facets of self that I valued most seemed frozen in space and time, unable to move forward or find expression in my life. And the facets that dominated my waking hours were unpredictable, unreliable and inadequate for the healing, growth and transformation I intuited was possible. I felt enslaved by internal and external barriers I could barely understand, let alone begin to resolve. Then, as I learned to nourish myself in areas I had been unwilling or unable to in the past, those frozen facets I so highly valued began unfolding, filling the space created for them in my life. With continued interior discipline, things that had once only been a hope or the hint of a dream slowly began to permeate each successive moment. And when, over time, I did come to understand the nature of my own barriers to wholeness, I suddenly discovered that I had the tools to overcome them. As those barriers gave way before my newly focused intentions, the secret Self unleashed within began to energize my interpersonal exchanges, interactions with my environment, and my relationship with the Universe itself. When I became more fully nourished, harmonizing loving intentions with constructive actions, I entered a beneficial mode of being as natural as breathing. All the fears, doubts, pain and unhelpful impulses in my life were not vanquished, but they were subordinated and made light by a greater force. They were consumed in a *blessing presence*.

What does a blessing presence look like, and what concrete, observable effects does it have in our lives? Well, for anyone tuned into the characteristics of authentic love, the blessing presence will encompass and evidence many of them. A blessing presence generates energy for ourselves and others to be fully nourished, to generously explore each processing space, to readily engage in ever-broadening arenas of affection with a discernment that helps keep all of our efforts on-target. A blessing presence will naturally encourage personal and societal evolution, edifying self and others in profound and unexpected ways. This isn't something that is always recognized, however, especially within cultural attitudes that might prefer comfort and consolation over authentic love. Nor do such edification and evolution hold much immediate sway in the gruff, rushed and tumbled world of crisis and survival. So in some ways, a blessing presence may go altogether unnoticed, especially in the short run. But over longer spans of interaction and experience, certain consequences are inevitable. If you are a steadily blessing presence, children will want to spend more time with you. People who are fearful or aggressive will, after a few false starts, open up and share their hearts with you. Friends and family will feel deeply appreciated and supported; not always in the moment, of course, because true love is not always expressed as soft, kind, generous or gentle – but over time the continuity of goodwill will shine through and loving choices will be vindicated. Animals – wild and domesticated, unfamiliar and familiar – will tend to hover nearby, comfortable to be within your circle of energy. Kind-hearted strangers will approach you to ask for help or advice, and offer you the same without hesitation. These are just a few of the more obvious evidences.

There is another consequence of a blessing presence that can be more challenging. Just as those who are innocent, kind or loving will be drawn to you, those who are emotionally wounded, self-destructive, or who have hardened their hearts to love may feel threatened, rebellious and reactive. Over time, even these interactions will be transformed, because that is the irresistible, permeating nature of a blessing mode of being. But initially, hurt, fear, anger and even hatred may rocket to the surface of anyone and anything around you that is groping blindly through a dark, dank period of denial. A little light neither inspires nor consoles someone who is lost in a maze of shadow, especially if they have willfully acclimated themselves to their own ignorance. In these situations, it is always good to remember our own incompleteness, our own failings and misunderstandings, and to refresh a great compassion for those parts of ourselves that struggle to emerge from their own chilly depths of night. Then the affectionate compassion necessary to maintain a blessing presence when we are being berated, threatened or abused is a bit easier to muster, and the resolve required for self-preservation or the protection of others will be grounded not in defensive anger, but in love.

Of course there are other, less tangible evidences of a blessing presence. A tendency to inadvertently awaken curiosity, insight and questioning in others, for example. Or to unconsciously find appropriate words of encouragement that balm the heart and inspire the spirit. To reflexively see through the outer trappings of a complex situation to its relevant core. To spread joy without thinking or kindle lasting affection with a glance. Perhaps to upset the status quo by accidentally undermining comfortable habits or perceptions. All of these are not deliberate, of course, they flow out of a certain way of being that is shaped by years of holistic nourishment. What is sometimes disorienting and unnerving is that these unbidden reflexes have cascading consequences, a catalyzing effect that catapults a single impulse into waves of disruptive but ultimately healing influence. Sometimes our loving resonance in one instant creates profound, enduring realignments beyond our perception or understanding. These are evidences we cannot always readily observe, but sometimes we can intuit them, or they can be relayed to us through the observations of others.

I have experienced many of these things. I have both lost friendships and been offered gratitude and love, felt both empowered and silly, been both admired and ridiculed, demonstrated catalyzing effects and endured my own futility. But more important than any of these externals is the quality of my internal life as a blessing presence grows within me. Where I had no peace, I now have more peace. Where I was wounded, I am now healing. Where I was grieving a loss, I have found renewed love. Where I was confused or deluded, I now have more clarity. Where I was spiritually unconscious, I am now increasingly conscious and connected. Where every resistance to my own will once disrupted equanimity, I can now more often acquiesce in the face of turmoil. At long last I have become more contented with my own ordinary, frail humanness and the vast unpredictability of existence. I have translated distraction, agitation and dissipation into a more focused and constructive passion. These internal qualities of heart, mind and spirit are really the greatest evidences of transformation through integral practice. Everything else is just, well, a delightful windfall; an unexpected blessing. I share all this merely to assure you that persistent effort holds tremendous promise for anyone and everyone.

What if Integral Fruits Aren't Evident?

What if we believe we are nourishing ourselves in every dimension, but are still experiencing evidence of depletion or even starvation? What if we remain physically ill, depressed, in conflict with others, struggling with addiction, codependent or unhappy about our life? Then there are still barriers to nourishment we have yet to work through. Perhaps we haven't recognized them yet, or the approaches we have taken so far to address our barriers have been incomplete, or perhaps we haven't been patient enough with our own learning process. That does not indicate failure, just a new opportunity for adjustment and growth. I have worked with people who have suffered so many years of inadequate nourishment, illness, fatigue, anguish and frustration that their own wholeness and well-being seem perpetually out of reach. They were at the end of their rope, ready to give up entirely. Within just a few weeks of initiating integral practice, most found a way to relieve the acuteness of their own suffering and plot a course toward well-being. And within a few months of continuing their *Integral Lifework Plan*, they began to operate on an entirely different level of self-sufficiency. Some have returned later on to collaborate on some subtler angle of wholeness or a newfound barrier, but they have confidence in new tools or insights being available because of their past experience. This is the faith we must keep whenever we stumble or fall.

Remember also that the progression of nourishment ranges from starvation through transformation, allowing several levels in between and even subtler states and fluctuations along the way. Who among us has reached a consistently transformative level of self-nourishment in all twelve dimensions? I have encountered very few individuals who would claim to have achieved this – I certainly don't claim it for myself. It is a worthwhile goal, to be sure, but consider that how we are nourished changes over time as well. A bit of fumbling and undernourishment is probably necessary for us to realize that we need to reassess or realign. Life itself is an ever-changing landscape of new challenges, opportunities and setbacks. We cannot remain static or calcified in our habits and insights and expect to adjust to the unanticipated events unfolding around us. So we practice, and we get a little better, and then we are reminded of the need for humility and renewed vigilance once again. Self-nourishment should not be limited to a frantic, short-term effort, but rather become a relaxed and continuous way of being. And once we learn to recognize everything we encounter as some type of energy exchange, we will always be moving forward regardless of what obstacles or missteps darken our well-lit path.

Remember also that there may be some structural limitations that continue to curtail our choices or our ability to nourish in certain areas. If we are over thirty-five and have poor vision, becoming a commercial pilot is probably not an option for us. In more serious instances, we may have a life-threatening condition that will shorten our time on Earth. In the same way, there will be hard limits to self-care that we must work around instead of through. But if we address those areas head-on, consciously embracing and integrating our structural limitations instead of fighting or denying them, then we will begin experiencing many of the fruits of an integral life despite them. If we focus on what we can achieve within the dimensions most readily accessible to us, we will also find we have added strength and endurance to deal with any structural limitations we face elsewhere. In my own case, despite a strong desire to perform great physical feats when I was young, my body just wouldn't cooperate, and in my zeal I continually injured myself instead of refining my skills. When I learned to accept my limitations, I had the energy and time to explore other strengths, and in fact discovered I was actually neglecting aspects of my being while obsessing over physical prowess. I was, in effect, substituting. Once I realized this, however, I could not neglect my physical well-being either. I found ways to strengthen myself, increase my flexibility and achieve the aerobic exercise I needed without endangering my health. And this enhanced the energy I required to pursue nourishment for all other facets of self.

Transforming Patterns of Imbalanced Undernourishment

The fruits of unbalanced undernourishment are all around us in the world. Hostility, destructive competitiveness, acquisitive narcissism, a lack of empathy and compassion, the self-destructive patterns of addiction and ever more desperate searches for new substitutions. The modern world is replete with suffering because so many cannot adequately nourish themselves or expand their arenas of affection. And if we are forever struggling with our own equilibrium, how could we sustain love for anything beyond a limited, self-absorbed horizon? However, merely calling attention to these consequences does not in itself have a transformative effect. In fact, it is often the case that when we are reminded of our shortcomings, the illogic of a particular belief, or the dysfunctional depths of our own addictions, we will in fact renew efforts to reinforce our position with heightened fervor. A recent study by political scientists Brendan Nyhan and Jason Reifler seems to support this idea with respect to political ideology. Ask most smokers if data on lung cancer, emphysema and the efforts of tobacco companies to make cigarettes more addictive has had any impact on their smoking habits, and they'll likely reply, "Yeah, when I hear that stuff it stresses me out, and I have to go calm myself down with a cigarette." The same is true when our self-limiting patterns of thought and emotion or our predilection for substitute nourishment are brought into question. Guilt won't cure eating disorders or problems managing strong emotions. Shame can't dissuade us from falling in lust with someone else's spouse or stealing from our employer. Knowing what is right and how what we are doing is destructive won't deliver us from the perpetual unhappiness of unhealthy habits.

Cognitive dissonance has much to do with this. When our established habits and beliefs are challenged with new information, we will tend to resist that new information and defend our existing patterns by rationalizing them. Why? Because we perceive that they have provided us with some level of nurturing, even though that nurturing may not be authentic or complete. And the more we are cornered by overwhelming contradictory evidence, the more entrenched we can become in our defensiveness. Remember, some part of us really believes that what we are doing is nourishment, that it somehow satisfies our fulfillment impulses and primary drives in some way – and in fact there may be some truth in that. Let's return to smoking. Many young people begin smoking to gain acceptance by their peers, hastening a common foundation of shared experience. Later on, adult smokers continue to find comforting camaraderie in sharing a smoke together. So, among other things, the Supportive Community nourishment dimension is being facilitated by this choice, with ongoing reinforcement outside of the shared activity. In a more temporary sense, the cigarette might also control their appetite for food, elevate their mood, and enhance certain cognitive functions – substituting nourishment across several dimensions at once. That seems like a pretty good deal, doesn't it? Especially if their nutrition is poor, other avenues of social integration are absent, and going too long without a cigarette creates anxiety or interferes with mental concentration. In this immediate context, smoking really doesn't seem like such a bad deal – except for the longer term consequences of cancer, heart disease, emphysema, premature death and so on – so we will tend to reject the delayed downside and cling to the immediate gratification of our habit.

What can help us change? The only reliable way to shift away from undernourishment and unhealthy substitutions is to experience appropriate, full-spectrum energy exchanges that meet all of the same perceived needs. The social acceptance piece, the appetite control, the mental clarity, the positive feelings, and everything else; that is, a conscious combination that satisfies multidimensional nourishment. Once we experience the real deal, we will internalize that there is a better way to achieve the nourishment we know we need – just as we once internalized a substitution habit like smoking as beneficial.

How do we transition from imbalanced to balanced nourishment? Ongoing transition processes are inherent to *Integral Lifework*. When we ground ourselves in compassionate affection, we constantly examine our real levels of nourishment in each channel of energy exchange, identify what barriers are preventing wholeness and begin managing them, and concurrently fall in love with those parts of our being we have been neglecting. Then we can infuse our lives with high quality nourishment that make our previous, incomplete efforts at self-care obsolete. And once this effort gains momentum, it reinforces itself with new synergies and burgeoning vitality. We experience contentment that sustains us and empowerment that inspires us to continue. We lavish affection on the thirstiest parts of our being, and no longer feel the urge to cling to inferior substitutes. What those who engage in integral practice often find is that the allure of previous substitutions, distortions and depleting habits simply fades away, and any impulse to revisit those past impulses leaves them feeling unfulfilled and empty. Once we have sampled ambrosia, lesser nourishment leaves a bitter aftertaste.

AFTERTHOUGHT

Integral Lifework is intended to provide enduring answers to some of life's most challenging and intriguing questions: Why do we suffer? How can we heal? What is love? What does healthy relationship look like? How can we feel more empowered? Where should we go for answers? When will we know we have discovered solutions that apply uniquely to our current situation? Such questions are as endless as they are relevant. And when we turn away from external dependence, when we disrupt our habit of consuming answers from authorities and traditions outside ourselves, we can begin to look inward. There, in the depths of our being, is everything we need to soften our most potent fears, relinquish our most disruptive impulses, heal from our most jagged wounds, and actualize our most precious dreams. Why would we ever look elsewhere when such power and grace reside within?

However, the promise of external solutions erupts perpetually around us, and the impulse to worshipfully embrace them is aggressively reinforced. The cultural and institutional pressures to rely on externals and motivate every action with dysfunctional dependence are as pervasive as they are resistant to change. But that way lies madness. External projections of hope are a tonic not for healing, but for a perpetuation of every malady. Science and technology, for instance, cannot rescue us from ourselves but only replace one set of challenges with another. The free market can commoditize innovation and creativity, but it cannot solve any of our most difficult societal problems. Religious dogma cannot escape its orbit around dominant cultural memes, but instead conforms to them over time, no matter how innovative its foundations may have been. And the heady heights of acquired knowledge – even those insights that can truly set us free – are not the same as the deliberate, steady and disciplined effort of self-emancipation. There is in fact nothing completely outside of our fragile vessel that will deliver us from our barriers to well-being or create a transformative existence on our behalf. We do not bear this burden alone, but we alone are accountable for our choice to heal, grow and evolve. The answers, resources and rewards are all inside us.

What is it that resides within? What part of us promises real freedom, strength and transformation? It is our capacity to love, to affectionately and compassionately care for all that we are – as individuals, as a collective, as part of the biological and energetic systems of the Earth, as part of the fabric of the Universe itself. Once we begin to embrace our own essential substance, turning away from the superficial conformities and verisimilitudes of everything we think we want and everything we think we know, we encounter the solid bedrock of existence. And when we touch that solid ground, when we feel its boundless energy and concrete importance, there is no turning back. We can either attempt to deny our soul, or embrace the inevitable momentum of love-consciousness and its evolutionary consequences.

Integral practice is of course also subject to this dynamic. As you read through this book and sample its exercises, some latent seeds in the recesses of your being may be jogged loose. Or perhaps a spring of water may be reawakened in some dry, untended dimension of self. Or you will simply find additional resources for the journey on which you have already intentionally embarked. But you provide the soil of consciousness and the sunlight of life-giving love. Your intention, attention and follow-through will cause this garden to grow and flower. You are the gardener of your own life and the sole purveyor of conscious evolution.

A friend of mine recently asked: "Do people really change?" I think to answer this question we must first realize that many culturally sanctioned modes of being have conditioned us to live in contradiction to who and what we are. So what feels like positive change may really just be letting go of that conditioning, disabusing ourselves of a false identity, and disconnecting our ego and willfulness from those old habits. What draws us towards our genuine center is the discovery that gratitude and love are already there within us; they are part of our nature – dominant parts that can govern all other aspects of self if we allow them to. Through mindful interior awareness we will find this truth and unveil an abiding connection with the ground of being, informing all loving action with insight and wisdom. Thus real, substantive transformation is mainly a returning to Self, a gradual *disillusionment* that discards substitutions in favor of authentic nourishment. Do people really change? Yes, absolutely. With true love as our compass, we will become more and more ourselves.

INDEX OF EXERCISES

Please note that many other exercises can be found throughout various sections of the book, particularly in The Twelve Dimensions in Depth chapter.

ENDNOTES

[1] Health Risks of Sleeping Pills, see
http://health.ucsd.edu/news/2002/FNbookPILL.pdf

[2] Impact of Parenting Style on Child Development, see
http://www.parenting.cit.cornell.edu/documents/Parenting%20Styles%20and
%20Adolescents.pdf

[3] Ibid

[4] Stress Hormones & Cancer, see
http://www.jbc.org/cgi/content/full/282/41/29919

[5] Tobacco Litigation Final Finding of Fact Summary, see
http://www.usdoj.gov/civil/cases/tobacco2/index.htm

[6] Tobacco Marketing Strategy, see
http://www.americanheart.org/presenter.jhtml?identifier=11226

[7] Breast Feeding Health Outcomes in Developing Countries, see
http://www.ncbi.nlm.nih.gov/books/bv.fcgi?rid=hstat1b.section.106751

[8] IGBM Report on Infant Formula Marketing, see
http://www.infactcanada.ca/crakcode.htm

[9] U.S. Infant Formula Usage, see
http://www.breastfeeding.com/reading_room/what_should_know_formula.ht
ml

[10] Perchlorate Exposure Health Risks from Infant Formula, see
http://www.nature.com/jes/journal/vaop/ncurrent/abs/jes200918a.html;
Fluoride Health Risks from Infant Formula, see
http://www.fluoridealert.org/health/news/09.html; Infant Death Risks from
Infant Formula, see
http://www.ncbi.nlm.nih.gov/pubmed/15121986?dopt=Abstract.

[11] Union Carbide Plant in Bhopal, see
http://www.amnesty.org/en/library/asset/ASA20/005/2005/en/dom-
ASA200052005en.html

[12] Bhopal Aftermath, see http://bhopal.org/index.php?id=22

[13] Charleston Chemical Plant Leak, see
http://www.wvgazette.com/News/200903170887

[14] DuPont Teflon Issues, see http://www.health-
report.co.uk/teflon_poisoning_denied.htm

[15] 3M Discontinues PFCs, see
http://www.motherjones.com/politics/2001/09/coming-clean

www.ingramcontent.com/pod-product-compliance
Lightning Source LLC
Chambersburg PA
CBHW020522270326
41927CB00006B/409